Self-Identity after Brain

An injury to the brain can affect virtually any aspect of functioning and, at the deepest level, can alter sense of self or the essential qualities that define who we are. In recent years, there has been a growing body of research investigating changes to self in the context of brain injury. Developments in the cognitive and social neurosciences, psychotherapy and neurorehabilitation have together provided a rich perspective on self and identity reformation after brain injury. This book draws upon these theoretical perspectives and research findings to provide a comprehensive account of the impact of brain injury on self-identity.

The second half of this book provides an in-depth review of clinical strategies for assessing changes in self-identity after brain injury, and of rehabilitation approaches for supporting individuals to maintain or re-establish a positive post-injury identity. The book emphasizes a shift in clinical orientation, from a traditional focus on alleviating impairments, to a focus on working collaboratively with people to support them to re-engage in valued activities and find meaning in their lives after brain injury.

Self-Identity after Brain Injury is the first book dedicated to self-identity issues after brain injury which integrates theory and research, and also assessment and intervention strategies. It will be a key resource to support clinicians and researchers working in brain injury rehabilitation, and will be of great interest to researchers and students in clinical psychology, neuropsychology, and allied health disciplines.

Tamara Ownsworth is a teaching and research academic in the School of Applied Psychology at Griffith University in Brisbane, Australia, with 18 years of experience as a clinician and researcher in the brain injury field. She is also a chief investigator on the NHMRC Centre of Research Excellence in brain recovery.

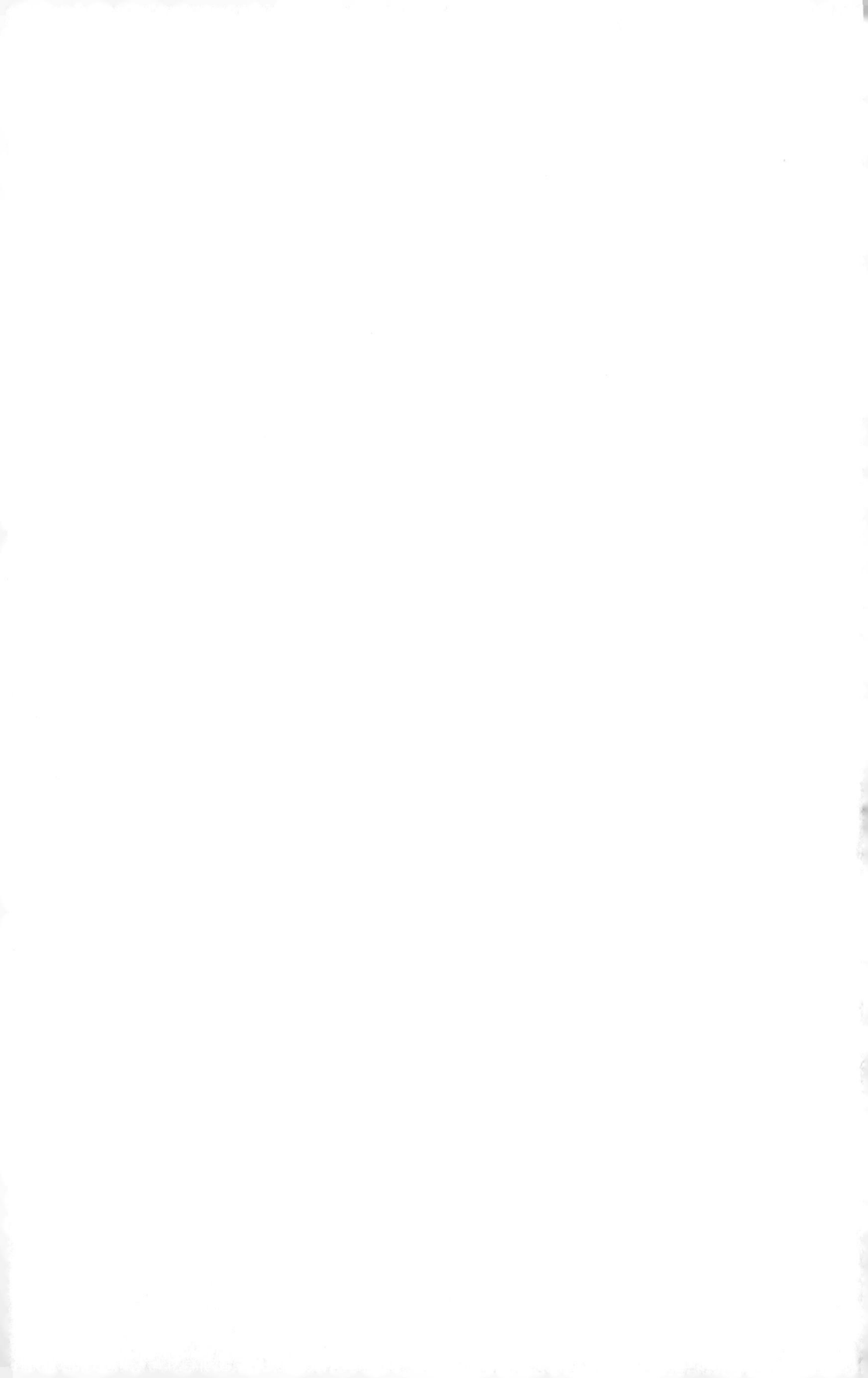

Self-Identity after Brain Injury

Tamara Ownsworth

Ψ Psychology Press
Taylor & Francis Group
LONDON AND NEW YORK

First published 2014
by Psychology Press
27 Church Road, Hove, East Sussex BN3 2FA

and by Psychology Press
711 Third Avenue, New York, NY 10017

Psychology Press is an imprint of the Taylor & Francis Group, an informa business

© 2014 Psychology Press

The right of Tamara Ownsworth to be identified as author of this work has been asserted by her in accordance with sections 77 and 78 of the Copyright, Designs and Patents Act 1988.

All rights reserved. No part of this book may be reprinted or reproduced or utilised in any form or by any electronic, mechanical, or other means, now known or hereafter invented, including photocopying and recording, or in any information storage or retrieval system, without permission in writing from the publishers.

Trademark notice: Product or corporate names may be trademarks or registered trademarks, and are used only for identification and explanation without intent to infringe.

British Library Cataloguing in Publication Data
A catalogue record for this book is available from the British Library

Library of Congress Cataloging in Publication Data
Ownsworth, Tamara.
Self-identity after brain injury / Tamara Ownsworth.
    Includes bibliographical references and index.
    1. Brain damage – Patients – Psychology. 2. Brain damage – Patients – Rehabilitation. 3. Identity (Psychology) 4. Self-perception. I. Title.
    RC387.5.O96 2014
    617.4'81044–dc23   2013037764

ISBN: 978-1-84872-109-8 (hbk)
ISBN: 978-1-84872-320-7 (pbk)
ISBN: 978-1-315-81954-9 (ebk)

Typeset in Baskerville
by HWA Text and Data Management, London

Contents

List of figures		vi
List of tables		vii
Series preface		viii
Acknowledgements		x
1	Overview of self-identity after brain injury	1
2	What is the self? Historical and contemporary accounts of self and identity	5
3	Introduction to brain injury and consequences during childhood and adolescence	37
4	Psychological adjustment and self-identity changes after brain injury	55
5	Approaches for assessing changes to self after brain injury	79
6	Individual psychotherapy and neurorehabilitation approaches	106
7	Group and community-based interventions	137
8	Family and paediatric interventions	160
9	Summary and future directions	183
	Appendix A: Head Injury Semantic Differential III	189
	Appendix B: The Brain Injury Grief Inventory	190
	References	192
	Author index	224
	Subject index	228

Figures

2.1	A schematic representation of the global self-system and components supporting continuity and change	35
3.1	A biopsychosocial framework of factors contributing to brain injury outcomes	41
3.2	Formulation of Dan's self-identity after brain injury	53
3.3	Formulation of Jasmine's self-identity after brain injury	54
4.1	Perspectives on the impact of brain injury during the first few months post-discharge	56
4.2	Biopsychosocial framework of the inter-related processes of self-awareness, sense-making and coping that contribute to self-identity after brain injury	58
4.3	Cycle of appraisals, anxiety and avoidance and the impact on self-concept	64
6.1	Example values worksheet	118
6.2	Examples of Janelle's ABC diary entries	129
7.1	Early and long-term focus of interventions contributing to identity maintenance and change after brain injury	139

Tables

2.1	Characteristic patterns of self-construal and identity formation across the lifespan	14
2.2	Components of the self based on social neuroscience perspectives	27
4.1	Summary of studies investigating changes to self and identity after brain injury	72
5.1	Summary of measures assessing self-awareness, sense-making appraisals and coping after brain injury	82
5.2	Overview of approaches for assessing self-concept and identity change after brain injury	92
6.1	A summary of issues impacting the working alliance and strategies used by psychotherapists in brain injury	110
6.2	Case vignettes illustrating barriers to rapport and therapeutic strategies	111
6.3	Guidelines for providing client-centred feedback in brain injury rehabilitation	116
6.4	GAS levels and corresponding behaviour for the example of Bill	121
6.5	Summary of Level 1 and Level 2 evidence supporting the effectiveness of psychotherapy for people with brain injury	124
6.6	Recommended adaptations to psychotherapy for people with brain injury	130
7.1	Summary of community-based initiatives to develop sustainable social networks for people with brain injury	154
8.1	Overview of contextualised interventions focusing on child and/or parent emotional and behavioural outcomes after brain injury	176

Series preface

Rehabilitation is a process whereby people who have been disabled by injury or illness, work together with health service staff and others to achieve their optimum level of physical, psychological, social and vocational well-being (McLellan, 1991). It includes all measures aimed at reducing the impact of handicapping and disabling conditions and at enabling disabled people to return to their most appropriate environment (Wilson, 1997; World Health Organisation, 1986). It also includes attempts to alter impairment in underlying cognitive and brain systems by the provision of systematic, planned experience to the damaged brain (Robertson & Murre, 1999). The above views apply also to neuropsychological rehabilitation, which is concerned with the assessment, treatment and natural recovery of people who have sustained an insult to the brain.

Neuropsychological rehabilitation is influenced by a number of fields from both within and without psychology. Neuropsychology, behavioural psychology and cognitive psychology have each played important roles in the development of current rehabilitation practice. So too have findings from studies of neuroplasticity, linguistics, geriatric medicine, neurology and other fields. Our discipline, therefore, is not confined to one conceptual framework; rather, it has a broad theoretical base.

We hope that this broad base is reflected in this modular handbook. The first book was by Roger Barker and Stephen Dunnett, which set the scene by talking about *Neural repair, transplantation and rehabilitation*. The second title, by Josef Zihl, addressed visual disorders after brain injury. Other titles in the series include *Behavioural approaches to rehabilitation* by Barbara A. Wilson, Camilla Herbert, and Agnes Shiel; *Neuropsychological rehabilitation and people with dementia* by Linda Clare and a second edition of Josef Zihl's book *Rehabilitation of visual disorders after brain injury*. The latest book is Tamara Ownsworth's *Self-identity after brain injury*, a popular topic in current neuropsychological rehabilitation.

Future titles will include volumes on specific cognitive functions such as language, memory and motor skills, together with social and personality aspects of neuropsychological rehabilitation, as this is the kind of handbook that can be added to over the years.

Although each volume will be based on a strong theoretical foundation relevant to the topic in question, the main thrust of the majority of the books will be the development of practical, clinical methods of rehabilitation arising out of this research enterprise.

The series is aimed at neuropsychologists, clinical psychologists and other rehabilitation specialists such as occupational therapists, speech and language pathologists, rehabilitation physicians and other disciplines involved in the rehabilitation of people with brain injury.

Neuropsychological rehabilitation is at an exciting stage in its development. On the one hand, we have a huge growth of interest in functional imaging techniques to tell us about the basic processes going on in the brain. On the other hand, the past few years have seen the introduction of a number of theoretically driven approaches to cognitive rehabilitation from the fields of language, memory, attention and perception. In addition to both the above, there is a growing recognition from health services that rehabilitation is an integral part of a health-care system. Of course, alongside the recognition of the need for rehabilitation is the view that any system has to be evaluated. To those of us working with brain-injured people, including those with dementia, there is a feeling that things are moving forward. This series, we hope, is one reflection of this move and the integration of theory and practice.

References

McLellan, D.L. (1991). Functional recovery and the principles of disability medicine. In M. Swash & J. Oxbury (Eds.), *Clinical Neurology*. Edinburgh: Churchill Livingstone.

Robertson, I.H., & Murre, J.M.J. (1999). Rehabilitation of brain damage: Brain plasticity and principles of guided recovery. *Psychological Bulletin*, *125*, 544–575.

Wilson, B.A. (1997). Cognitive rehabilitation: How it is and how it might be. *Journal of the International Neuropsychological Society*, *3*, 487–496.

World Health Organisation. (1986). *Optimum care of disabled people* (report of a WHO meeting). Turku, Finland: WHO.

Barbara A. Wilson
Ian H. Robertson

Acknowledgements

I would like to thank my colleagues at Griffith University for supporting me during the book writing process and providing feedback. In particular, I am grateful to Toni Dwan, Elizabeth Beadle, Owen Lloyd, Cassandra Shields, and Analise O'Donovan. Special thanks are owed to Cath Haslam for her feedback and ideas for Chapter 7 and to Barbara Wilson for her encouragement. I am also very grateful to my family for their support on this journey. Finally, I would like to express my appreciation and admiration to the people with brain injury and family members I have seen clinically or as participants in my research.

1 Overview of self-identity after brain injury

This introductory chapter highlights the importance of addressing self-identity issues in brain injury rehabilitation and presents an overview of the book.

An injury to the brain can affect virtually any aspect of functioning. At the deepest level it can alter one's sense of self or the unique and persisting qualities that define who we are. People with brain injury may perceive losing some fundamental part of their selves (e.g., 'I'll never be a patch on who I was'). Close family members and friends may grieve the loss of the person and the relationship they once had. Changes to self after brain injury are complex and not readily observable or easy to address in rehabilitation. Neuropsychological rehabilitation broadly aims to assist people to manage the everyday consequences of brain injury and to live a meaningful and fulfilling life. All rehabilitation approaches contribute in some way to rebuilding a person's self-identity regardless of the aspect of functioning focused on (e.g., mobility, speech or memory). However, people do not reconstruct their sense of self from objective functional gains per se, but rather the *personal meaning* they derive from their everyday experiences after brain injury.

The importance of self in rehabilitation has long been recognised, with neurorehabilitation and psychotherapy approaches used in combination to facilitate identity transition after brain injury (Ben-Yishay et al., 1985; Wilson et al., 2009; Ylvisaker, McPherson, Kayes & Pellet, 2008). Despite growing interest in self-identity after brain injury (Gracey & Ownsworth, 2008), there are few evidence-based guidelines to support identity-oriented assessment and intervention practices.

Research investigating changes to self in the context of brain injury has only emerged in the literature over the past few decades, stimulated largely by the seminal work on self-concept by Tyerman and Humphrey (1984). The interface between social psychology and cognitive neuroscience (i.e., social neuroscience) allows for a more advanced understanding of how sense of self emerges as a product of our neurobiology, culture and their interaction (Feinberg, 2011a; Jetten, Haslam & Haslam, 2012; Rochat, 2011; Walsh, Fortune, Gallagher & Muldoon, 2012). Neuropsychological models offer accounts of how cognitive and emotional subsystems of the brain work together to create an ongoing sense of self that actively constructs meaning in our day-to-day experiences (Conway & Pleydell-Pearce, 2000; Damasio, 1999; LeDoux, 2000).

In a keynote address at the Annual Brain Impairment Conference in Brisbane in 2010, Professor Barbara Wilson identified that research on self-identity after brain injury was one of the top ten cutting-edge developments in the field. In an article based on the address, she noted that: 'Contemporary models such as Conway's (2005) "self-memory system" and Haslam et al.'s (2008) work on social identity theory provide a means of thinking about the interplay between brain systems, cognition, personal and social identity' (2011, p. 35). In light of such progress, it was timely to write the first book dedicated to self-identity issues after brain injury. This volume seeks to highlight recent developments in theory and research relevant to self-identity and consider the implications for clinical practice, thus providing a useful resource for students, clinicians and researchers in the field.

This book aims, firstly, to provide a context for understanding self-identity changes after brain injury by reviewing different theories of self and identity that derive from psychology, sociology and cognitive neuroscience. The second aim is to provide a comprehensive account of the impact of brain injury on self-identity. Thirdly, the book aims to review clinical strategies for assessing self-identity processes and interventions for supporting individuals to re-establish a positive identity after brain injury. The book's final aim is to summarise the main areas of progress in self-identity and brain injury research and identify directions to advance the field.

Overview of the book

Before considering the impact of brain injury on self-identity it is important to understand what is meant by 'self' and 'identity'. Chapter 2 provides an overview of historical perspectives and more contemporary theories that contribute to our current understanding of self-identity. This discussion draws initially on the ideas of early philosophers such as Aristotle and Locke, whose insights bear remarkable similarity to social neuroscience perspectives on self-identity today. The chapter then focuses on theoretical advances during the 19th and 20th centuries, including perspectives from psychoanalytic, developmental, humanistic and social psychology which collectively highlight the influence of biology, socialisation and culture. A discussion of more contemporary accounts of self and identity in the 21st century follows, based on cognitive and social neuroscience developments. In the final section of the chapter these perspectives are integrated into a framework which supports readers to consider the potential for changes to self after brain injury.

To introduce brain injury, Chapter 3 summarises the main causes and functional consequences and provides a developmental perspective. The diverse factors contributing to brain injury outcomes are conceptualised within a biopsychosocial framework, which recognises the interactive influence of pre-morbid, neurological, social environmental and psychological factors. The second half of this chapter focuses on the impact of sustaining a brain injury early in life and implications for emerging sense of self in childhood and adolescence. Empirical evidence regarding biological and social vulnerability and factors moderating the relationship between the neuropathology of brain injury and functional outcomes is discussed. The psychosocial consequences of brain injury for children and adolescents are reviewed, with a specific focus on the impact of metacognitive and social cognition impairments on emerging sense of self. Two case studies (Dan and Jasmine) illustrate the complex interplay of factors influencing identity formation after childhood brain injury.

Chapter 4 presents a comprehensive review of psychological adjustment and self-identity changes after brain injury in adulthood. Psychological adjustment refers to the process of becoming aware of, making sense of, and adapting to changes in one's functioning and life circumstances. The inter-related processes of self-awareness, sense-making and coping are examined within a biopsychosocial framework. Building on this framework, research investigating self-identity changes after brain injury is specifically reviewed. Overall, this research indicates that premorbid characteristics and neuropsychological status influence perceived changes to self, and that opportunities to re-engage in meaningful activities and social roles are instrumental to rebuilding sense of self. An adaptive self-identity after brain injury is fostered by everyday experiences that provide personal meaning and reinforce self-worth.

Many different approaches are used in clinical practice to measure self-perceptions and other processes related to self-identity. The issues surrounding measurement of subjective phenomena are initially considered along with some caveats. Adopting the framework presented in Chapter 4, Chapter 5 initially reviews approaches for assessing self-awareness, sense-making appraisals and coping after brain injury. These approaches include self-report questionnaires, interviews and behavioural observation approaches. The focus then shifts to assessment of self-concept and changes in self-identity after brain injury, with an appraisal of methods developed specifically for the brain injury population. In the final section of Chapter 5, assessment approaches are considered for children and adolescents with brain injury. Approaches developed for the general paediatric population that have potential utility for brain injury are discussed with recognition that these methods require psychometric evaluation for this population.

The importance of focusing on identity issues in rehabilitation has long been recognised. Any intervention that aims to improve people's functioning and influence their self-perceptions contributes in some way to the identity reformation process. Chapter 6 reviews individual psychotherapy and neurorehabilitation approaches for adults with brain injury. Strategies for enhancing the working alliance and engagement in therapy are initially discussed. The application of and evidence base for diverse approaches, including psychoeducation and feedback, goal-directed interventions, cognitive and behavioural therapies and project-based learning are described. Further, the utility of technological aids for supporting sense of self by enhancing attainment of goals and recall of everyday experiences is considered. Chapter 6 advocates for approaches that systematically integrate psychotherapy and neurorehabilitation to support emotional and cognitive functioning and participation in valued activities and relationships.

Chapter 7 emphasises the key influence of social factors and peer support in the identity reconstruction process, and provides a review of group, holistic and community-based interventions. The characteristics and efficacy of structured group interventions and comprehensive holistic rehabilitation programmes that create a therapeutic milieu are considered. A major challenge for clinicians is to support people with brain injury to maintain their gains after rehabilitation and build upon these outcomes through sustainable networks of support. Community initiatives that can provide a sense of belonging, achievement and contribution include paid work, volunteering, leisure activities, advocacy, group projects and leadership opportunities. Chapter 7 concludes with a discussion of the potential for social media to enhance social functioning and well-being of people with brain injury.

The effects of brain injury are far reaching, and can destabilise the entire family unit and the relationships and identity of its members. An essential aspect of rehabilitation involves supporting family members to adjust to the impact of the brain injury on their lives and well-being. The first section of Chapter 8 discusses the impact of brain injury on 'family identity' and reviews three main approaches to supporting family members. Approaches include: 1) involving family members in therapy for the person with brain injury, 2) interventions designed specifically for family members, and 3) family system interventions. The second part of Chapter 8 summarises rehabilitation approaches for children with brain injury. Despite a general absence of interventions that focus specifically on self-identity issues for children, related approaches in the literature include holistic neuropsychological rehabilitation, parenting or family-based interventions, and multi-component context-sensitive approaches (e.g., home, school and work).

The final chapter summarises and integrates leading developments in the self-identity and brain injury literature and provides directions for future research. Key advances in the field include: a) brain imaging studies mapping the neural correlates of self-related processing and social identification; b) theoretical accounts depicting the impact of brain injury on self-perceptions and identity; c) research revealing the role of biopsychosocial factors in identity reconstruction after brain injury; d) development and preliminary validation of measures assessing changes to sense of self; e) emerging evidence to support the efficacy of individual, group and community-based interventions for enhancing psychological adjustment to brain injury; and f) family-based therapy and contextualised approaches for supporting people with brain injury and their family members. Priority areas for future research include: validating paediatric assessment tools, modelling the identity transition process over time and evaluating the efficacy of individual, group and family-based interventions for improving self-concept after brain injury. The chapter concludes the book by identifying future research directions along these lines.

Conclusion

A brain injury is a life-altering experience that leads to changes in people's abilities and social situation. The most complex consequences entail changes in selfhood, which are perplexing for individuals, family members and professionals. Understanding and managing changes in self-identity is an integral part of rehabilitation. Although this has long been recognised, systematic research investigating changes to self in the context of neurological disorder has only emerged in the literature over the past two decades and such research is in its infancy. The focus on self and identity reformation therefore represents a relatively new frontier in brain injury research. It is hoped that this book stimulates research and clinical innovations that will enrich the lives of people with brain injury and their families.

2 What is the self?
Historical and contemporary accounts of self and identity

*Before we consider the impact of brain injury on self-identity it is important to understand the concepts of 'self' and 'identity'. An in-depth account of the philosophy and scientific study of the self could easily fill several volumes, as indeed many have (see Brinthaupt & Lipka, 1992; Leary & Price Tangney, 2003). A journal (*Self and Identity*) devoted to this area attests to the strong level of scholarly interest in understanding who we are and what makes us different from, or the same as, others. This chapter provides an overview of key terminology, historical perspectives and psychological and social neuroscience contributions to understanding self and self-identity. An integration of these perspectives at the end of the chapter provides a framework for considering the potential for changes to self after brain injury and the processes for rebuilding self-identity in this context.*

Definitions of self and identity and related terminology

'The self' has been referred to as that conscious being and agent responsible for unique thoughts and actions, or the essential nature of a person that endures over time (Brinthaupt & Lipka, 1992). This encompasses the collective characteristics we think of as our own, including bodily experiences and internal psychological states (Dumont, 2013). The self is often referred to as a cognitive structure (e.g., a mental schema or theory) that is multi-dimensional and hierarchical in nature (Feinberg & Keenan, 2005). Other authors refer to the self as a narrative sequence or language-constructed metaphor (Freeman, 1992). The self possesses both consistent characteristics and those continually under construction. Thus, sense of self reflects our past and present selves as well as our possible selves, or who we might become (Markus & Nurius, 1986). The term *self-construal* refers to an individual's sense of self in relation to others. Two main types of self-construal co-exist: independent self-construal, or one's perceived uniqueness and separateness from others, and interdependent self-construal, based on our relationships with others (Markus & Kitayama, 1991).

The self encompasses many inter-related concepts including self-awareness, self-concept, self-esteem, self-efficacy and identity. *Self-awareness* refers to the capacity to experience ourselves as distinct from others and the environment and to consciously perceive our own abilities and internal states (Damon & Hart, 1982). *Self-concept* is commonly described as the overarching thoughts and feelings a person has about him- or herself in order to arrive at a definition of self (Rosenberg, 1965). Self-concept encompasses awareness of one's unique and stable characteristics, values and behaviour (existential self-concept) and self-identification based on comparison with other people (categorical self-concept) (Harter, 2012). *Self-esteem* has been referred to as the evaluative component of self-concept, or the judgements that an individual makes about his or her own worth, value or competence (Schweitzer, Seth-Smith, & Callan, 1992). The two terms are closely interrelated, and it has been found that people with low self-esteem typically have a less stable and well-defined self-concept compared with those with high self-esteem (Setterlund & Niedenthal, 1993). There is also overlap between these concepts and self-efficacy. *Self-efficacy* refers to sense of personal agency, or a person's evaluation of and beliefs about his or her ability to perform particular tasks or cope with certain situations (Bandura, 1989). Each term can refer to a global set of beliefs regarding one's self-worth and competency (i.e., global self-concept or general self-efficacy), or specific domains and behaviours, as covered in Chapter 5.

The term *identity* is derived from the Latin word 'identitas' which refers to sameness, or relating only to itself. In the social sciences, identity refers to perceptions of the unique and persisting qualities that distinguish self from others (Dumont, 2013). Self-identity is often conceptualised as part of personality formation. Both entail characteristics within the individual, including typical ways of thinking, feeling and behaving; however, self-identity refers more specifically to awareness of one's inner sameness and continuity (Allport, 1961). Others can observe and describe someone else's personality (e.g., 'she is outgoing and adventurous'), whilst self-identity is subjectively constructed and experienced (e.g., 'I am hardworking and family oriented'). However, this does not imply that self-identity is separate from one's social context. Social identity has been defined as 'the sense of self that people derive from their membership in social groups' (Jetten, Haslam, & Haslam, 2012, p. 4), which places more emphasis on understanding self on the basis of group membership (i.e., 'we' and 'us') than distinctive personal attributes (e.g., 'I' and 'me'). Social identity forms in relation to a virtually countless number of group memberships, including age, gender, religion, class, nationality, ethnicity, sports, political views, leisure and work. Therefore, one's social identity is multi-faceted and potentially changeable, according to the situational context. Social identity and self-identity are closely interrelated aspects of the self-system, or one's working model of self. The notion that identity is both subjectively and socially constructed will be constantly revisited in this book.

There are many competing perspectives on what constitutes self-identity, which parallel debates on what it means to be human. Mathews, Bok, and Rabins (2009) considered the philosophical and neuroscientific underpinnings of self-identity in their book *Personal Identity and Fractured Selves*, using case studies of people with altered self-identity in the context of neurological conditions. Despite opposing views that stem from the study of morality versus science, there was consensus that self-identity entails a personal account or self-narrative that strives to be clear, consistent and organised (Mathews et al., 2009). It is the philosophy of this book also that a richer understanding can be gained by examining self-identity through the lens of diverse epistemological positions to gain greater insight into one of the biggest mysteries that people contemplate in their lives, that of 'who am I?'

Historical perspectives on self-identity

There is an extensive body of literature on the philosophy of the self and many ancient notions relevant to self and identity have endured over time. Aristotle (383–322 BC) provided one of the earliest influential accounts of self, referring to the soul as the core essence of a person and an integrated function of the body (Hett, 1936). Aristotle highlighted the importance of self-knowledge and relationships with others in forming sense of self. He viewed self-knowledge as the start of all wisdom, but claimed that 'we are not able to see what we are from ourselves' (Magna Moralia, 1213a15–16, cited in Cooper, 1999). Hence, we need to look to others for a less distorted account, and come to know ourselves and personal qualities through interacting with others and observing their reactions to us (Nicomachean Ethics, 1169b33–35, as cited in Bartlett & Collins, 2011). Aristotle believed that all objects have a 'telos', or a purpose that reflects its real nature and potential. As humans we are compelled to understand ourselves, discover our destiny and fulfil this potential. Human potential becomes fully realised through social activity, in the shared discussions of one's thoughts and perceptions (Stern-Gillet, 1995). Aristotle also recognised the importance of activity ('handiwork') and occupation for personal development and reaching one's potential through actions. These early observations foreshadowed the concept of 'self-actualisation' which Maslow (1943) developed into a formal theory in the 20th century.

Descartes (1596–1650) highlighted the importance of reason and conscious thought processes to support the existence of self. His famous quote, 'I think, therefore I am' (*Discourse on Method*, 1637; cited in Clarke, 2006) has been literally interpreted as: I think and thought cannot be separated from me, therefore, I exist (Clarke, 2006). Most philosophers following Descartes have argued that self-knowledge requires persisting notions of self and understanding one's nature and character traits, which differs from our knowledge about the world external to us. Locke (1632–1704) specifically linked this view to self-identity, proposing that the self requires continuity of consciousness and gradually emerges through sense perception and reflection on one's own experiences (Locke & Winkler, 1996). He advanced the fundamental notion that sense of self requires consciousness of one's past *and* future thoughts and actions as well as to be aware of these processes in the present moment. This view stresses the importance of memory to sense of self which will be revisited later in this chapter.

In summary, an important early notion that has endured over centuries is that sense of self forms through self-knowledge, interpersonal interaction and activity. Self-identity requires continuous consciousness or an integrated sense of one's past, present and the future. The desire for greater self-understanding and to reach one's full potential is a basic human drive.

A further major contribution of early philosophers was the development of basic assumptions about humans that set the scene for ongoing debate in the literature as well as advancement of scientific methods. These assumptions are often expressed as polarised views on nature versus nurture, uniqueness versus universality and freedom versus determinism, although most authors take a relative rather than absolute stance on each.

Of particular relevance to self-identity, the *nature* versus *nurture* debate concerns the relative influence of heredity or inborn characteristics and environmental factors on human experience. Advocates for hereditary would argue that the self is strongly influenced by pre-determined genetic and biological factors and that, once established, is relatively stable (unless one's biological state is disrupted through injury or illness). Supporters of the role of the environment would contend that sense of self is continually under construction throughout our lives, as shaped by life events, people and other environmental influences (Dumont, 2013). In the context of self-identity, the latter perspective poses the question of how we maintain consistency in our self-perceptions over time given changes in the physical and social environment. Thus, to what extent is self-identity influenced by predetermined factors that support stability over time, as opposed to a dynamic or reactive phenomenon?

A second basic philosophical assumption, *uniqueness* versus *universality*, relates to whether (or the degree to which) people are unique or distinct from others, or essentially share the same characteristics. Self-identity, or the global impression we have of ourselves, marks what is different or sets us apart from others. Social identity refers to our collective identities or those we share with others on the basis of social membership (Jetten et al., 2012). Thus, we have many social identities through membership in different social groups and roles (e.g., Australian, parent, neuropsychologist). A further question that arises from this assumption is whether we have a single 'true' overriding identity or multiple identities that can be assumed in different situations.

The third assumption, *freedom* versus *determinism*, questions the extent to which individuals have conscious control over their thoughts and behaviour, as well as understand the motives for these. That is, do we mainly react to external events or the conditions of our environment, or are we the agents of our own experiences, consciously acting on our own initiative to influence our circumstances? The influence of cognitive and motivational processes outside conscious awareness also warrants consideration.

These philosophical themes and the questions they pose influenced the development of many early psychological theories, which in turn provided the foundations for contemporary perspectives on self and identity.

Psychological perspectives on self-identity

In the earliest recognised textbook of psychology, *The Principles of Psychology* (1890), William James defined the self as 'all that [a person calls] Me' (p. 21). James argued that we have two aspects of the self, the *I* (subjective self) and the *Me* (objective self), and proposed that the Me is experienced in three forms: the *Material Me* (body and possessions), the *Social Me* (as perceived by one's peers) and the *Spiritual Me* (one's inner or subjective being). An overall self-evaluation is based on all forms of the Me; however, these are subjectively weighted in terms of their importance, with those most important reflecting 'the strongest, truest, deepest self' (James, 1890, p. 310). James proposed that we have an internal frame of reference or 'self-system' by which we interpret our experiences, judge the value of our accomplishments and form our aspirations. Therefore, self-esteem 'depends entirely on what we back ourselves to be and do' (James, 1890, p. 310). Similar to Locke, James argued that self-identity requires a sense of sameness and continuity of self between the present and the past, as follows:

> The identity which the *I* discovers, as it surveys this long procession, can only be a relative identity, that of a slow shifting in which there is always some common ingredient retained. The commonest element of all, the most uniform, is the possession of the same memories.
>
> (James, 1890, p. 372)

The notion that memories play a central role in creating sense of self and identity forms the basis of contemporary models of self (see Conway, 2005). Since James, many psychological theories have emerged that contribute to contemporary views on self-identity. Given the considerable breadth of psychological literature on self and identity, the following review focuses mainly on leading theoretical accounts with selective insights from empirical research.

Psychoanalytic perspectives on self and identity

As the founder of psychoanalytic theory and psychoanalysis, Freud (1856–1938) pioneered the systematic study of personality, and placed major emphasis on the role of unconscious processes and psychosexual stages of development. Freud sought to understand how events from an individual's past influence adult personality characteristics, and particularly how the disruption to development at an earlier stage may lead to 'fixation', causing psychological problems in adulthood. Of particular relevance to understanding self, Freud wrote *The Ego and the Id* (1923) in which he described three dynamics within the self: id (the it), ego (the I) and superego (the above I). The id represents our biologically-driven and unconscious instincts which motivate us to seek pleasure and avoid pain through reflexive actions and immediate gratification of our needs. The ego emerges from the id, and acts as an intermediary between the id and the external world, seeking to meet its demands in a realistic and appropriate manner. Within the inner core of the ego is the superego, which represents our higher moral standards and idealised views that develop through socialisation. The superego seeks perfection and provides our moral conscience, producing feelings of guilt, shame and self-criticism when the ego does not curb actions driven by the id. The superego also produces positive feelings of pride and self-satisfaction when our actions are consistent with our ideal self-image (Freud, 1923).

In Freud's model the ego strives to find a balance between the id and the superego in order for a well-adjusted personality to form. However, there is frequent conflict between the id and the superego where the self becomes divided by two dynamic forces; one seeking immediate satisfaction and the other promoting a rigid moral code for behaviour (Brunner, 2002). In order to manage this tension and anxiety (e.g., fear of losing control or fear of punishment), Freud proposed that the ego develops defense mechanisms (e.g., denial, rationalisation, repression), which represent ways of protecting ourselves from threats to self. These are proposed to operate unconsciously, or outside of our awareness and serve to distort reality and reduce threat. These strategies are often adaptive and creative ways of coping with excessive anxiety, although when employed too often these can be unhelpful and exacerbate problems (Cramer, 2000).

Despite Freud's many critics (see Richards, 1990), his theory has remained an influential model for understanding human behaviour, with empirical research supporting various concepts of psychoanalytic theory (Bornstein, 2005). In particular, Freud's emphasis on the importance of recollection for self-understanding has influenced life history and narrative approaches to studying self (Freeman, 1992). The development of psychoanalysis and its techniques has transformed the treatment of emotional problems. For Freud, psychoanalysis entails an ongoing self-discovery process through which a person gains insight into and develops his or her personality and learns to resolve past conflicts and fixations. The goal of psychoanalysis is to become one's 'best self', or what one would have become under optimal conditions (Freud, 1917).

Carl Jung (1875–1961), a previous member of Freud's psychoanalytic society, developed analytic psychology and was greatly influenced by Eastern religions and mythology. He believed that a mature personality is formed by integration and harmony within the self, rather than by interpersonal relations (Jung & De Laszlo, 1959). The human 'psyche' encompasses both conscious and unconscious processes and strives towards harmony, self-actualisation and 'individuation', or knowing oneself as well as possible. The ego is part of the conscious mind and responsible for providing coherence and continuity of self; yet, according to Jung this is not where the true centre of our personality lies. Jung distinguished between our personal unconscious, which is organised into 'complexes' or unique patterns of thoughts, feelings and memories that cannot be fully accessed, and our 'collective unconscious'. The latter refers to qualities we share with others based on our common experiences of living in a society that is comprised of social groups and roles. It is through our collective unconscious that common beliefs, emotions, concepts and symbols (e.g., language) are inherited or passed down the generations, contributing to one's cultural and ethnic identity. These predisposed representations include 'archetypes' or universal forms of thinking and responding that emerge as ways of experiencing our humanity. He described four main archetypes: the persona, the shadow, the anima and the self (Jung & De Laszlo, 1959).

The *persona* refers to social roles or representations ('masks') of oneself in public. Personas vary across situations, according to how we want to be viewed by others and perceived social expectations. The *shadow* reflects our base impulses or socially unacceptable thoughts, feelings and actions that are incompatible with social and moral standards. The persona and shadow reflect the duality of human nature, and both are necessary parts of our psyche. Jung proposed that by understanding and appropriately expressing the shadow, we can experience greater fulfilment in life. The *anima/animus* archetype refers to the feminine side of the male psyche and masculine side of the female psyche respectively. The *self* is the centre of our personality and unites both conscious and unconscious aspects. According to Jung (1954), an ultimate goal of human existence is to develop and know all aspects of ourselves.

A particularly influential adaptation of psychoanalytic theory is object relations theory (Kohut, 1971; Mahler, 1975), which posits that one's self-structure is largely shaped by interactions with significant others. During the first three years of life 'separation' (distinguishing oneself from caregivers) and 'individuation' (forming one's own skills and personality) occur to support an emerging 'core identity' (Mahler, 1975). This psychological development is influenced by the quality of relationship or emotional bond between the infant and their caregiver/s, with supportive and empathic relations contributing to autonomous self (Kohut, 1971). With its focus on early relationships and parenting, object relations theory stimulated the emergence of attachment theory (see Bowlby, 1977), a leading socio-emotional developmental framework for understanding individuals' characteristic responses during interactions with others. Attachment styles entail working models of the self and others that develop during infancy and childhood and persist into adulthood.

Key theorists in the social psychology movement of psychoanalytic theory more generally emphasise the integral influence of interpersonal relations, family and culture in psychological development. For example, Adler (1954, 1964) believed that we construct our identity through conscious awareness and self-examination of our own experiences within a social world. Sullivan (1953) proposed a six-stage model in which the first stage centres on the fulfilment of one's immediate needs during infancy, and the final stage refers to establishment of culturally sanctioned adult social and occupational relationships. Three of the stages relate to adolescence, highlighting this period as a pivotal one for forming mutual relationships and one's self-image.

In a more contemporary psychoanalytic account, Fonagy, Gergely, Jurist and Target (2004) propose a social biofeedback model in which links between affect regulation, mentalisation and development of the self are emphasised. Affect mirroring is the mechanism through which a child's affect regulation develops and his or her attachment security (or lack of security) is reinforced. Sensitive and responsive caregivers react to their young child's display of emotions with 'contingent marked mirroring' or exaggerated facial, vocal and gestural cues that both reflect and distinguish the child's emotional expression. Affect mirroring supports children to learn to recognise and modulate their own affect. Mentalisation, or the ability to 'envision mental states in self and others' (Fonagy et al., 2004, p. 23) emerges through the parent mirroring the child's affect and the parent relating to the child as an independent subject. Through affect mirroring and mentalisation infants develop 'intersubjectivity', learning to differentiate their inner self from the external world. Over time, children learn to distinguish pretence, appearance and false beliefs from reality. Their social biofeedback model has been applied to account for psychological dysfunction, proposing that too much or too little affect mirroring can lead to insecure attachment and developmental psychopathology.

The notion of different selves is an important concept of psychoanalytic theory. Horney (1950) made an important distinction between *real self* and *idealised self*. Our real self reflects who we truly are: a realistic appraisal of our abilities and potential. Our idealised self is what or who we believe we *should* be, or our ego-ideal and preferred persona. Excessive focus on the idealised self and denial of one's true self can lead to 'tyranny of the should' and a strong drive for meeting these standards. Hence, a greater discrepancy between one's real and idealised selves causes anxiety, guilt and other negative emotions. Those with greater self-awareness, or more accurate perceptions of one's real self, have greater opportunity to achieve their goals and reach their full potential. Based on Horney's conceptualisation, Markus and Nurius (1986) examined the nature and function of *possible selves* and their influence on self-concept. Possible selves refer to how individuals perceive their potential or future self, which stems from and is connected to past and current selves. These include our idealised or hoped-for selves, as well as feared selves. We have a repertoire of possible selves derived from our goals, wishes and fears; some of which are more salient or personally compelling than others (e.g., a single person who deeply wishes to be in a relationship may have a clear vision of themselves happily married). Many of our possible selves are strongly influenced by social comparison, including images in the media, and the desire to become like others we admire or, alternatively, unlike those we wish to avoid becoming (e.g., lonely in older age). The concepts of real, idealised, and possible selves are closely related to self-schema, which will be discussed in the section on cognitive theories.

Overall, the major contributions of psychoanalytic theory to understanding self and identity include the notion that the self is an integral part of the human psyche and comprised of conscious and unconscious processes. Innate drives and urges outside conscious awareness motivate our behaviour whilst the expression of these needs is influenced by perceived social standards and ideals. One's self-structure is shaped by interactions with significant others, particularly early caregivers' affect mirroring and learning to regulate one's own affect. We develop defense mechanisms to distort the reality of an unpleasant situation, manage threats to our self-esteem and maintain a positive self-image. We have many selves, including real self, idealised self, and possible selves, and the discrepancies between these influence our global self-concept.

Developmental psychology perspectives on self and identity

Psychologists have proposed various models to explain the development of self and identity over the lifespan. Attention has particularly been drawn to childhood and adolescence as significant developmental phases for constructing sense of self (Harter, 2012). One of the most influential theorists on identity was Erikson (1902–1994), who provided an ego-analytic perspective on development. Erikson (1963) believed that the ego has an adaptive function of maintaining well-being and effective performance, and recognised the interactive influence of biological, cognitive, emotional and socio-cultural factors on identity formation. Erikson described psychosocial stages of development with ego strengths forming at each phase, providing the foundation for the next more complex phase. His lifecycle framework depicts an individual's active efforts to understand others and relate to the world, and the corresponding ego strengths or virtues formed at each stage. A mature positive identity is proposed to form when these stages are successfully resolved and negotiated, with ego-strengths continuously nurtured and affirmed (Berk & Andersen, 2000). Building on Erikson's theoretical stages of identity development, Table 2.1 summarises characteristic patterns in self-construal and identity formation that emerge across the lifespan.

During the first few months of life, babies learn to detect social stimuli and contingencies, or relationships between their own actions and the environment. In particular, a parent's response to an infant's emotional displays (i.e., affect mirroring) influences the infant's emerging affect regulation and mentalisation skills (Fonagy et al., 2004). The capacity for self-recognition develops between 15–20 months of age and is based on stable features of one's physical self and bodily movements (Damon & Hart, 1982; Harter, 2012). 'Existential self' is the most basic part of one's self-schema and forms when children recognise that they are a separate and stable entity from others. Use of self-descriptive statements about one's body, action capabilities and sense of control that reflect self-awareness is generally observed around 2 years of age, which is also when children begin to process the intentions of others (Harter, 2012). Children aged 2–3 years can recognise that they are an object in the world and have properties they can categorise, usually in concrete terms. The emergence of 'categorical self' is greatly supported by language and representational thought (Harter, 2012). Imitative play and changes in self-description indicate a lack of constancy of self during this stage (Damon & Hart, 1982).

Physical attributes and action capabilities remain the key basis for understanding self during early childhood. Self-definitions of children aged 3–5 years are largely based on how they act on the environment and activities they engage in, although they start to distinguish their own private thoughts and beliefs from those around them, and thus in a momentary sense become aware of 'inner self'. Young children's self-representations are typically unrealistically positive (i.e., overestimating personal abilities) as they lack the ability to distinguish between real and ideal selves (Harter, 2012). They also lack perspective-taking skills and therefore do not incorporate the views of others (i.e., egocentrism) or engage in social comparison. Their excessively positive views or age-appropriate narcissism may serve as an emotional buffer to foster positive development (Harter, 2012). The beginnings of cognitive self-concept form with autobiographical memory supporting extended sense of self through temporal comparisons with self at a younger age. As a young child's autobiographical memory develops they begin to form a sense of continuity, initially focusing on the permanence of physical attributes, and supported by language. Self-knowledge of one's thoughts, actions, feelings and attributes (i.e., the I-self and Me-self distinction) is essential to support autobiographical memory and development of personal narrative, which is supported by parents' recollections (Harter, 2012).

Children aged 5–7 years refer to a more elaborate taxonomy of attributes than very young children, typically focusing on specific competencies (e.g., 'I am good at drawing', 'I am better at running than my best friend') rather than global self-evaluations. There is more recognition that others evaluate the self (i.e., social comparison) and social standards begin to act as a self-guide to influence behaviour, although their perspective-taking skills are still limited (Harter, 2012). Metacognitive self-awareness emerges through an array of self-descriptors that reflect gender and cultural norms, and awareness of future plans or projecting self into the future.

Table 2.1 Characteristic patterns of self-construal and identity formation across the lifespan

Developmental stage	Erikson's psychosocial stages and ego strengths	Characteristic self-construal and patterns in self-identity formation
Infancy (< 2 years)	Trust versus mistrust (hope)	Self-recognition and existential self – knowledge of self as a separate and permanent entity (15–18 months), as demonstrated by infants' reactions to their mirror images. Self-recognition is based initially on contingency cues (bodily movements) and then specific perceptual features
Toddler years (2–3 years)	Autonomy versus shame and doubt (will)	Categorical self – use of concrete descriptors of how self differs from others (e.g., gender, big and small); however, awareness of characteristics as constant aspects of self is yet to form
Preschool years (3–5 years)	Initiative versus guilt (purpose)	Inner self – awareness of private thoughts and imagination and able to distinguish between inner thoughts and the physical world, although children are unable to recognise these as stable characteristics
School years (6–11 years)	Industry versus inferiority (competence)	Psychological self – increasing awareness of stable psychological characteristics that distinguish self from others. Domain-specific self-concepts typically emerge around age 8 as children are able to evaluate their competencies across different domains to form higher-level self-representations (i.e., global self-concept)
Adolescence (12–18 years)	Ego identity versus role confusion (fidelity)	Interpersonal self – recognition that one's behaviour and personal characteristics vary according to situational influences, with definitions of self particularly influenced by one's peers and social groups; different identities are often experimented with before one's true identity begins to form
Young adulthood (18–24 years)	Intimacy versus isolation (love)	Different identity statuses emerge, including those characterised by diffusion (non-directed), foreclosure (prematurely formed by others), moratorium (searching) and achievement (secure commitment). Typically the period in which a more organised, unified, and consistent identity forms that is comprised of broader goals and values in life (e.g., employment and relationships)
Adulthood (25–64 years)	Generativity versus stagnation (care)	Maturation of self – involving extension of sense of self (interest in other's welfare) and self-objectification (a realistic view and acceptance of self), and a unifying philosophy of life. Self-esteem has been found to reach a peak around age 60
Maturity (65 years to death)	Ego integrity versus despair (wisdom)	Ageing self – transition from midlife to old age is found to be associated with a decline in self-esteem due to the instability of this period, including role changes (retirement, children leaving), loss of relationships (e.g., spouse death) and decline in health. However, positive changes also emerge, as many older adults age successfully and derive positive meaning and wisdom from their life experiences

However, they lack the ability to form higher-level representations concerning their own traits or global self-esteem (Harter, 2012). Self-representations are still mostly positive and reflect all-or-nothing thinking with respect to characteristics (e.g., 'I'm smart at reading'). In early to mid-childhood children still have largely inaccurate self-appraisals and overestimate their abilities, hence failing to distinguish between real and idealised self.

Around 8 years of age children can distinguish between their mind and body, recognising that they not only look and act different, but also have different characteristic thoughts and feelings to others that can be both positive and negative (Damon & Hart, 1982). Psychological aspects become more important for distinguishing self as a stable entity from others in mid-childhood, as 'psychological self' emerges. Self-descriptions are increasingly based on social characteristics such as family and friends (i.e., peer comparison). This shift in self-understanding coincides with the development of more flexible, organised and logical cognitive skills. Harter's research found that children under 8 years of age have difficulty evaluating their competence in different areas (see Harter, 2012). Children aged 8 and older were able to make distinct and more accurate evaluations of their competence (i.e., both positive and negative) across cognitive, social and physical abilities, suggesting that domain-specific self-concepts emerge around this time. Additionally, they were able to draw on these domains of competence to define their self-worth in more generalised terms (i.e., global self-concept). The influence of one's peers and social ideals become more evident as self-descriptions become interpersonal in nature (e.g., helpful, kind, popular), and the child's own experiences are more prominent in their autobiographical memory than parents' accounts. Harter (2012) noted that cognitive developments (e.g., memory and perspective-taking skills), an increase in social comparison (e.g., appearance, behaviour, school performance) and the ability to distinguish between real and idealised self-attributes pose liabilities for children's self-esteem, as more accurate and potentially negative self-perceptions emerge.

Adolescence is recognised as a momentous time for identity formation in which physical development coincides with social and emotional maturation, which allows adolescents to simultaneously identify with their peers and appreciate their own individuality and self-sameness (Lenz, 2001). During this peak period of identity formation, adolescents often experience heightened self-consciousness and absorption and may experiment with different identities, goals and values. In line with Erikson's (1963) model, late adolescence and early adulthood are common periods in which *role confusion* arises, whereby individuals struggle to relate to the values of their society and culture and fulfil expected roles. An *identity crisis* occurs when a person cannot establish a clear and stable identity.

However, for most adolescents a more unified self-system emerges with self-definitions based on both psychological (e.g., beliefs and ideology) and social characteristics. In particular, adolescents incorporate significant others' views, or how they perceive that others perceive them, into their own self-concept; a concept referred to by sociologists as the 'looking glass self' (Cooley, 1902) and 'generalised other' (Mead, 1934), as discussed in more detail later in this chapter. Peer evaluation and the reactions of close friends become increasingly important sources of self-definition. The capacity to reflect on one's past and future selves and recognise both conscious and unconscious thought processes forms in adolescence, enabling more complex notions of self to emerge (Damon & Hart, 1982). Cognitive development in perspective taking and abstract reasoning skills contributes to the changing structure of self. During early adolescence there is often oscillation between positive and negative attributes of self, depending upon the relational context. In later adolescence positive and negative qualities are recognised in unison, and a more balanced and integrated sense of self forms that is governed by personal standards and notions of self in the future (Harter, 2012).

Research supports that self-concept becomes increasingly differentiated with age (Marsh, 1989). A decline in self-concept typically occurs in early to middle adolescence, which corresponds with the transition from primary to high school. Indeed, students in early high school have been found to have lower self-esteem than students at other levels of schooling (Crain, 1996). The lower self-esteem observed during early adolescence has been attributed to conflicting role demands and complex peer and romantic attachments than can rapidly form and change during this period (Orth, Trzesniewski, & Robins, 2010). Academic self-concept has been found to gradually increase throughout high school (Bolognini, Plancherel, Bettschart, & Halfon, 1996), whilst physical self-concept decreases with age (Lau, 1990). Studies on gender differences have identified that males typically report more positive self-concept regarding physical competence, while females place more emphasis on cognitive competence or academic self-concept, and also develop greater attachment and intimacy in their relationships (Lau, 1990; O'Koon, 1997). Early episodic memories have a key influence on the formation of self-identity, particularly those formed during adolescence and early adulthood, which are important developmental periods from both a social and biological perspective (i.e., maturation of the prefrontal cortex) (Rathbone, Conway, & Moulin, 2011).

Marcia's (1980) research on identity development of young adults identified the following four different identity statuses: *identity diffusion*, a lack of direction or commitment to particular occupations or ideology; *identity foreclosure*, premature commitment to a ready-made identity formulated by others; *moratorium*, a short-term delay in forming an identity as individuals search to identity the occupations and ideology in which to invest; and *identity achievement*, in which individuals have undergone decision-making processes, and resolved any crises in order to securely commit to occupations and ideology. The latter two identity statuses are viewed as more adaptive, with research supporting that young adults in these categories have higher self-esteem, report greater convergence between their ideal and real selves, have more advanced moral reasoning skills and assume greater personal responsibility over their lives (Marcia, 1980). Difficulty forming and maintaining personal relationships and establishing one's career can particularly affect the identity and self-esteem of young adults (Orth et al., 2010). While adolescence and early adulthood are common periods in which role confusion and so-called 'identity crises' occur, such experiences of frustration and despair can occur at many points throughout life.

Longitudinal research in adulthood highlights that despite overall consistency in self-concept, changes in sense of self occur throughout the lifespan. These changes are influenced by individual characteristics (e.g., coping mechanisms and IQ), life events and shifts in relationship status (Cramer, 2003). A cohort-sequential longitudinal study (the American's Changing Lives Study; Orth et al., 2010) examined changes in self-esteem of 3,617 young and older adults (aged 25–104 years) over a 16-year period. Self-esteem was found to follow a quadratic trajectory, with an increase during young and middle adulthood, a peak around 60 years of age and then a decline in older age. The increase in self-esteem during the midlife period may occur because most people have established their work, family and romantic relationships, and derive satisfaction from these roles, thus feeling a sense of control and mastery. Orth et al. (2010) found that women had lower self-esteem than men overall, although their self-esteem trajectories converged in old age. In terms of ethnicity, White and African-American individuals had similar trajectories during young and middle adulthood; however, a greater decline in self-esteem was experienced by African-Americans in older age. Socioeconomic status and physical health were dynamic moderators in the relationship between age and self-esteem. Specifically, the decline in self-esteem in older age was related to a reduction in socioeconomic status (i.e., income and employment status) and deterioration in physical health.

Despite empirical evidence of a decline in self-esteem in older adulthood, perspectives on successful ageing concur that older adults can maintain positive psychological well-being through use of effective coping and social resources and by maintaining a productive and active lifestyle (Young, Frick, & Phelan, 2009). The concept of wisdom is universally recognised, with definitions typically encompassing attributes such as knowledgeable, pro-social behaviours, emotional stability, insight and social reasoning. Neuroimaging studies have identified that neuroanatomical correlates of 'wisdom' include the prefrontal cortex (dorsolateral, ventromedial and anterior cingulate areas), limbic striatum and amygdala. The integration of these areas is proposed to support self-referential processing (Jeste & Harris, 2010).

The notion of self maturing with age is reflected in Allport's (1961) concept of 'proprium' or the functions of self that evolve from infancy to adulthood. According to Allport, maturity entails an extension of sense of self (i.e., an interest in others and their welfare), self-acceptance of one's abilities and shortcomings and an appreciation of how these attributes differ from other people. A mature person also displays self-objectification, which includes a realistic view of one's skills and responsibilities, and a sense of humour regarding personal weaknesses and self-contradictions as well as those common to all humanity. Finally, maturity entails having a unifying philosophy of life and a sense of greater purpose and meaning in one's existence. Allport (1955) believed that we are always in the process of 'becoming', which is the main premise of humanistic psychology.

Overall, developmental perspectives on self and identity emphasise how greater self-understanding and identity emerges across the lifespan, coinciding with development of physical, cognitive, and socio-emotional competencies. Adolescence and young adulthood are viewed as key periods for identity formation, during which sense of self is influenced by peer relationships and the start of independent and working lifestyles. Although self-identity is relatively stable across the lifespan, changes in self-esteem and self-concept can occur and are influenced by life events and one's personal and social resources.

Humanistic and existential perspectives on self and identity

Consistent with Allport's (1955) notion of 'becoming', humanistic and existential psychology perspectives on self emphasise the capacity for people to grow, self-actualise and find meaning in their life experiences. Although not strictly humanistic or existential in focus, perspectives on self from occupational therapy, phenomenology, and personal construct theory share some common principles and will also be briefly reviewed within this section. Maslow (1970) proposed a hierarchy of human needs, which encompasses physiological needs (at the base), safety, belonging and love, self-esteem and self-actualisation (at the pinnacle). According to this framework, when the lower four needs have been sufficiently satisfied an individual has the opportunity to fulfil his or her highest and unique potential. Conditions that foster the fulfilment of self-esteem and self-actualisation needs include close and supportive relationships, positive learning experiences and satisfying employment or occupation.

A further contribution of Maslow's theory was the concept of 'peak experience', which involves intense focus and engagement in an activity to the extent that there is a loss or 'transcendence' of self. While absorbed in this activity, individuals feel a sense of completeness, unity and meaningfulness. This concept is similar to Csikszentmihalyi's (2000) notion of 'flow' which refers to complete absorption in an activity or merging of action and awareness, which can become the basis for a creative approach to life. Achieving a state of flow is an important concept in meditation and different schools of Zen Buddhism. Unlike many theorists who predominantly stress the importance of interpersonal relations, Maslow also recognised that sense of self is derived from occupational activities. His work influenced the development of more contemporary theories, including Self-Determination Theory (Ryan & Deci, 2001), which proposes that humans have an innate drive to fulfil their potential and overcome adversity. Maslow's views are consistent with the existential focus on 'being' and positive psychology principles of engagement and meaningfulness. The field and science of positive psychology is dedicated to understanding and building human strengths to support individuals and communities to thrive. Positive well-being entails satisfaction with the past, flow and happiness in the present, and optimism and growth in the future (Seligman & Csikszentmihalyi, 2000).

Existential psychology has many parallels with humanistic psychology due to its emphasis on meaning and human potential. A sense of meaning, purpose and choices in life are viewed as central tenets of existential well-being. Existentialism focuses on the structure of a person's existence and what it means to be human or a self (May, 1953). The only reality or truth in our existence is what we *do* and what we are conscious of and relate to ourselves. Existential perspectives focus on understanding self at the level of 'being' or experiencing life in the moment. Humans are viewed as continually emerging or in the process of becoming and rediscovering selfhood (i.e., reflecting on one's values, making choices and pursuing new possibilities). A self-actualised individual is one who can experience life, accept his or her circumstances and live according to personal values that guide choices and actions. By understanding that we are responsible for our own lives we may better confront life (being) and avoid the threat of 'non-being' or a meaningless existence (May, 1953).

The therapeutic discipline of mindfulness is based on principles of existential and humanistic psychology as well as Buddhist meditation, teaching people to consciously bring awareness to the here-and-now experiences and accept their thoughts and emotions without judging or challenging them (Harris, 2006; Kabat-Zinn, 1990). The broader approach of acceptance and commitment therapy (ACT; Hayes, 2002) aims to support people to create a rich and meaningful life by being guided by their personal values and taking effective action. The core principles and techniques of ACT are reviewed in Chapter 6.

Along a similar vein, occupational therapy perspectives emphasise the following dimensions to a meaningful existence and life well lived: *doing* (purposeful action), *being* (living in the moment), *belonging* (affiliation and affirmation), and *becoming* (self-actualisation) (Hammell, 2004; Wilcock, 1998). Occupational activities and social roles support each dimension of existence by providing the opportunity to develop our interests and competencies and to learn about personal strengths and limitations from others and the environment. Occupation also encourages us to adapt and cope with challenges and to gain a sense of mastery and autonomy within our environment. Engagement in meaningful activities enhances mood and self-worth and can be an important avenue for interpersonal interaction to foster a sense of belonging and reduce loneliness (Dumont, 2013). More broadly, occupation provides structure and routine in life and can reinforce our value to others and contribution to society. The activities and roles we choose are guided by our sense of self (i.e., values, beliefs and motivation), but also strengthen who we are and shape who we become. Ultimately, occupation creates a sense of consistency, coherence and meaning in our lives (Dumont, 2013). However, the meaning of occupation is subjectively derived, and thus can only be understood from the insider's perspective (Hammell, 2004).

The field of phenomenology and study of the structure of human experience has contributed greatly to our understanding of self and subjective experience. This field and its related approaches emphasise the importance of understanding phenomena from the individual's lived experience and reality (see Patton, 2002). Humanistic psychologist Carl Rogers (1951) was greatly influenced by phenomenology, proposing that a person is the only one who is aware of, and able to understand his or her own experiences. His theory of self proposes that people learn only what they perceive as most significant to them, in order to maintain or enhance their sense of self. If people receive information that challenges their self-concept, and feel under threat and judged, they are likely to resist, deny or distort this information. Individuals raised in an environment with unconditional positive regard are more likely to form a positive self-concept and have the opportunity to fully actualise. Roger's person-centred principles concerning the importance of openness, empathic understanding, being non-judgemental and creating a non-threatening environment for learning and self-discovery have been applied in many contexts including education and therapy (Rogers, 1951).

Also adopting a phenomenological perspective, Freeman (1992) defined the self as an ongoing story or narrative that is tied to one's life history and subject to enhancement or exaggeration. He proposed that self-understanding is inextricably bound to language and constructed by inner dialogue: 'Simply stated, on some level we *are* the stories we tell about ourselves. This is so whether the tales are accurate (roughly speaking) or inaccurate' (p. 25). Self is viewed as a meaning maker or interpretive creation that links together what we have been, what we are now and what we imagine we will become (Freeman, 1992). Therefore, human perceptual and cognitive processes define all experiences, including sense of self.

Kelly's personal construct theory (Kelly, 1955) is also based on the premise that events are open to many different interpretations (i.e., constructive alternativism) and that the world does not automatically make sense to us. Therefore, we create our own meaning and reality of the world by developing personal constructs, which are similar to schemas and act as hypotheses to allow us to predict what is going to happen and feel a sense of control over events. We examine how well these constructs fit with our subsequent experiences, holding on to them if they are realistic and adaptive in helping us to cope with the world. Alternatively, if these constructs are not supported by our experiences or are unhelpful in terms of how we cope with or manage situations, we strive to alter the misleading construct for a more accurate and adaptive way of construing the world (Kelly, 1955). The 'self-construct' reflects perceived patterns in one's own behaviour, which constitute attributes (e.g., kind, friendly and warm) and develop through social interaction. Kelly viewed therapy as a means of reconstruction, which assists clients to identify their own conceptual framework that created and maintains their psychological difficulties and to consider alternative interpretations. Kelly's view of people as active agents who create their own reality is consistent with many cognitive theories, as discussed in the next section.

In summary, humanistic and existential perspectives focus on understanding an individual's internal frame of reference and the meaning of experiences and realising one's unique potential. Related disciplines or approaches include occupational therapy, phenomenology and personal construct theory.

Cognitive theories on self and identity

Influenced by many of the approaches and theories previously outlined, cognitive theories of self posit that thought processes determine the reality and meaning of everyday experiences, including one's view of self and the world. Similar to humanistic theories, cognitive theories tend to adopt an optimistic view of people's capacity to change and reach their potential, and have led to major advances in counselling and therapy approaches (see Chapter 6). The review of cognitive theories in this section incorporates social cognitive perspectives, which span developmental, cognitive and social psychology.

Bandura's (2001) socio-cognitive theory of personality proposes that we simultaneously construct and are constructed by our social context. The concept of personal agency refers to our capacity to act on intentions, anticipate outcomes, self-reflect and modify our goals and actions accordingly. We begin to form an 'agentic self' as infants from observing causal relations between our actions and the social environment. Bandura viewed cognitive processes as the subfunctions or personal determinants of a 'self-system' integral to perception and regulating our behaviour. Cognitive processes influence what we attend to, how we perceive and respond to events, use of symbols (e.g., language) and the ability to anticipate the consequences of our actions.

Self-efficacy, or personal beliefs about our ability to perform behaviours to achieve desired outcomes, is the central mechanism of personal agency which directs our thoughts, motivation to learn and our choice of goals (Bandura, 2001). Self-efficacy regarding different skills, roles and life domains develops throughout the course of our lives and can be altered by life events and our relative perceptions of success and failure (e.g., the experience of a car accident altering people's self-efficacy as a driver). The concept of self-efficacy is distinct from but related to 'locus of control' (Rotter, 1954), an attribution style that refers to the extent to which we believe our own actions can influence outcomes (internal locus), or are governed by external factors (external locus). People with an internal locus of control assume more responsibility for their actions and outcomes and experience more positive social and psychological adjustment, including coping better with illness and stressful events (Elkis-Abuhoff, 2003).

Traditional cognitive theories propose that underlying schemas or core beliefs can account for different emotional states and behavioural reactions that people may experience in the same situation (see Beck, 1967; Ellis, 1962; Lazarus, 1966; Markus, 1977). According to Beck's cognitive theory, throughout our lives we develop schemas, or fundamental beliefs and generalisations about the world, other people and ourselves (self-schemas). Early harmful experiences in life (e.g., loss or rejection in relationships) and other stressful life events contribute to negative self-schemas, which may reflect fear of loss, rejection, failure and threats to one's safety. Individuals with a particularly strong desire for close and supportive relationships (i.e., sociotrophy) and those who excessively strive for personal achievement and independence (i.e., autonomy) may be more vulnerable to psychological distress if threat is posed to these core life dimensions (Eisenstadt, Leippe, & Rivers, 2002). Individuals with a negative 'cognitive triad' (or pessimistic views of self, the world and the future) have characteristically unhelpful thinking styles and sequences, which serve as interpretive filters in daily life. Unlike the self-enhancing thinking styles of individuals without depression, depressed individuals tend to have more realistic self-appraisal of their abilities and the outcome of events (i.e., depressive realism), or alternatively perceive threat, failure or problems when there is little evidence of these (Beck, 1967).

Self-schemas have a pervasive impact on how self-related information is processed. New information about self is more likely to be processed in a manner that is congruent with an existing self-schema (Markus, 1977). People therefore look to confirm or verify existing beliefs about themselves from both a motivational and cognitive perspective. Most people have an inherent motive for self-enhancement, thus positive feedback and recall of events favourable to self are more readily accessed in non-depressed individuals (Eisenstadt et al., 2002). Hence, adaptive self-schemas contribute to optimistic self-expectations, positive attentional biases and mood-congruent recall of events. Conversely, maladaptive self-schemas (e.g., 'I'm worthless and unlovable') lead to negative self-expectations, biases in information processing (i.e., cognitive distortions) and mood-congruent recall of events (Eisenstadt et al., 2002). People's trait self-esteem influences how they incorporate new information about self into their existing self-schema. In particular, people with high self-esteem more readily assimilate positive feedback into their self-schema, whilst those low in self-esteem more readily assimilate feedback about failure (Stake, Huff, & Zand, 1995).

Given the deep-seated nature of self-schemas and the notion of self-identity as one's sense of sameness and continuity over time, this poses the question of how changes in self occur. Continuity and stability of self is typically adaptive for individuals to perceive that the world and their own actions are predictable. Nonetheless, changes in self-concept and identity can occur, and appear to be precipitated by four main conditions. First, as considered later in more depth, a neurological disorder can disrupt the neural networks that support sense of self (Feinberg, 2011b; Mathews et al., 2009). Second, changes in self-concept and identity have been reported across the lifespan in response to life events and transitions (Crain, 1996; Cramer, 2003; Orth et al., 2010). An extensive body of literature attests to the impact of major stressful life events on sense of self and how trauma can 'shatter' one's world views, particularly views regarding one's vulnerability and self-image (see Gluhoski & Wortman, 1996). Both negative and positive changes in self can result from such experiences, as covered in more detail in Chapter 3. Third, changes in self-concept and schemas occur more gradually through self-relevant situational feedback and the development of self-discrepancies, as discussed in the next section on social psychology perspectives. Fourth, people's capacity to alter their self-schemas is a fundamental assumption guiding psychotherapy practices. Therapy approaches and conditions conducive to schema change are covered in Chapter 6 on individual therapy approaches.

In summary, cognitive theories of self focus on the role of cognitive processes including global beliefs and processing biases about self in the world. We simultaneously construct and are constructed by our social context and develop self-schemas based on early life experiences. These are continually updated throughout our lives, affecting how self-related information is processed. Change in self-schemas can occur as a result of neurological disorders, major life events, self-relevant feedback and participation in therapy.

Social psychology and sociological perspectives on self and identity

As emphasised throughout this chapter, self-identity is neither developed nor experienced in a vacuum. The related disciplines of social psychology and sociology have made an immense contribution to understanding the influence of social interaction and culture on self-identity. Sociological perspectives broadly propose that self is the product of social factors (Durkheim, 1960). Symbolic interaction theories explain how we interpret the actions and intentions of others during social interaction, and how these in turn influence views of ourselves. For example, Cooley (1902) described the concept of 'the looking glass self' whereby our sense of self is influenced by the impressions we have of what others think of us (i.e., reflected appraisals). Extending this view, Mead (1934) proposed the notion of 'generalized other', suggesting that sense of self truly emerges when we assume the view that others take towards us (or what other people generally think of us). Goffman's (1956) dramaturgical approach likened social interaction to playing a role or acting. He emphasised the human tendency for 'impression management' whereby people are motivated to present themselves in the most favourable light, often using 'props' to create a positive image (e.g., designer clothing and impressive books on a coffee table). People have both a front stage (i.e., the image they want to project to others) and a back stage (i.e., a more relaxed and authentic self-presentation) as they play these roles, with some 'actors' convincing their audience more than others. Sociological perspectives therefore aim to depict the influence of the social world on our self-image and the impressions we convey to others.

Social psychology perspectives on self highlight the role of social processes such as self-categorisation and social comparison in shaping self-concept. According to social identity theory (Hogg & Abrams, 1988; Jetten et al., 2012; Tajfel & Turner, 1979), our social identity forms from the knowledge that we belong to a social group or category. People strive to establish and maintain a positive sense of self by differentiating their own group from others. Two key processes are involved in forming one's social identity: *self-categorisation*, which involves evaluating one's own characteristics on the basis of perceived similarities or differences with others, and *social comparison*, or selectively focusing on personal attributes that are favourable or unfavourable in relation to others (Stets & Burke, 2000). A downward social comparison involves the tendency to perceive one's self as better off than those less fortunate. An upward social comparison involves the tendency to identify one's self more closely with others who are deemed to have more positive qualities or social advantages (Suls, Martin, & Wheeler, 2002). People form broad cognitive representations on the basis of the perceived characteristics of one's own group (i.e., self-stereotyping) and those of other groups.

Social identity perspectives share some assumptions with identity theory, which proposes that in addition to social group membership, sense of self is formed through identification with roles and their associated meaning and expectations (Stets & Burke, 2000). Roles provide a link between individuals and their social world, creating a sense of position and responsibility and access to certain resources. Roles also enable participation in socially meaningful and valued activities. Therefore, views of self are shaped by both socially-based and role-based identities. Having a particular social identity means being like others and viewing things from a shared perspective, while role identity is based on different perceptions and behaviours related to assuming certain roles. In both respects, identities are activated within certain situations, motivating individuals to act in accordance with identity standards (e.g., norms and expectations), a process commonly referred to as self-verification (Stets & Burke, 2000). However, given that we typically have multiple roles and social group memberships, it is unclear whether we have one single 'true identity', or multiple identities that may be assumed in different situations. The activation of a particular identity in a situation depends on psychological 'salience' or the perceived importance and relevance to one's goals of group membership (Stets & Burke, 2000).

A corollary of existing in a social world is that people regularly receive feedback about themselves from others and the environment. Such feedback may relate to physical or psychological attributes, or be based on performance of specific behaviours in a situation. According to self-comparison theory (Eisenstadt & Leippe, 1994), self-relevant situational feedback may serve to alter or verify one's self-concept. This information is initially processed at a shallow level, with changes in affect relating to the valence of the information, such that one can instantly feel pleased or shaken up by feedback. However, more in-depth analysis of the meaning of the feedback and its relevance to self often follows, in which the information is appraised according to three cognitive representations of self. These include the *actual self* or qualities one genuinely perceives one has, the *ideal self* which relates to qualities one desires but does not feel one has, and the *rejected self* which includes undesirable qualities one does not want to possess. Feedback relevant to self is initially compared with actual self, and if a match is not found the information is examined against the other two selves. If a match does not occur, this serves to highlight a *self-discrepancy* which requires further investigation, such as searching one's self-knowledge base or autobiographical memory and recalling relevant experiences to examine the credibility of the feedback. Effortful cognitive processing is required to resolve the self-discrepancy and either accept or dismiss the feedback. If the feedback is accepted, this updates one's self-knowledge and alters self-concept in either a positive or negative way. For example, accepting feedback that is in line with one's desired self, or dismissing feedback that relates to one's rejected self would serve to enhance or maintain a positive self-concept (Eisenstadt et al., 2002).

Self-discrepancy theory (Higgins, 1987) overlaps with self-comparison theory, proposing that the level of congruence or discrepancy between the actual self, ideal self, and ought self influences a person's emotional state. The *ought self* reflects self-expectations based on self-imposed standards for behaviour. Self-discrepancies occur when a person's assessment of actual self is discrepant from either the ideal self or ought self. Self-discrepancy can also occur between one's actual self and the self a person perceives that others want them to be (ideal-other self) or feel they ought to be (ought-other self). Therefore, the outcome of events or feedback on self that gives rise to self-discrepancies can contribute to positive or negative changes in self-concept.

Cultural and non-Western conceptions of self

Social constructionist perspectives broadly highlight the impact of social, cultural and power relations on identity (Gergen, 1991). Foucault (1980) emphasised the influence of power relations and authority on the creation and maintenance of knowledge and discourse in all facets of life including, for example, subjective understandings of one's own health and sanity. He argued that identity does not intrinsically exist within people themselves but is socially constructed and internalised through social discourse and power regimes and their influence on society (e.g., through media representations).

Cultural theorists similarly propose that sense of self is deeply embedded within one's culture and relations with others and that culture provides a model that prescribes how to manage one's self in everyday living (Lehman, Chiu, & Schaller, 2004). Supporting this view, cross-cultural research highlights how conceptualisations of self vary considerably across cultures, particularly in relation to the salience of private and inner aspects of self and public and relational aspects of self. People with more independent self-construal define themselves by their internal attributes (e.g., traits, abilities and values), while those with more interdependent self-construal define themselves by their relationships or connection to others (Markus & Kitayama, 1991).

In many Western cultures, the importance of positive self-esteem, asserting oneself and appreciating distinct personal qualities is emphasised (i.e., independent views of self). Western notions of self are characterised by a sense of personal agency, inwardness and individuality which is influenced and affirmed by one's social context (Markus & Kitayama, 1991). Self-actualisation largely occurs through personal accomplishment, or fulfilling one's own unique potential. Conversely, in many Asian cultures (e.g., Japanese, Chinese, Thai, Indian) harmonious relations with others and looking after and fitting in with members of one's group is most valued (i.e., interdependent views of self). Relationships, reciprocal concern and being connected to others are more central to self and identity than personal achievements (Markus & Kitayama, 1991). The value placed on interdependent self as part of a collective was proposed to account for the finding that Asian American students reported lower self-esteem than White American and Black American students (Bachman, O'Malley, Freedman-Doan, Trzesniewski, & Donnellan, 2011). The influence of culture on self-construal has been demonstrated at a neural level. Specifically, Zhu, Zhang, Fan, and Han (2007) found that the same neural substrate (i.e., ventromedial prefrontal cortex) was activated for Chinese participants when they made judgements about both their own traits and traits relating to their mothers. For Western participants, the activation of this region was specific to judgements about traits related to self (Zhu et al., 2007).

Culture also influences sense of self through language, which is the main symbolic tool for expressing one's cultural identity (Yihong, Ying, Yuan, & Yan, 2005). The primary language we speak supports self-construal through inner speech and social discourse, including the personal stories we tell (Bucholtz & Hall, 2003). It is therefore relevant to consider whether people who speak the same language share a common identity. Although this view may be supported in some instances (e.g., expatriates bonding through language and gang members using specific slang as a form of code), the ideology and practices of individuals who speak the same language can differ immensely within or between countries (Bucholtz & Hall, 2003). Nevertheless, studies of bilingualism support that self-identity changes may be experienced when people learn another language. Yihong et al. (2005) found that a significant proportion of Chinese college students who learnt English reported that although they maintained their native cultural identity, they experienced some changes in their behaviour, values and beliefs. Further, a subgroup reported experiencing conflict or confusion over their cultural identity due to learning English.

The Western notion of self is not universal and the emphasis placed on strengthening one's self-concept is not shared by many non-Western traditions (e.g., Hinduism, Buddhism and Taoism). In fact, in the teachings of Zen Buddhism the self does not exist (Mosig, 2006). Rather, existence is characterised by impermanence or change (anicca), suffering (dukkha), and nonself (anatta). The main goal of Zen is enlightenment or being 'awakened' to the reality that everything in the universe, including mental states, exists because of necessary conditions and causal interconnections (i.e., dependent origination). We are all part of a process that continues indefinitely; thus, birth is not the start, death is not the end (Rahula, 1974). A person is composed of five elements: form (body), feelings, perceptions, impulses and consciousness. Because self is an illusion created by perceptions and the language used to describe these, if you remove these elements nothing remains. The focus of Buddhist psychology is to alleviate suffering brought about by the belief that self is a separate entity. For example, belief in the existence of a separate self can bring about greed, conceit, selfishness, cravings, alienation, hatred and many other negative states. Without the boundaries that self can impose, a person becomes an interconnected part of the universe (Mosig, 2006).

Naturally, this book is based on the premise that the self *does* exist and is an integral part of our humanity. The predominantly Western views reflected in the literature reviewed and my own background is important to acknowledge because notions of self are culturally relative. In spite of this, cross-cultural perspectives recognise a universal tendency for people to seek to grow and fulfil their potential and that this may occur in diverse ways, including personal achievement and the betterment of one's community and culture (Miller, 2006). People's religious beliefs and spirituality are closely tied to their sense of self in this respect. Whilst religion relates to 'a search for significance in ways related to the sacred' (Pargament, 1997, p. 32), spirituality is a broader concept that entails fundamental questions about the meaning or purpose of life and 'transcendence' of self or one's place in the world (see Collicutt McGrath, 2011). Transpersonal psychology perspectives similarly adopt this view by seeking to understand how a deeper or wider sense of who we are and our humanity can be experienced through connecting with others, nature, spirituality and religion, which is consistent with insights from Eastern traditions (see Jennings, 1999). Research in the burgeoning field of social neuroscience highlights how culture and neurobiology interact to produce our experience of self in the world.

Cognitive and social neuroscience perspectives on self and identity

Most authors agree that despite its subjective and non-materialistic nature, self emerges from the brain as a product of both one's biology and culture (Mograbi, Brown, & Morris, 2009). Various conceptualisations of self have been developed in the social neuroscience literature (Damasio, 1999; Feinberg, 2011a; Gallagher, 2000; Neisser, 1988; Ward, 2012), and are summarised in Table 2.2. Despite proposing different components of self, these frameworks broadly agree that self entails *bodily self* or one's sense of agency and embodiment, *relational self* as defined by interpersonal interaction, relationships and shared culture, and *narrative self* or an ongoing sense of self supported by memory, personality and motivation (Feinberg, 2011b). Bodily self is viewed as the core of our self-awareness, and encompasses sense of control over our own actions and awareness of body sensations (i.e., tactile perception, internal states) and the body's location in space (Christoff, Cosmelli, Legrand, & Thompson, 2011). Damasio's (2003, 1999) influential model of consciousness refers to multilayers of self, namely, *proto-self* (bodily and sensory-motor functions), the transient and constantly recreated *core self* (moment-to-moment awareness of internal and external

Table 2.2 Components of the self based on social neuroscience perspectives

Feinberg (2011a)	Gallagher (2000)	Neisser (1988)	Damasio (1999)	Ward (2012)
Bodily self: sense of self located in the body (embodiment) and control of one's own thoughts and actions (agency)	*Minimal self:* body ownership and control of our own actions, mental contents of self	*Ecological self:* being located in one's body	*Proto-self:* bodily self based on sensory-motor functions (non-conscious life functions)	*Sensorimotor self:* sense of agency or being in control of one's own actions; sense of embodiment or ownership over one's body
Relational self: sense of self related to both one's mental processes and the external world; culturally determined aspects of self: groups, social roles, beliefs and practices	*Narrative self:* social identity and autobiographical memory extending over time to provide a conscious sense of unity or self-harmony	*Interpersonal self:* feelings of self tied to emotion and social interaction	*Core self:* processing of stimuli related to self and the external world (moment-to-moment awareness)	*Cultural/collective self:* group memberships and shared beliefs, skills and rituals
Narrative self: continuity and uniqueness of self: our own personal memories and history and stable characteristics		*Conceptual self:* semantic self-knowledge, social roles and identities	*Autobiographical self:* one's subjective experience of self over time and episodic memory, linking past, present and future	*Ongoing self:* personal memories, personality traits and motivation to maintain self-esteem
		Private self: self-awareness, ability to reflect on and own one's conscious experiences		
		Extended self: self existing over time		

phenomena supported by thalamo-cortical loops), and *autobiographical self*, which requires extended consciousness of the past, present and future and is continually revised by new experiences.

Like many other psychological concepts, the study of self and self-identity poses many challenges for cognitive neuroscience. Feinberg and Keenan (2005) identified three main reasons why the self is largely an enigma for neuroscience. Firstly, the self is proposed to be a unified single entity; however, the brain is divided into millions of neurons and hence the unification of self in a divisible brain is difficult to account for. Secondly, self is subjectively experienced, and is therefore not easy to measure objectively. Thirdly, and related to the two former issues, the location of self in the brain is complex to determine in the context of other forms of consciousness and cognitive and emotional processes. Despite these challenges, the neurobiological underpinnings of self have been considered on many levels, including behavioural genetics, neuroanatomical structures and their interconnectivity and models of neuropsychological processes. Some leading theoretical and empirical advances in cognitive and social neuroscience over the past decade provide insight into the neural processes and brain structures supporting our experience of self in the world.

Evidence from the field of behavioural genetics supports the role of heredity in many human characteristics, including IQ, memory, personality traits and gender identity (Loehlin, 1992). Although research has yet to specifically investigate the role of heredity in self-identity formation, there are some noteworthy findings concerning self-esteem. For example, Neiss, Sedikides, and Stevenson (2006) investigated genetic influences on level and stability of self-esteem using 183 pairs of adolescent twins and found that the contribution of heredity was substantial for both level and stability of self-esteem. However, self-esteem was also uniquely influenced by non-shared environmental factors which had the greatest overall impact on level and stability of self-esteem. Consistent with this finding, Rochat (2011) concluded that the self is a phenotype emerging from an interaction between one's genotype and the environment.

Neuroanatomical connectivity supporting self

Self is often viewed as synonymous with, or a prerequisite for, consciousness (Feinberg & Keenan, 2005). The experience of a unified and conscious self requires an integrated neural network. Feinberg (2011a) proposed a nested hierarchy comprised of three interconnecting systems represented in concentric rings. These include the outer exterosensorimotor system (i.e., primary sensory-motor cortices and unimodal association cortex), the integrative self system (i.e., medial heteromodal association cortex and medial paralimbic structures), and the interoself system at the core, which is phylogenetically the earliest to evolve, and includes brain stem and medial limbic structures. Feinberg (2011a) proposed that medial and orbitomedial prefrontal regions support the integrative self system which produces internal representations of self and mediates the relationship between self and the external world.

Several empirical studies have endeavoured to localise self in the brain by examining the neural processes of healthy individuals, or alternatively examining the experience of 'loss of self' in people with various forms of neuropathology or disorders of consciousness (see reviews by Feinberg, 2011b; Mathews et al., 2009; Northoff, Qin, & Feinberg, 2011). In such research, it has been necessary to define self in measurable terms, which has typically involved examining specific types of self-referential processing. For example, self-recognition tasks using facial stimuli and other self-relevant or self-related stimuli (e.g., pictures, one's own name and other personally salient words) versus non-self-specific stimuli have often been used. These approaches are based on the premise that people become aware of self when required to make a judgement on, or respond to self-related stimuli (Northoff et al., 2011). Such techniques have been applied to investigate awareness of self for people in altered states of consciousness (Qin et al., 2010). For example, research conducted on patients in a persistent vegetative state revealed neural activity in the anterior cingulate cortex when individuals heard their own name, and these signal changes were correlated with level of consciousness. Their findings suggest that full consciousness may not be required for particular types of self-referential processing (Qin et al., 2010).

The conceptual and methodological issues associated with experimental studies of self were considered extensively in a review by Northoff et al. (2011). Their meta-analysis identified that despite different methodologies, the neuroanatomical substrate most consistently implicated in self-referential processing was an integrated subcortical–cortical midline system; however, the processing of self-specific stimuli appears to be more distinctly associated with activation of the anterior paralimbic and midline regions (perigenual anterior cingulate cortex and insula). Interestingly, this same paralimbic region is found to be more active in the resting state for people with depression, which is a disorder known to be characterised by excessive self-focus and rumination (Grimm et al., 2009). The paralimbic and insula regions have also been implicated in the processing of self-related and emotional stimuli (Northoff et al., 2011).

The ability to perceive changes to self over time is important for identity formation across the lifespan (see Table 2.1). D'Argembeau and colleagues (2008) examined the neural correlates of self-reflection over time, requiring subjects to reflect on their own psychological characteristics for the present and past, and also those of an intimate other for present and past. Although cortical midline structures were recruited for each of the four reflective tasks relative to the control condition, the degree of activity varied significantly within this neural circuitry across the conditions. Specifically, the ventral and dorsal medial prefrontal cortex and posterior cingulate cortex were recruited more when reflecting on the present self than when reflecting on the past self or the other person. These findings suggest that cortical midline structures support the ability to differentiate our present and past selves and thus maturation of self-identity over time.

At the neural level, the discovery of the mirror neuron system provided a major advance in understanding the basis of core social abilities, such as imitation and empathy, as well as possible insight into how we form our self-other identity. A key early finding was that the same group of neurons in the premotor cortex of monkeys was found to respond when they observed others perform a task as when they performed the task themselves (Rizzolatti, Fadiga, Gallese, & Fogassi, 1996). In humans, the mirror neuron system is believed to be located in the inferior frontal, ventral premotor and inferior parietal regions. Specifically, externally focused processes (i.e., those based on one's own or others' physical features and actions) rely on lateral fronto-parietal networks which are activated, for example, by observing different hand and lip movements for imitation purposes. Mirror neurons have also been implicated in understanding the intentions and emotional states of others (Rizzolatti & Craighero, 2005). Internally oriented processes that focus on one's own or others' mental states rely on cortical midline structures. For example, personally experiencing or observing disgust reactions in others has been found to activate the insula region, suggesting that this region is involved in both experiencing emotion and sharing another person's emotional state (see also the 'as-if-loop'; Damasio, 2003). More generally, there is converging evidence that the insula is activated when we share the emotional experiences of others and process self-referential information, suggesting that this region supports how we form our sense of self in relation to others.

Brain lesion studies have identified that damage to different areas of the brain produce distinct patterns of disturbance in self. 'Neuropathologies of the self' refer to disorders characterised by a profound alteration or disturbance in personal identity or relationship between self and the world (Feinberg, 2011b). Feinberg proposed a four-level hierarchical model to account for neuropathologies of self, which depicts different mechanisms contributing to these disorders. At the first and lowest level, various cognitive or functional deficits (e.g., sensory loss, perceptual disturbance, amnesia, executive dysfunction) serve as bottom-up factors that play a role in altering sense of self. At the second level, self-related deficits including impaired self-awareness (i.e., anosognosia), loss of body relatedness and loss of autobiographical memory contribute more directly to loss of identity and neuropathologies of self. The third level represents various defence mechanisms or ways in which the person tries to adapt to or cope with cognitive and self-related deficits. The person's own basic psychological defences (e.g., denial, projection) and unconscious motives may create an altered reality or a breakdown in ego boundaries and ego functions. At the fourth and highest level, various syndromes emerge from the interaction between these lower levels, including somatoparaphrenia (e.g., delusional denial of ownership of a limb), confabulation and Capgras syndrome (Feinberg, 2011b).

Based on a review of lesion studies, Feinberg identified that neuropathologies of self are most likely to occur after lesions to the right hemisphere, particularly damage to the medial-frontal or orbitofrontal regions. A key implication of Feinberg's four-tier model is that selective disturbances in self may occur based on the pattern of underlying cognitive and self-related deficits in addition to the person's own psychological defences and motivation.

Neuropsychological processes supporting self and identity

Self-identity requires awareness of one's inner sameness and continuity, and awareness of self in relation to others and the external world. Yet, self-identity is also continually under construction. Many different neuropsychological models are relevant to understanding sense of self, including broad models of hierarchical and interacting subsystems (e.g., Feinberg, 2011a; Teasdale & Barnard, 1993) and specific models of consciousness and autobiographical memory (Conway, 2005; Conway & Pleydell-Pearce, 2000; Damasio, 1999; Tulving, 1985; Zeman, 2002), emotion (Damasio, 2003; LeDoux, 1996), and executive function and metacognition (Stuss, 2007; Shallice & Burgess, 1996). The following review draws on these models to consider processes that support inner sameness and continuity of self and potential mechanisms underlying changes to self and identity.

Tulving's (1985) model of memory systems and consciousness proposes three different memory systems that correspond to different types of consciousness or levels of self-knowing. Procedural memory is associated with *anoetic* or implicit consciousness, which is bound to one's current situation and environment (i.e., perceptual registration and raw response to internal and external stimuli). Semantic memory is linked to *noetic* consciousness, which allows us to be aware of and perceive relationships between objects and events and symbolic representations of the world formed in the past (e.g., the names of friends from school). Episodic memory corresponds with *autonoetic* consciousness, and reflects an integrative process that allows us to recall events from our past and link these to notions of self in the future, thus providing extended consciousness. There are some parallels between this model and Damasio's (1999) account of proto-self, core self and autobiographical self (Table 2.2). However, core self is present only in the moment and reflects one's conscious experience of internal representations and the external world temporarily held in short-term memory (e.g., responding to a question someone has just asked). Autobiographical self entails extended or autonoetic consciousness, integrating past memories of self with one's ongoing experiences and future intentions and aspirations.

Conway and Pleydell-Pearce's (2000) model of the self-memory system suggests that memories relating to the self are motivated ongoing constructions that are prone to bias and error. The self-memory system consists of *autobiographical knowledge* (i.e., semantic and episodic memories) which is hierarchically organised around specific life-defining themes (e.g., work and relationships), and the *working self*. The latter component reflects a person's goals and motivation and serves to direct his or her thoughts and behaviour through online monitoring and control processes. The autobiographical knowledge and working self components interact to construct memories of one's past that are closely linked to personal goals and motivation, and support the maintenance of self-schemas. The central executive plays a key role in updating self-knowledge and implementing plans consistent with one's current goals and inhibiting thoughts or responses that conflict with or disrupt these plans. The working self is nevertheless constrained by one's autobiographical knowledge concerning what may be realistic goals to pursue.

Research has demonstrated an overlap in the neural activity involved in remembering our past and imagining our future, suggesting that we have a 'remembering–imagining' system that supports both personal accounts (Rathbone et al., 2011). The processes of reflecting on one's past and considering self in the future engage autobiographical memory circuitry (e.g., left hippocampus and posterior visuospatial regions), whilst reflecting on current self is more distinctly associated with activation in the medial prefrontal cortex (D'Argembeau et al., 2010). Through this integrated system we create a coherent life story that draws upon memories of our past and projects the self into the future through goals and plans. Ultimately, self-identity is closely linked to one's memories, beliefs and goals (Conway, 2005). Emotions play a critical role along with cognitive processes in supporting sense of self.

The emotions elicited by past memories and those linked to new experiences are processed via the amygdala and connecting thalamic and cortical pathways. This network represents an evaluative system that determines the emotional salience of our experiences, providing an emotional colouring or 'felt sense' to new memories formed (LeDoux, 1996). Research has mainly focused on the role of the amygdala in fear processing, highlighting two main pathways that operate to detect and respond to threat from internal stimuli (e.g., self-critical thoughts) and external stimuli (e.g., negative feedback from others). Firstly, the innate and fast-acting thalamo-amygdala pathway bypasses the cortex and produces autonomic, endocrine and behavioural responses according to simple stimulus features (e.g., intensity). This emotion-driven system is adaptive for survival and can interrupt ongoing activity to divert attention to the presence of threat or danger. Secondly, our conscious experience of fear depends on the slow-acting thalamo-cortical-amygdala pathway to cognitively appraise the meaning of stimuli within the context (LeDoux, 1996, 2000).

In an emotionally charged situation (e.g., an argument with a close friend), the fast-acting and non-conscious threat response system can initially dominate or disrupt higher order goal systems, performing a quick analysis of the emotional meaning of the situation. Cognitive representations form that link external stimuli (e.g., an angry face) with internal affective and physiological states (e.g., fear and autonomic reactivity), and are retrieved when triggered in relevant situations (Damasio, 1999). Immediate and emotionally driven responses often precede more carefully thought out reactions that are congruent with one's goals and social needs. Working memory has an integral role in supporting the conscious processing of incoming information, serving as a mental workspace to consider the personal salience of our experiences by drawing on stored representations from long-term memories (LeDoux, 2000). The working memory system registers that the self is under threat (i.e., activation of the fear system) and supports processing of information at the implicational level, to determine what this may mean for one's self and the future to guide goal-directed behaviour (e.g., effective communication to maintain harmony in a valued relationship).

Gainotti (2012) proposed a further pathway for unconscious processing of emotions and memories. Specifically, there is converging evidence from experimental research and lesion studies that unconscious processing of emotional information is mediated by the right hemisphere via a subcortical pathway involving the right amygdala. The right hemisphere more generally has a greater role in the comprehension and expression of emotions, supporting rapid discrimination between pleasant and unpleasant or threatening stimuli. It has also been proposed that the right hemisphere may be involved in repression and denial, or the unconscious distortion of reality to protect self from negative emotional states (Gainotti, 2012). However, the left hemisphere also plays a critical role in supporting sense of self, both in terms of language functions (e.g., inner speech) and providing unity and conscious processing of ongoing experiences.

Teasdale and Barnard's (1993) model of information processing distinguishes between propositional and implicational meanings relevant to self. Propositional meanings refer to the literal meaning of language and our store of semantic or declarative knowledge which is largely mediated by the left hemisphere. Propositional level of knowledge about self refers to objective physical and biographical information (e.g., age, height, place of birth). Implicational meanings refer to more abstract themes and schematic mental models of human experience. These include metaphor, imagery and narrative, and are closely tied to emotion. Personal metaphors and self-narrative elicit certain emotional, motivational and bodily states and guide one's actions (Ylvisaker & Feeney, 2000). For example, a woman who views herself as strong and resilient as an oak tree in a storm may persist with her goals despite setbacks. The right frontal lobe has been identified as the site of convergence for neural processes supporting higher level self-representations (e.g., self-metaphors) and self-reflective capacity (Stuss, Picton, & Alexander, 2001).

Various higher cortical functions support the experience of self and interactions between self and the world. These are mediated by two major functional systems, the executive control system supported by the dorsolateral prefrontal cortex (DLPFC), and the behavioural/emotional self-regulatory system supported by the ventromedial prefrontal cortex (VMPFC). According to Stuss's framework (2007), executive control functions of the DLPFC include planning, monitoring, switching and inhibition, and help to coordinate and direct our thoughts and behaviours. Behavioural/emotional self-regulation occurs via the VMPFC to support the processing of emotions (i.e., reward-based learning) that guide effective decision-making in accordance with one's goals. Activation regulating functions (i.e., superior medial frontal) support drive, or the ability to generate, organise and sustain activity to pursue goals. Stuss referred to metacognitive processes as higher level integrative functions, which are essential for self-identity and personality formation. These abilities have been linked to the frontal polar region (particularly right frontal) and include self-awareness, autonoetic consciousness, and social cognition (Platek, Keenan, Gallup, & Mohamed, 2004). As highlighted throughout this chapter, sense of self is largely derived from social interaction and our ability to relate to others. Our self-reflective capacity is central to maintaining or updating our self-schema concerning new experiences (e.g., goal achievement, feedback) that reinforce or alter existing notions of self.

Neuropsychological mechanisms underlying changes to self

The neuropsychological accounts described so far depict the interaction between cognitive and emotional systems that support both the stability and ongoing construction of self-identity. The process of updating self-knowledge and self-schemas is important to consider in more detail, particularly given the focus of this book. As previously discussed, social psychology perspectives highlight that self-comparison and self-discrepancy processes may alter self-concept regarding personal competencies or attributes (Eisenstadt & Leippe, 1994). The corresponding neuropsychological functions that support these processes are unclear. One possible explanation lies in the concept of a 'comparator mechanism', which may be responsible for updating self-knowledge and beliefs based on perceived goal success and feedback from others.

Agnew and Morris (1998) proposed the Cognitive Awareness Model (CAM) to account for anosognosia and the notion of 'petrified self' in Alzheimer's disease (Mograbi et al., 2009). However, this model has broader utility for understanding changes in self-concept and identity. The CAM proposes that self-appraisal of one's cognitive abilities is based on perceptions of relative success or failure on activities (note: this could be extended to psychological attributes and social skills). New information relevant to self is continually monitored and either temporarily stored in short-term memory or consolidated in long-term memory. The Personal Data Base (PDB) represents our storehouse of personal semantic information derived from experience. The PDB is updated by a set of comparator mechanisms within the central executive system, which detect a mismatch between the PDB record and experiences of success or failure (i.e., self-discrepancy). The capacity to consciously perceive a mismatch relies on signals being sent to the Metacognitive Awareness System (MAS), to produce explicit awareness of one's performance, which is compared against existing self-knowledge in the PDB. New information about self may also bypass the MAS and guide behaviour through implicit awareness of performance failure or success (Agnew & Morris, 1998). Importantly, the PDB record is shaped by social and cultural expectations (i.e., general semantic knowledge). Hence, self-perceptions of ability or goal success are influenced by social standards or expectations of significant others (e.g., family or peers).

Although not specifically accounted for by the CAM, emotional and motivational factors are likely to influence the extent to which a mismatch between one's performance and existing self-knowledge is consciously perceived. Emotional factors interact with conditions in the environment and affect cognitive processing. Specifically, when an individual feels under threat there is typically a narrowing of attention and reduction in the availability of information from the current situation due to selective attention, and relevant past experiences due to selective recall (Teasdale & Barnard, 1993). Negative feedback and goal failure may activate threat-based coping reactions. Some individuals may be excessively motivated to protect their self-image or manage their social impression, and thus employ defense mechanisms to deny or distort information (Feinberg, 2011b; Ownsworth, 2005). Others may selectively attend to their errors (i.e., magnification) or readily perceive information as a threat to self (e.g., perceiving criticism in others' neutral comments).

According to Rogers (1951), individuals may react in three possible ways to new experiences in life, namely, they may: 1) ignore the information because it is perceived to have no relation or significance to self; 2) perceive, symbolise and assimilate the information in relation to self; or 3) deny the relevance or distort the meaning of information because it presents a threat to one's desired self-image. Perceived threat in the environment and lack of emotional safety is likely to impair self-monitoring and self-reflective processes conducive to updating self-knowledge and modifying self-schema (Harter, 2012; Rogers, 1951). In contrast, openness, empathy, building of trust and positive regard from others creates a supportive context for learning about self.

In summary, sense of self forms and is maintained and updated by a coordinated neural network. At a basic level, information about self is registered through sense organs and undergoes perceptual processing to form higher level representations of the external world and our internal states (i.e., affective and bodily reactions). Working memory supports the encoding and retrieval of this information in autobiographical memory in accordance with a person's goals, motivation and emotional state. Executive processes support the abstraction of patterns or themes about self across specific autobiographical memories. Metacognition and social cognition processes support online monitoring and appraisal of one's performance during activities and social interaction. A comparator mechanism detects changes in self (i.e., self-discrepancies) and updates self-knowledge. However, coping mechanisms and various contextual factors (e.g., emotional support) influence how new information relevant to self is perceived and the extent to which it modifies self-schema or broader notions of self.

An integrated account of self and relevance to brain injury

Based on the diverse theories considered throughout this chapter, a schematic representation of self-identity is presented in Figure 2.1. Self-identity is represented as a unified and global self-system comprised of multiple identities which are tied to specific social roles and relationships and generalised self-attributes. Some identities are more salient and compelling in certain situations than others, as reflected by the broken lines. Collectively, these identities and their personal significance contribute to a coherent life story or self-narrative. Our global self-system provides continuity of self by integrating awareness of one's past and present (i.e., who we are) with the future (i.e., who we might be or hope to become). Self-identity is continually under construction with cognitive and emotional processes interacting to update self-knowledge and shape sense of self.

This broad framework provides a structure for considering the impact of brain injury on self-identity. Accordingly, subsequent chapters of this book seek to address the following questions:

- What impact does brain injury have on self-identity at different phases of life (e.g., childhood, adolescence, and adulthood)?
- How do acquired physical, cognitive, behavioural and socio-emotional impairments influence sense of self? Related to this, does the inability to update

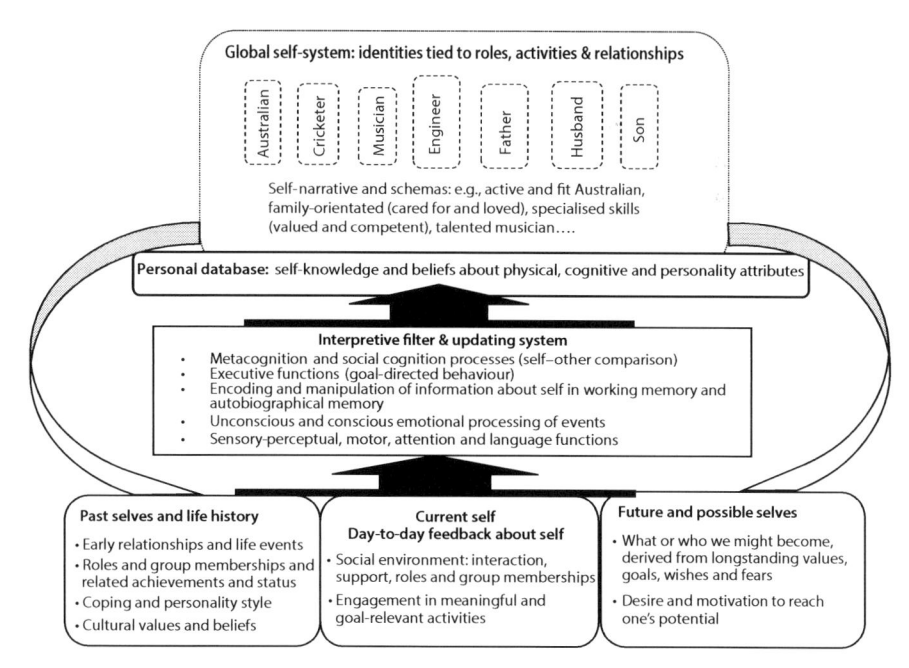

Figure 2.1 A schematic representation of the global self-system and components supporting continuity and change

self-knowledge or perceive negative social reactions reduce threats to self and protect one's self-image? Alternatively, do these impairments pose a barrier to reconstructing an adaptive identity?
- What pre-injury, neuropsychological and social factors influence sense of self after brain injury?
- How are changes in self-identity after brain injury best identified or measured?
- How can rehabilitation best support individuals to maintain or rebuild a positive self-identity after brain injury?
- How do family members cope with changes to their loved one and the impact of brain injury on their own lives?

Conclusions

Chapter 2 introduced the key concepts of self and identity and related terminology relevant to this book. Historical perspectives and leading psychological and sociological accounts of self and identity provided a foundation for contemporary social neuroscience perspectives that will be drawn upon in the chapters that follow. Chapter 3 presents an introduction to brain injury and the consequences during childhood and adolescence. Theories and research on adjustment to brain injury and self-identity changes in adults are discussed in Chapter 4. In-depth consideration is given to clinical approaches for assessing self-identity processes in Chapter 5, and individual, group and family-based interventions are the focus of Chapters 6, 7 and 8 respectively. Chapter 9 summarises leading developments and recommendations for future research in this field.

3 Introduction to brain injury and consequences during childhood and adolescence

This chapter provides an introduction to brain injury and summarises the main causes and functional consequences. The diverse factors contributing to outcomes after brain injury are conceptualised within a biopsychosocial framework which highlights the interactive influence of pre-injury, injury and post-injury characteristics. A developmental perspective of the consequences of brain injury for children and adolescents is presented that draws on the biopsychosocial framework to identify vulnerability and protective factors influencing adjustment. Two case studies illustrate the impact of sustaining a brain injury early in life on developing sense of self.

Overview of the causes and consequences of brain injury

This book focuses on *acquired* brain injury, which refers to damage or disease processes that disrupt brain functioning after birth and produce persisting physical, cognitive and behavioural impairments. This term encompasses neurological damage caused by diverse mechanisms including non-progressive and progressive processes, those with sudden and gradual onset, and both internal and external mechanisms. The focus here is on non-progressive causes of brain injury, due to extensive coverage elsewhere on the impact of progressive neurological disorders on sense of self (see Clare, 2008). Although this book is chiefly concerned with the impact of brain injury on adults, the consequences of childhood brain injury are reviewed in this chapter to provide an account of how brain injury disrupts developing sense of sense.

The most common causes of non-progressive brain injury include stroke, traumatic brain injury (TBI), lack of oxygen (e.g., near drowning, cardiac arrest), infection, poisoning and brain tumour. However, it is noteworthy that people with brain tumour can experience further decline in function after the initial diagnosis due to inoperable tumours, re-occurrences, and the impact of treatment on neurological functioning. Focusing on the two most common causes of brain injury, estimated worldwide incidence rates for stroke and traumatic brain injury are approximately 15 million and 10 million respectively, with rates varying according to socio-economic status, age and gender (Corrigan, Selassie, & Orman, 2010; Feigin, Lawes, Bennett, Barker-Collo, & Parag, 2009; Rutland-Brown, Langlois, Thomas, & Xi, 2006). Across the lifespan the incidence of stroke was recorded as 94 per 100,000 for high income countries in comparison to 117 per 100,000 for low to middle income countries (Feigin et al., 2009).

A large cohort study in the UK by Wolfe et al. (2011) found the incidence of stroke to be considerably higher for adults over age 65 (approximately 70 per cent), and was equally common in men (51 per cent) and women (49 per cent). However, another study found a greater incidence of stroke for men than women up to age 75, no difference in rates for men and women in the 75–84 age bracket, and greater incidence for women in the 85 years and older age bracket (Rosamond et al., 2007). Wolfe et al. (2011) found that ischaemic strokes were most common (77 per cent), followed by primary intracerebral (14 per cent) and subarachnoid haemorrhage (6 per cent).

Corrigan et al. (2010) reported that incidence of TBI is highest for people at the extremes of the lifespan, with 900 cases per 100,000 for children (< 10 years) and 659 cases per 100,000 for older adults (> 74 years). Falls represented the main cause of injury in both age groups. Most studies have found a greater incidence of TBI for non-white ethnicity than white ethnicity groups (Corrigan et al., 2010; Thompson, McCormick & Kagan, 2006). TBI is more common for men than women, particularly in the 18–25 year age bracket where a ratio of 3:1 is commonly reported and road traffic accidents are the leading cause (Australian Institute of Health and Welfare [AIHW], 2008). The overall higher prevalence of TBI for men has been attributed to males engaging in more risk-taking behaviour and activities (Corrigan et al., 2010). Low socio-economic status (SES) has also been found to be a general risk factor for TBI. However, a study in New Zealand by McKinlay, Grace, Horwood, Fergusson and MacFarlane (2009) found that other pre-injury factors were more predictive of TBI than SES for children aged 0–15 years. The strongest unique predictors included the presence of other adverse life events and punitive parenting style, with the greater risk of injury attributed to family stress and reduced supervision. Overall, these population-based studies highlight that the risk of sustaining brain injury is greater for some individuals than others, and that post-injury outcomes need to be considered in the broader context of pre-injury functioning and social factors.

Brain injury outcomes can be broadly summarised using the International Classification of Functioning, Disability and Health, or ICF framework (World Health Organisation, 2001), which delineates consequences at the level of body functions (i.e., impairments or loss of function), activities (i.e., limitations performing tasks or actions) and participation (i.e., restrictions in involvement in a life situation). The ICF framework recognises that a person's functioning arises from a dynamic interaction between the health condition/s and contextual factors (i.e., personal and environmental factors). Environmental factors relate to the physical, social and attitudinal aspects of one's living environment (e.g., climate, legislation, social attitudes, access to health care). Personal factors include individual characteristics such as age, gender, ethnicity, occupation, personality traits and coping behaviours which affect how the health condition is subjectively experienced.

The ICF framework has been used to develop comprehensive core sets for many major health conditions including TBI and stroke (see Bernabeu et al., 2009; Geyh et al., 2004). The core sets present a classification system or checklist that can be used to create a profile of a person's functioning and health. For example, Koskinen, Hokkinen, Sarajuuri and Alaranta (2007) applied the ICF checklist to examine level of functioning and barriers or facilitators in the environment for adults with TBI in post-acute rehabilitation. Impairments in body functions were most common for the following: mental functions (e.g., memory, higher level cognitive functions, attention, emotional functions, energy and drive functions, and language), sensory functions and pain, and neuro-musculoskeletal and movement related functions. The most common activity limitations and participation restrictions related to the following: learning and applying new knowledge, communication, mobility, domestic life, interpersonal interactions and relationships and major life areas (e.g., employment). Environmental factors impacting post-injury adjustment included problems with services, systems and policies, support and relationships, and products and technology.

Follow-up studies of TBI and stroke highlight persisting problems with cognitive, emotional and behavioural functioning. For example, at a three-year follow-up after TBI, Tate et al. (2006) found that the most common problems were attention (53 per cent), memory (61 per cent), problem-solving (52 per cent) and indifference (37 per cent). In the first 12 months post-TBI the rate of depression has been found to be as high as 53 per cent (Bombardier, Fann, Temkin, Esselman, Barber, & Dikmen, 2010); however, most studies report rates around 30 per cent for TBI (Ownsworth, Fleming et al., 2011) and stroke (De Wit et al., 2008). Wolfe and colleagues (2011) identified that global cognitive impairment (18 per cent) and levels of anxiety (35 per cent) and depression (31 per cent) remained high over 10 years post-stroke. Australian data indicate that the cognitive and emotional aspects of functioning are the most common areas warranting long-term support for people with brain injury (AIHW, 2008). Fleminger and Ponsford (2005) also emphasised that the neuropsychiatric sequelae of TBI contributed more to long-term disability than neurophysical sequelae.

Participation in valued activities, life roles and relationships is often greatly impacted by brain injury. The transition from hospital to home is a peak time during which people with brain injury strive to regain independence and resume their pre-injury lifestyle (Nalder et al., 2012; Turner, Ownsworth, Cornwell, & Fleming, 2009). Research examining community reintegration outcomes has highlighted that return to some level of independence in the home and community is typically achieved by most individuals in the first 6 months. Nalder et al. (2012) found that 89 per cent of their mixed brain injury sample ($n = 90$) reported that they were able to be left at home alone for a period of at least 4 hours within the first 6 months post-discharge, with most people achieving this soon after discharge. Furthermore, 78 per cent of the sample regained their ability to independently access the community and use public transport in the first 6 months (Nalder et al., 2012). Community reintegration outcomes that require higher level cognitive functions, such as return to work or study, and return to driving were less commonly achieved in the first 6 months post-discharge. Specifically, Nalder et al. (2012) found that 62 per cent of participants returned to work or study in the first 6 months, which is higher than the return to work rates of 40–50 per cent typically reported in the literature (Kreutzer et al., 2003). Nalder et al. (2012) identified that approximately half of their brain injury sample (55 per cent) returned to driving in the first 6 months post-discharge.

In addition to reduced productivity, people's social group memberships and support networks are known to diminish after brain injury and there is often heavy reliance on close family members to provide long-term care and support (Degeneffe,

2001; Haslam et al., 2008). Interactions and relationship dynamics within the family often drastically change as particular members assume a caregiver role, as discussed in more detail in Chapter 8. For example, children may support a parent with brain injury, a wife or husband may care for their spouse, and parents may resume caring for an adult child who had previously left home and achieved independence. Such role adjustments can place considerable strain on relationships (Gervasio & Kreutzer, 1997; Marsh, Kersel, Havill, & Sleigh, 2002). Nalder et al. (2012) found that 18 per cent of people with brain injury experienced a relationship breakdown with a family member or partner in the first 6 months post-discharge. However, much higher rates have been reported in the longer-term with 49 per cent experiencing separation or divorce from their partner at 5–8 years post-injury (Wood & Yurdakul, 1997). As noted by Prigatano (1989), the complex impairments arising from brain injury compromise people's ability to engage in 'work, love and play'; the fundamental aspects of normal life.

Overview of factors influencing outcomes of brain injury

The outcomes of brain injury differ for every person due to a unique combination of pre-injury factors, injury-related factors and post-injury circumstances. Many authors have applied a biopsychosocial framework to consider the multitude of factors that interact to influence psychological well-being and social outcomes (e.g., Ownsworth & McKenna, 2004; Ownsworth & Oei, 1998; Pepping & Roueche, 1991; Yeates, Gracey, & Collicutt McGrath, 2008). As well as guiding empirical research, these frameworks can assist clinicians to develop a working model or formulation that guides assessment and treatment efforts (Gracey, Evans & Malley, 2009; Wilson et al., 2009). Factors related to outcome are typically clustered into the subsets of pre-injury characteristics, neuropathology, psychological factors and the social environmental context, as depicted in Figure 3.1. Although an in-depth review of these factors is beyond the scope of this chapter, the following section provides an overview of empirical findings concerning the impact of pre-injury characteristics and neuropathology on outcome. The role of psychological factors and the social environmental context is considered later in this chapter for children and adolescents, and is the main focus of Chapter 4 on psychological adjustment and self-identity changes.

In terms of pre-injury characteristics, a person's biology, social background and previous life circumstances are essential to consider when interpreting outcomes after brain injury. Pepping and Roueche (1991) referred to these as 'pre-existing assets and liabilities'. Other authors have similarly highlighted that not only are particular people at greater risk of sustaining a brain injury in the first place, but some are more likely to experience poor outcomes (McKinlay et al., 2009; Thompson et al., 2006). At the genetic level, there is some empirical support that apolipoprotein E (Apo E) genotype is associated with poorer long-term functional outcomes after controlling for age and injury severity (Friedman et al., 1999; Ponsford et al., 2011). With regards to age, in the adult brain injury literature, Senathi-Raja, Ponsford and Schönberger (2010) found that older adults with TBI had poorer cognitive outcomes than younger adults when compared with matched controls.

```
┌─────────────────────────────────┐      ┌─────────────────────────────────┐
│   Pre-injury characteristics    │      │         Neuropathology          │
│ - Genotype, age, gender,        │      │ - Cause and mechanisms of injury│
│   ethnicity, occupation,        │      │ - Severity, location, recurrence│
│   health, cognitive and         │      │ - Treatment type and            │
│   physical abilities            │      │   effectiveness                 │
│ - Psychological and social      │      │ - Direct effects on functioning │
│   resources                     │      │                                 │
└─────────────────────────────────┘      └─────────────────────────────────┘

                    ┌──────────────────────────────────┐
                    │     Outcomes of brain injury     │
                    │    Physical, cognitive, social,  │
                    │     emotional and behavioural    │
                    └──────────────────────────────────┘

┌─────────────────────────────────┐      ┌─────────────────────────────────┐
│      Psychological factors      │      │       Social environment        │
│ - Personal appraisals and       │      │ - Concurrent stressors          │
│   reactions (personality,       │      │ - Access to resources (physical,│
│   self-awareness, coping        │      │   financial, information, social│
│   strategies, motivation        │      │   support and rehabilitation)   │
│   and goals)                    │      │                                 │
└─────────────────────────────────┘      └─────────────────────────────────┘
```

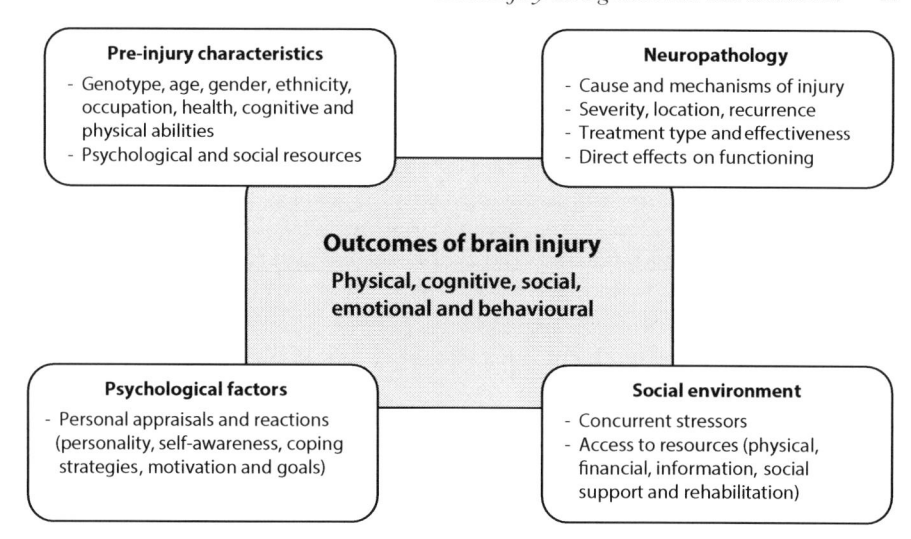

Figure 3.1 A biopsychosocial framework of factors contributing to brain injury outcomes

Some studies suggest that women experience better outcomes than men after TBI due to the neuroprotective role of oestrogen and progesterone (e.g., Roof & Hall, 2000); however, the reverse has been found for stroke (Falcone & Chong, 2007). Overall, the evidence for gender differences in cognitive and functional outcomes is mixed (Ownsworth & McKenna, 2004; Thompson et al., 2006). Research by Sherer et al. (2003) highlighted the influence of ethnicity on occupational outcomes after TBI. Individuals' ethnicity was significantly related to their pre-injury productivity, education and cause of injury; however, after adjusting for the influence of these predictors, African Americans and other ethnic minorities still had significantly poorer occupational outcomes than Whites.

Premorbid cognitive functioning, psychological status and social resources have also been investigated as predictors of outcome after brain injury. Withall, Brodaty, Altendorf and Sachdev (2009) found that individuals with higher premorbid IQ experienced better functional outcomes after stroke than those with lower premorbid IQ. Kesler, Adams, Blasey and Bigler (2003) identified that irrespective of TBI severity, individuals with greater total intracranial volume demonstrated lower pre-post injury intellectual decline. Total intracranial volume and education both predicted post-injury IQ category (< 90 or ≥ 90). The authors proposed that people with a larger premorbid brain volume and higher education level are less vulnerable to cognitive deficits after TBI. Also supporting the notion of cognitive reserve, higher estimated premorbid IQ has been found to correlate with lower levels of depression after brain tumour and TBI (Ownsworth, Hawkes, Chambers, Walker & Shum, 2010; Salmond, Menon, Chatfield, Pickard & Sahakian, 2006). Although the factors underlying the relationship between premorbid IQ and brain injury outcomes are unclear, the role of pre-existing psychological and social resources is important to consider.

In line with this view, Bombardier et al. (2010) found that premorbid psychological status (i.e., diagnosis of depression and lifetime alcohol dependence) was the best predictor of diagnosis of major depression after TBI. Pre-existing stressors, family dysfunction and social disadvantage have also been found to be important predictors of outcome following childhood TBI (Anderson, Godfrey, Rosenfeld & Catroppa, 2012; McKinlay et al., 2009). More generally, the factors contributing to mental health, cognitive functioning and occupational or educational achievement prior to brain injury are likely to have a key influence on well-being after brain injury (Ownsworth & Oei, 1998; Sherer et al., 2003). This issue will be revisited in the context of childhood brain injury in the next section.

In addition to pre-injury characteristics, brain injury outcomes vary according to the underlying neuropathology, as indicated by injury mechanisms and the location, extent and severity of damage. For example, survival rates and functional outcomes are typically poorer for haemorrhagic stroke than ischaemic stroke, in part due to greater advances in treatment for the latter such as thrombolytic therapy (Fleminger, 2009). In the case of TBI, injuries that involve acceleration and deceleration forces (e.g., a high speed motor vehicle accident), typically produce poorer functional outcomes than more focal lesions due to diffuse axonal injury or widespread shearing and tearing of axons and blood vessels (Levin, 2012). However, focal damage to the prefrontal cortex and temporal poles is also particularly common following TBI, and can disrupt higher order cognitive processes and emotional and behavioural regulation. These impairments are found to be associated with poor occupational and social outcomes (Fleminger & Ponsford, 2005; Ownsworth & McKenna, 2004). Hypoxic-ischaemic injuries, brain infections and surgery for intractable seizures most commonly affect the medial temporal lobes, with the extent of damage to the hippocampus and parahippocampal gyrus found to correspond with the degree of memory impairment (Stefanacci, Buffalo, Schmolck & Squire, 2000; Yonelinas et al., 2002).

Although damage to the same brain region typically produces similar functional effects, different mechanisms of injury have been found to produce varied impairment profiles. For example, Anderson, Damasio and Tranel (1990) compared the neuropsychological functioning of individuals with stroke matched closely to individuals with brain tumour on the basis of lesion location, and found differences in neuropsychological profile. In the case of brain tumour, although the site of tumour growth is often related to the symptoms (e.g., expressive communication deficits arising from tumours in the left frontal region), due to compression and displacement effects the tumour may produce more widespread damage within the brain as a result of midline shift, obstruction of the ventricle system and increased intracranial pressure. Hence, global cognitive decline may be experienced, particularly for large tumours (Mellado-Calvo & Fleminger, 2009). Nonetheless, there are converging findings from lesion studies and brain imaging studies of brain–behaviour relationships with respect to sensory-perceptual, motor, language, cognitive and emotional functions (Fleminger, 2009). It is also well established that disturbances in self and self-regulation are most consistently associated with damage to the right prefrontal region, particularly the medial and orbito-medial areas (Feinberg, 2011a; Stuss et al., 2002).

Severity of injury for both TBI and stroke has been found to be a relatively reliable predictor of many outcomes such as survival, global functional status and cognitive outcomes (Anderson et al., 2012; Falcone & Chong, 2007; Fleminger, 2009). However, injury severity is less consistently related to psychological outcomes, including emotional adjustment (Fuentes, Ortiz, Sanjose, Frank, & Díez-Tejedor, 2009). Furthermore, the neurological characteristics of brain tumour (e.g., type, location and size of tumour) do not reliably account for differences in quality of life and emotional status following brain tumour (Ownsworth, Hawkes, Steginga, Walker & Shum, 2009).

Overall, despite evidence that premorbid and neurological characteristics influence the outcomes of brain injury, such factors alone cannot account for differences in functional status and emotional adjustment. The contribution of psychological characteristics (e.g., self-appraisals and coping reactions) and social environmental factors (e.g., access to information, rehabilitation and social support) to sense of self after brain injury will be considered in detail in Chapter 4. The following section considers the impact of sustaining brain injury early in life and the implications for emerging sense of self.

Brain injury during childhood

The outcomes of brain injury differ for children and adults, in part due to brain maturation processes which affect the timing in which functional skills emerge. In particular, the development of sensory, language, cognitive, physical/motor and emotional and social skills depends on neural processes supporting the integrity of brain structures and connective pathways. Brain structures have the general appearance of those of an adult by age 2 years, and all main fibre tracts are evident by age 3 years. A rapid increase in grey matter volume is evident up until 4 years of age (Johnson, 2001). The second wave of synaptogenesis occurs during ages 6–12 years. Pruning of cells and synapses occurs between 12–25 years of age and increases in white matter and myelination occur throughout adolescence and into adulthood. These maturation processes occur earlier in the posterior regions of the brain while the prefrontal cortex and connective pathways are the last to mature (see Gogtay et al., 2004; Johnson, 2001). Therefore, when brain injury occurs during childhood it can disrupt skills that are developing as well as those yet to develop (Ewing, 2006; Ewing-Cobbs et al., 2006). In contrast, damage to the adult brain is more likely to lead to a loss or decline in skills previously acquired.

Recovery after childhood brain injury can reflect many trajectories, including an initial decline and then recovery to premorbid levels, a consistent lag in comparison to normal children, and the delayed emergence of problems (Babikian & Asarnow, 2009; Levin, 2012; Taylor, Yeates, Wade, Drotar, Stancin, & Minich, 2002). Although the relationship between age and outcome from brain injury is complex, it is generally recognised that sustaining a severe brain injury during early childhood (e.g., before the age of 7) is associated with poorer outcomes than an injury during later childhood. Early damage to the prefrontal cortex can lead to the delayed emergence of problems with emotional and behavioural regulation (orbital), initiation and drive (ventromedial) and executive control (dorsolateral). These difficulties can become more evident or emerge with changes in environmental structure and increased expectations of independence and behaviour regulation, which often occurs as children transition from primary school to high school (Cronin, 2001; Ewing, 2006).

In a meta-analysis of neurocognitive outcomes of paediatric brain injury, Babikian and Asarnow (2009) synthesised findings of 28 studies according to injury severity (mild, moderate, severe), age at injury (0–5 years, 6–16 years) and time post-injury (0–5 months, 6–23 months, ≥ 24 months) for 14 neurocognitive domains. They found negligible overall differences in most neurocognitive domains for children with mild TBI as compared with controls, with the exception of processing speed and verbal fluency skills which evidenced small to moderate effects and were greatest at ≥ 24 months. For children with moderate TBI overall differences from controls were negligible for most cognitive domains. However, small and consistent differences were found for attention and problem-solving at each time point, and large effects emerged at ≥ 24 months for processing speed and inhibition. Conversely, large early effects for IQ decreased by later time points. The pattern for children with severe TBI was quite distinct from the trends for mild and moderate TBI, with gaps in cognitive performance increasing over time and denoting significant deficits in most neurocognitive domains relative to controls. This was especially marked for IQ, verbal memory, processing speed, attention, fluency and problem-solving. The most striking finding was that children with severe TBI evidence a slower rate of development, which contributes to an expanding gap in cognitive performance over time relative to age peers (Babikian & Asarnow, 2009).

In terms of behavioural outcomes, a systematic review by Li and Liu (2012) found that approximately 30–50 per cent of children developed attention, hyperactivity and inhibitory control difficulties (note: approximately 20 per cent had a premorbid history of these issues), and that oppositional defiant disorder or conduct disorder emerged for 20–40 per cent of children. Aggressive behaviour was less common, and was typically linked to pre-injury aggression and impairments in self-regulation and social problem-solving. In terms of internalising disorders, novel depressive disorders developed in 10–15 per cent of school-aged children within the first two years after TBI. Rates of new-onset mood or anxiety disorders were found to be higher after TBI (46 per cent) than orthopaedic injury (14 per cent) (Luis & Mittenberg, 2002). The emergence of novel externalising and internalising disorders was linked to neuro-cognitive sequelae across many studies, particularly lesions to the left inferior frontal, right medial frontal, orbitofrontal cortex and left temporal lobe.

Li and Liu's (2012) review indicated that family environmental factors such as socio-economic status and parenting style influence children's behavioural outcomes. However, research by Yeates, Taylor, Walz, Stancin and Wade (2010) suggests that this relationship may vary over time. For example, permissive and authoritarian parenting styles were related to few behavioural problems soon after injury, but poorer behavioural outcomes in the longer term (Yeates et al., 2010). The influence of parenting style on behavioural outcomes may be greatest for children with severe TBI. Specifically, after controlling for key demographic and premorbid variables (e.g., socio-economic status, parental distress, family functioning and pre-injury behaviour), Wade, Cassedy, Walz, Taylor, Stancin and Yeates (2011) found that parental warm responsiveness was associated with fewer internalising and externalising behavioural problems after severe TBI, whilst greater parental negativity was associated with more externalising behaviours. Wade et al. described a model of reciprocal influences whereby the child's early emotional and behavioural dysregulation is responded to with criticism and harsh discipline, which in turn contributes to 'a cycle of mounting parental negativity and escalating child behaviour problems' (p. 130). Their finding that parenting style contributes to the emergence of new behavioural problems highlights the need for family-centred intervention (see Chapter 8).

Paediatric brain injury research indicates that age at injury and severity of injury are both important prognostic factors for cognitive, behavioural and social outcomes (Anderson, Catroppa, Morse, Haritou, & Rosenfeld, 2005; McKinlay et al., 2009). In a long-term follow-up study of children who sustained mild TBI before age 10, McKinlay, Dalrymple-Alford, Horwood and Fergusson (2002) found greater evidence of hyperactivity, attentional and conduct problems at ages 10–16 years when compared with uninjured peers. These problems were largely found to persist into adulthood, and were more marked for children who sustained their injuries before age 5 (McKinlay et al., 2009). Ylvisaker and Feeney (2007) also found that long-term communication disability was more evident for children who sustained a severe brain injury at a younger age, and was related to underlying impairments in executive, cognitive and behavioural functioning. Further, Anderson et al. (2005) identified that children who sustained a severe TBI at a younger age (i.e., < 8 years) were more likely to experience poor cognitive outcomes at 12 and 30 months post-injury than older children. Such findings support the 'double hazard' model concerning the heightened vulnerability of children who sustain early and severe brain damage (Anderson et al., 2005).

A link has also been demonstrated between early severe injury, white matter disruption and poor functional recovery. Specifically, in a sample of children aged 2–7 years, severity of TBI and white matter volume was predictive of IQ at 10-year follow-up (Anderson et al., 2012). Children's intellectual, adaptive, executive and social functions were mainly in the low average to average range; however, those with more severe TBI had significantly poorer adaptive functioning and speed of processing. Pre-injury ability was most predictive of adaptive functioning whilst family functioning was the best predictor of social and behavioural outcomes.

Taylor et al. (2002) examined short-term and long-term (4 years post-injury) behavioural and educational outcomes of children with mixed injury severity. Children with severe TBI displayed poorer behavioural, adaptive and academic functioning than orthopaedic controls; however, social disadvantage (e.g., family socio-economic status and stressors) also predicted poorer outcomes and moderated the relationship between injury severity and outcome (i.e., mathematical ability). Children with severe TBI from dysfunctional social backgrounds were found to be doubly disadvantaged and had less 'catch-up growth'. The authors proposed that the social environments of these children were less conducive to recovery, with parents having limited personal and social resources for providing the stimulation and support to facilitate experience-dependent recovery.

It is therefore evident that family and social factors contribute to both the risk of injury (McKinlay et al., 2009) and extent of recovery, particularly from severe

TBI. Taylor et al. (2002) inferred that recovery of certain functional skills (e.g., mathematical ability) may be more dependent on 'environmentally mediated neural reorganisation' (p. 22). Levin (2012) highlighted that the mechanisms of TBI may also influence neuroplasticity in young children. For example, he noted that there is likely to be more potential for reorganisation of cerebral function following early focal vascular lesions as compared with severe and diffuse white matter injuries that involved greater acceleration and deceleration forces.

Overall, most research to date has focused on cognitive, behavioural and social outcomes of paediatric brain injury. Very few studies have examined psychological consequences or effects on self-concept for children and adolescents. The literature reviewed in Chapter 2 indicates that the development of self-awareness and sense of self occurs as a product of both one's biology and socio-cultural context. Specifically, children learn about themselves and form their self-concept through social interaction and by developing age-appropriate competencies, as supported by brain development. A developmental perspective of identity and self-concept formation (Erikson, 1963; Harter, 2012) may suggest that children who sustain a severe injury at a very young age would have more difficulty developing a positive sense of self, due to the greater impact on their physical, cognitive and social competencies and disparity in performance from their peers.

However, some literature suggests that self-awareness and cognitive impairments influence children's capacity to recognise and appraise the effects of their injury, and assimilate this knowledge into their developing self-concept. Furthermore, if children are injured before they have formed a stable self-concept it is possible that the brain injury will have less detrimental psychological effects because they are less likely to experience self-discrepancy, or unfavourable comparisons between current self with past or ideal selves (Higgins, 1987). Social environmental factors, such as parental responsiveness and parenting style have been found to influence behavioural outcomes (Wade et al., 2011; Yeates et al., 2010). For example, efforts to shield a child from information about their injury or from experiencing a sense of failure may protect against the negative effects of deficits on self-esteem. Ylvisaker, Feeney, and Szekeres (1998) also noted that the high level of support and accommodations (e.g., reduced expectations and assistance on tasks) often provided by family and professionals could help to ensure that young children mainly experience success in their pursuits at home and school, rather than exposing them to their difficulties and associated emotional reactions. However, in the long term such social responses may exacerbate adjustment problems for young children or those with significant cognitive deficits, who may struggle to make sense of their difficulties in relation to their peers as these emerge over time.

Children with brain injury have been found to display a lack of knowledge about their injury as well as impaired self-awareness of the functional effects (Beardmore, Tate, & Liddle, 1999; Jacobs, 1993). Qualitative research by Jacobs (1993) identified four factors influencing children's (7–15 years) understanding of brain injury, namely, their knowledge of normal brain and body functioning, access to information about their own injury, a clear account of how their injury occurred, and the extent of their cognitive impairments. Children had more accurate understanding of the observable physical changes (e.g., mobility and appearance), and tended to describe parts of their body as 'handicapped' rather than themselves. Children were typically less aware of learning problems, although problems with reading and memory were more commonly identified than other cognitive deficits (i.e., subtle language and social and behavioural problems). Overall, children showed a lack of self-understanding about their brain injury and its consequences, which was attributed to a combination of developmental and social environmental factors (e.g., hospital staff not checking their understanding or providing information about their injury).

Beardmore et al. (1999) found that children aged 9–16 years with brain injury reported significantly fewer problems than their parents, particularly regarding changes in attention and behaviour. Children's knowledge of their TBI (e.g., understanding of the accident, brain injury and coma) was significantly and positively related to their memory ability. Furthermore, lack of awareness (i.e., a greater discrepancy between the child and parent's ratings on a checklist) was associated with higher self-esteem on the Piers–Harris Children's Self-concept Scale. Overall, these findings suggest that memory problems affect children's ability to accurately recall information about their TBI and that lack of awareness of changes in functioning may serve to protect their self-esteem. Adopting different methodology to assess metacognitive functioning, Hanten, Bartha and Levin (2000) found that children with severe TBI overestimated their accuracy in being able to learn and recall new information over time; however, the association between performance appraisal and self-esteem was not examined.

Hawley (2012) assessed the self-esteem of 91 children with TBI who were approximately two years post-injury. She found that children with TBI reported significantly lower self-esteem compared with their peers. Self-esteem was positively correlated with IQ and memory functioning and negatively correlated with anxiety, depression, parental stress and maladaptive behaviours. The link between self-esteem and social functioning was evident in a study by Andrews, Rose and Johnson (1998), who found that children with TBI reported lower self-esteem, greater loneliness and poorer social adaptive functioning (e.g., more aggressive and antisocial behaviour) compared with controls.

Numerous studies have found that children with TBI display social information processing deficits, reduced social competence and poorer socio-emotional outcomes (Dennis et al., 2013; Snodgrass & Knott, 2006). Impaired executive control has been proposed to contribute to poorer social functioning through related impairments in communication and social problem-solving (Levin, Hanten & Li, 2009). Children with TBI have also been found to demonstrate impaired emotional prosody and facial emotion recognition (Schmidt, Hanten, Li, Orsten & Levin, 2010) and use fewer positive or assertive strategies in social problem-solving situations (Ganesalingam, Yeates, Sanson & Anderson, 2007; Warschausky, Cohen, Parker, Levendosky & Okun, 1997). Together, these impairments in the ability to 'read people' and use effective strategies during social interaction may underlie various maladaptive behaviours that arise from TBI. In turn, the experience of peer rejection and social isolation is likely to contribute to a further decline in or disruption to social skill development.

Although it is clear that many children with TBI display metacognitive and social cognition impairments, it is less clear how these difficulties influence a child's emerging self-concept. On the one hand, poor self-awareness and lack of social awareness (e.g., reduced ability to perceive criticism or negative social reactions) may to some extent counteract the effects of severe TBI and functional impairments on a child's self-concept. Furthermore, children injured before their stable self-concept emerges (i.e., around age 8) may potentially form a more positive self-concept as adults than children injured during later childhood or adolescence. This is because they may be less likely to experience self-discrepancies or unfavourable temporal comparisons between their pre-injury, post-injury and future selves. However, children who sustain a severe brain injury earlier in life are also more likely to have persisting functional impairments (McKinlay et al., 2002; Schmidt et al., 2010). These impairments are likely to affect their ability to interact positively with their peers, perform well at school and develop the cognitive, social and emotional competencies that contribute to an adaptive identity in adulthood.

Long-term follow-up studies of childhood brain injury have yet to shed light on this complex issue. For example, a follow-up study of 123 adults who sustained TBI during childhood identified that those with severe TBI were most vulnerable to poor psychological and social outcomes, irrespective of age at injury (Anderson, Brown, Newitt & Hoile, 2009). However, 85 per cent of the sample were aged 6–12 years (only 3 per cent were < 6 years and 12 per cent were > 12 years), and the impact of age at injury on self-concept was not specifically examined. Overall, it is likely that many factors influence the impact of childhood brain injury on psychological adjustment, including age, premorbid functioning, social background, mechanisms and severity of injury, the neural circuitry disrupted and associated functional impairments, and the presence of positive social supports and a stimulating environment to facilitate experience-dependent recovery (Anderson et al., 2012; Levin, 2012; McKinlay et al., 2009; Taylor et al., 2002; Ylvisaker et al., 1998).

Brain injury during adolescence

Similar to brain injury in early childhood, persisting cognitive and behavioural impairments have been documented for adolescents which affect their ability to re-engage in school, work and their social life (Stancin, Drotar, Taylor, Yeates, Wade, & Minich, 2002; Wilson, Donders & Nguyen, 2011). As described in Chapter 2, adolescence is an important developmental period for identity formation, in which adolescents strive to become more independent, form their career paths and establish intimate relationships (Lau, 1990; O'Koon, 1997). Brain injury disrupts both biological and social maturation processes involved in establishing self-identity.

Some authors suggest that in comparison to younger children, adolescents often have uneven ability profiles with 'hidden deficits' that are less likely to be recognised due to their other intact skills and more rapidly recovering abilities (e.g., speech and mobility) (Hawley, 2005; Hux & Hacksley, 1996). Some of these less observable changes relate to complex cognitive and behavioural difficulties, which can have delayed onset and be influenced by the level of structure and support within the environment (Ewing, 2006; Hawley, 2005). Similar to younger children, adolescents have been found to lack awareness of their post-injury changes. For example,

Stancin et al. (2002) found that at 4 years post-injury adolescents with severe TBI rated their health-related quality of life similar to orthopaedic controls, and that such ratings were significantly higher than their parents' ratings for the adolescent. Similarly, Wilson et al. (2011) found that adolescents with TBI typically reported fewer metacognitive and behavioural regulation problems compared with their parents, and that adolescents with severe TBI were more likely to underestimate their degree of executive dysfunction (e.g., impairments in working memory, planning and organisation skills) than those with mild TBI.

Consistent with the findings for younger children (e.g., Beardmore et al., 1999), Wilson et al. (2011) suggested that the cognitive and behavioural consequences of TBI may reduce adolescents' capacity to accurately appraise their post-injury impairments, thus protecting their self-esteem. However, adolescents are often self-conscious and feel a strong need to fit in with their peers because these represent a main source of self-definition. Awareness deficits may contribute to feelings of frustration and confusion regarding their lack of success on tasks and with peer relationships, and therefore have a negative impact on self-concept (Hux & Hacksley, 1996). Adolescents also typically have a stronger sense of their past and future selves than younger children and thus, despite the presence of awareness deficits, are likely to feel distressed when their dreams for the future are not realised (Bullock, Gable & Mohr, 2005; Harter, 2012). Many studies have focused on the school re-integration process due to its significance for social and cognitive development as well as providing a vocation and a sense of identity.

Qualitative research by Sharp, Bye, Llewellyn and Cusick (2006) identified that the two key phases of school re-integration involve 'organising the school return' and 'being back at school'. Adolescents with a longer absence from school found this transition more difficult, and the success of their re-integration was influenced by the visibility of the students' difficulties (i.e., noticeable or hidden) and the school's response to these issues. A major theme related to the challenge of 'fitting back in', with those who achieved this goal finding it easier to continue their schooling, while others who struggled to fit in considered leaving school. Students identified various negative reactions from their teachers and peers, including feeling pressured, singled out and misunderstood. Students perceived various losses, including abilities, friends, confidence in their direction in life and a loss of feeling 'the same'.

Kennedy, Krause and Turkstra (2008) found that adolescents with TBI often needed to put greater time and effort into their studies. However, despite this investment they were often unable to maintain their pre-injury level of academic performance and had to adjust their goals for study and work. The greater time required to compensate for learning problems reduced their ability to spend time with peers in social activities. Consequently, adolescents with TBI were considered at greater risk of anxiety and depression and social isolation.

Mealings and Douglas (2010) specifically focused on adolescents' experiences of returning to school after TBI and the impact on their identity. Three themes that emerged from their analysis included 'adolescent student sense of self', 'changes' and 'supports'. Various issues impacted on students' sense of self, including their experiences of school and ability to resume this part of a normal life. Many goals were tied to returning to school, including re-connecting with friends, pursuing their educational and work goals and re-gaining a sense of purpose and direction. Students were aware of various changes in their functioning and related activity limitations and they perceived both positive (e.g., pride in their achievements) and negative experiences (e.g., being singled out or treated differently) in their adjustment to TBI.

In terms of supports, the key role of family and friends was emphasised as well as the importance of forming a good relationship with 'integration aides' in the school system. For one student, positive support and relationships served as a buffer to help maintain his sense of self and social participation despite changes in functioning. For another student, behavioural problems and difficulty relating to his peers and supports contributed to a loss of social participation and thwarted goals which negatively impacted his sense of self. Overall, adolescents' ability to maintain or form a positive identity after brain injury was influenced by their relationships, sense of belonging and social acceptance, and the ability to pursue meaningful goals and a life path (Mealings & Douglas, 2010).

Qualitative research focusing on the transition from high school to work or university suggests that students linked in with transition support services and those with more positive attitudes (e.g., motivation, flexibility) are more likely to achieve successful post-secondary education outcomes (Todis & Glang, 2008). Students without this support were often reliant on their parents to advocate for work and study opportunities and provide ongoing support to maintain these positions (Backhouse & Rodger, 1999). Recommendations for supporting children with brain injury and their family and teachers are provided in Chapter 8.

Overall, it is well recognised that children and adolescents do not always experience a good recovery or favourable outcomes after brain injury (Anderson & Catroppa, 2006). To date, there has been very little research conducted on changes in self-concept or the impact of brain injury on identity formation for children and adolescents. The following two case studies highlight the influence of pre-injury, injury-related and post-injury factors on adjustment to brain injury in the context of early childhood and during adolescence.

Case illustrations

Dan's experience of encephalitis during childhood

Dan was 6 years old when he developed viral meningitis which lead to encephalitis and epilepsy. An early neuropsychological assessment indicated generalised intellectual decline (IQ in the low average range) and severe impairments in memory, processing speed, visuo-spatial skills and language. His mother perceived that Dan experienced few behavioural or emotional changes; however, because his seizures led to repeated hospitalisations, he developed anxiety about having seizures outside of home. As a result, he missed a considerable amount of schooling and was largely educated at home by his mother who was a teacher. Dan presented to an adult brain injury service at 21 years of age and was keen to have a neuropsychological assessment to guide his vocational training. The assessment indicated that his intellectual functioning was in the 'low average' range with relative strengths in verbal reasoning.

He displayed moderate to severe deficits in new learning and memory, which appeared to contribute to his difficulties with planning and problem-solving due to the need to hold information on-line to pursue a plan of action. The test results were consistent with his insightful descriptions of everyday forgetfulness and confusion as documented in a journal prior to attending an appointment:

> I can only recollect or hold one or two things in my brain at any time and I lose track of what I'm trying to achieve; (for example) take milk out of the fridge, put into coffee, then straight away go to repeat the same action – looking for the milk in the fridge when it's still on the bench.

Dan only had a faint recollection of life before his illness, although he was aware that he had learnt to read and write before he became unwell. His mother described his determination and persistence to relearn these skills, which took many years to achieve. Dan's literacy skills proved to be very important because he kept a diary every year to document his experiences, including his seizures. As an adult living with amnesia, these recordings appeared to have helped him to form his self-narrative. Reading over Dan's diaries in therapy, he was able to identify key themes of what he had learnt about himself and life growing up. He summarised his personal philosophy as follows:

> Everything I do through each day is a personal challenge. I try to think positively but at the same time I expect nothing; my idea being that high expectations sometimes carry great disappointments. I have a need to be accepted, but life has taught me that if people can't accept me for who I am, then that's their problem not mine. I must be true to myself and do the best that I can within my limitations.

Applying the self-identity framework developed in Chapter 2, various factors contributed to Dan's realistic and adaptive sense of self, including his past history of overcoming adversity and tangible accomplishments (e.g., literacy skills, completing high school and semi-independence) and access to information and feedback about himself in the present. He particularly valued praise from other people because this served to reinforce his skills and progress towards his plans and goals. Dan's severe memory impairment posed a barrier to making sense of and recalling his everyday experiences. However, through his extensive use of compensation (i.e., constant recordings of daily challenges and achievements) and supportive feedback from his mother and extended family, Dan had formed adaptive self-schemas. In particular, he had learnt that with persistence he was able to experience success on many tasks and gradually work towards the plans he valued in life. He recognised that achieving 'normal' aspects of life (i.e., working and being in a relationship) was harder for him than for other people, but also felt that he appreciated small achievements more than most people, as 'having low expectations often brings the nicest surprises'.

Dan was selective about his social interaction and avoided high-risk situations (e.g., travelling on public transport or going to a shopping centre alone) due to concerns about both his physical safety (i.e., having a seizure) and emotional safety (i.e., negative social reactions). He felt it was important to be surrounded by a small network of people whom he trusted and were encouraging of him. However, he acknowledged that this also restricted him from meeting new people and approaching prospective employers. Therefore, pursuing his goals of finding work and meeting a girlfriend would mean taking some 'risks'. Overall, Dan held realistic views about his challenges and due to his determination was highly motivated to learn ways to manage his anxiety and develop greater interpersonal skills (see Figure 3.2). Dan's therapy programme was largely successful in terms of improving his self-management of anxiety, supporting him to access an employment agency, and achieving a satisfying and durable job placement (part-time work in a newsagency). His desire to be in a relationship remained an ongoing goal for him.

Jasmine's experience of TBI during adolescence

Jasmine was 15 years old when she sustained a TBI in a motor vehicle accident. Her Glasgow Coma Scale score of 9/15 and duration of post-traumatic amnesia of 6 days indicated a moderate to severe injury. Neuroimaging indicated bilateral frontal lobe contusions that were most marked in the orbital prefrontal area. Jasmine made a rapid physical recovery and received extensive multi-disciplinary rehabilitation, with additional sessions funded by private insurance. At 6 months post-injury the results of a neuropsychological assessment indicated that her verbal and non-verbal intellectual functioning, basic attention, processing speed and memory were generally in the high average range for her age. Mild deficits were evident on tasks assessing more complex attention and behavioural regulation (i.e., switching, response inhibition and rule following). Jasmine also displayed emotion regulation problems, including frequent outbursts of anger and laughter, and reduced empathy and social concern. Jasmine was aware of physical and cognitive changes (e.g., 'I get tired easily and can't concentrate as well'), but lacked insight into her emotion and behaviour regulation problems.

When she was discharged home, Jasmine, her family and the teachers at her private school were optimistic about her graduated return to school because of her premorbid academic strengths, seemingly 'good' cognitive recovery and her determination to resume her studies. The school organised for additional tuition in the home and Jasmine's friends had maintained close contact with her since her accident. Her friends received education about the effects of TBI and understood that Jasmine was more likely to make tactless remarks and become frustrated and overexcited. Jasmine's mother and her friends viewed these changes as an extension of her previous personality, because she had always been 'headstrong' and liked things her own way. Despite her cohesive support network and extended rehabilitation programme, Jasmine developed depression within one month of returning to school. This appeared to be triggered by her becoming aware that she was no longer one of the strongest students in the class, and that despite the huge effort she invested in study and use of study aides she was unable to regain her former academic status (i.e., top of the class on exams and assignments).

Jasmine received ongoing psychological support to adjust to her post-injury changes. In therapy she identified that she was struggling with the vast differences she

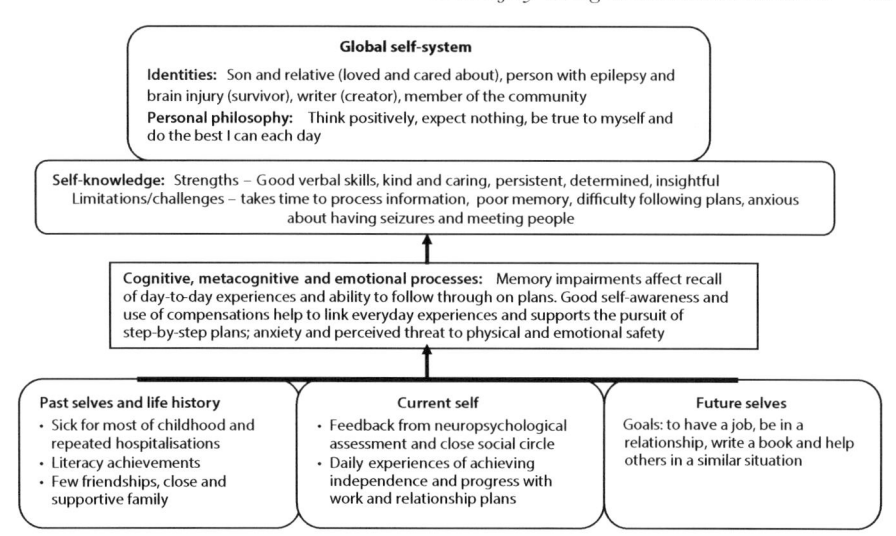

```
                    ┌─────────────────────────────────────────────────────────┐
                    │                    Global self-system                    │
                    │ Identities:  Son and relative (loved and cared about), person with epilepsy and
                    │ brain injury (survivor), writer (creator), member of the community
                    │ Personal philosophy:  Think positively, expect nothing, be true to myself and
                    │ do the best I can each day
                    └─────────────────────────────────────────────────────────┘
```

Self-knowledge: Strengths – Good verbal skills, kind and caring, persistent, determined, insightful
Limitations/challenges – takes time to process information, poor memory, difficulty following plans, anxious about having seizures and meeting people

Cognitive, metacognitive and emotional processes: Memory impairments affect recall of day-to-day experiences and ability to follow through on plans. Good self-awareness and use of compensations help to link everyday experiences and supports the pursuit of step-by-step plans; anxiety and perceived threat to physical and emotional safety

Past selves and life history	Current self	Future selves
• Sick for most of childhood and repeated hospitalisations • Literacy achievements • Few friendships, close and supportive family	• Feedback from neuropsychological assessment and close social circle • Daily experiences of achieving independence and progress with work and relationship plans	Goals: to have a job, be in a relationship, write a book and help others in a similar situation

Figure 3.2 Formulation of Dan's self-identity after brain injury

perceived between her pre-injury and current self in terms of school performance, and her greatest concern was that she would be unable to pursue her former plans to study forensic medicine. She felt that being an average student with an ordinary job would mean failure for her and that she was letting her family down. Jasmine's parents, teachers and guidance counsellor were involved in a coordinated plan to encourage her to work towards smaller milestones and explore various career options through work experience. She participated well in this process and enjoyed work experience as a laboratory assistant. However, she remained set on achieving her lifelong goal of going to university to study forensic medicine, with her interests (reading and television) focused on this career.

Unlike Dan, Jasmine really struggled to form a realistic and adaptive post-injury identity. She vacillated between feeling highly optimistic about her future and experiencing despair and a sense of failure when things did not go as planned (e.g., receiving an average mark or forgetting to complete a task). She found it difficult to balance her life between different interests (e.g., playing sports, socialising) and her parents, friends and teachers were concerned about her intense and sole focus on her studies. Her mother was worried that she was 'putting all her eggs in one basket, and what if it's the wrong basket?' The rehabilitation plan involved providing continuing support to Jasmine and her family throughout high school, and particularly during the transition from high school to university. As represented in Figure 3.3, her high personal standards and strong achievement drive were considered to place her at risk of poor psychological adjustment if these plans were not realised (i.e., getting accepted into a particular university degree and pursuing post-graduate studies). Jasmine successfully transitioned to university and commenced a biological sciences degree. However, she experienced ongoing psychological and social adjustment problems, including anxiety and difficulty relating to other students and her lecturers.

Global self-system

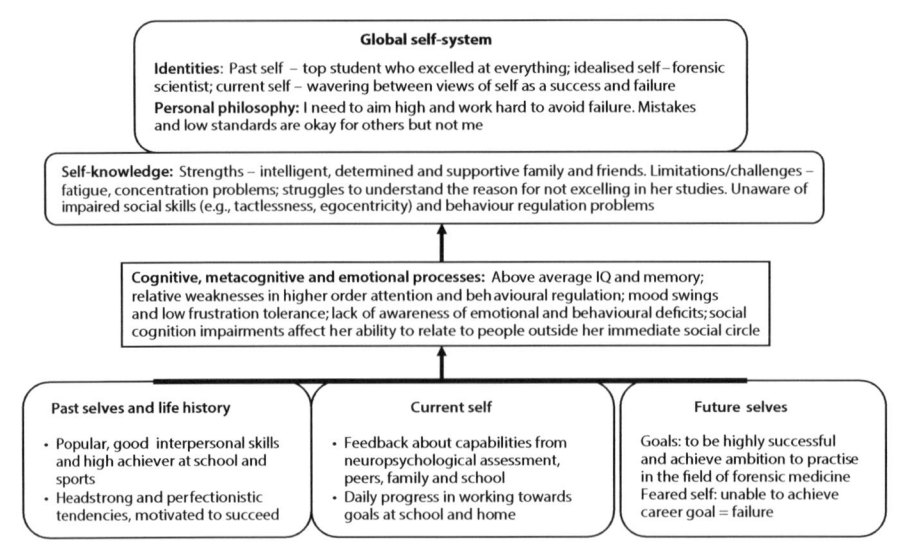

Identities: Past self – top student who excelled at everything; idealised self – forensic scientist; current self – wavering between views of self as a success and failure
Personal philosophy: I need to aim high and work hard to avoid failure. Mistakes and low standards are okay for others but not me

Self-knowledge: Strengths – intelligent, determined and supportive family and friends. Limitations/challenges – fatigue, concentration problems; struggles to understand the reason for not excelling in her studies. Unaware of impaired social skills (e.g., tactlessness, egocentricity) and behaviour regulation problems

Cognitive, metacognitive and emotional processes: Above average IQ and memory; relative weaknesses in higher order attention and behavioural regulation; mood swings and low frustration tolerance; lack of awareness of emotional and behavioural deficits; social cognition impairments affect her ability to relate to people outside her immediate social circle

Past selves and life history	Current self	Future selves
• Popular, good interpersonal skills and high achiever at school and sports • Headstrong and perfectionistic tendencies, motivated to succeed	• Feedback about capabilities from neuropsychological assessment, peers, family and school • Daily progress in working towards goals at school and home	Goals: to be highly successful and achieve ambition to practise in the field of forensic medicine Feared self: unable to achieve career goal = failure

Figure 3.3 Formulation of Jasmine's self-identity after brain injury

Her case manager supported her to access learning support services and she was able to maintain pass grades.

Despite strong social support and resources, Jasmine's post-injury adjustment was more complicated than Dan's, in part because of her previous high academic achievement and personality style and the nature of her injury (i.e., orbito-frontal damage). Dan sustained his injury at a younger age and had global cognitive impairment, thus placing him at risk of a poor long-term functional outcome. However, due to Dan's realistic views of his own strengths and limitations, good use of compensation and strong social support, he had developed a clear and constructive self-identity. Together, these case studies show how the combination of factors depicted in Figure 3.1 influence people's ability to form an adaptive self-identity after childhood brain injury.

Conclusions

Brain injury leads to diverse impairments that impact on people's everyday functioning and social roles. A biopsychosocial framework provides a useful approach to conceptualise factors influencing outcomes, and hence can guide assessment and treatment efforts. The impact of a severe brain injury early in life can greatly interfere with development of social, adaptive and behavioural competencies, although the long-term impact on self-concept and identity is unclear due to a lack of empirical research. Two case studies were used to highlight the interactive influence of premorbid, neuro-cognitive, social environmental and psychological factors on developing sense of self. Chapter 4 focuses on the process of psychological adjustment and empirical findings concerning changes in self-identity for adults with brain injury.

4 Psychological adjustment and self-identity changes after brain injury

Psychological adjustment after brain injury refers to the process of becoming aware of, making sense of and adapting to changes in one's functioning and life circumstances. This chapter presents a framework of the interrelated processes of self-awareness, sense-making appraisals and coping, and considers the interactive influence of premorbid, neurocognitive and social environmental factors on adjustment. Building on this framework, the chapter reviews studies that have examined changes to self and identity in the context of brain injury. Overall, this research supports that people's self-identity after brain injury is influenced by their pre-injury personality, neuropsychological impairments, self-appraisals and coping behaviours, social reactions and opportunities to re-engage in meaningful activities and roles.

An overview of psychological adjustment to brain injury

After a brain injury people are faced with the challenging process of making sense of and adapting to major changes in their functioning and lifestyle. Early stressors include the development of life-threatening symptoms, medical investigations and diagnosis of a neurological condition, treatment to save the person's life and ongoing procedures to monitor and stabilise the condition. The person with brain injury and family members often experience great uncertainty about the future in terms of prognosis for survival, recurrence and recovery. After the acute medical phase, the focus shifts from survival to recovery and rehabilitation efforts to maximise people's physical, speech and language and cognitive and behavioural functions. This typically involves a combination of approaches, including remedial or restorative efforts to regain or relearn skills, and compensatory strategies to manage persisting impairments (Wilson et al., 2009). Early onset mood disturbances are often managed through pharmacological, environmental and/or behavioural interventions (Fleminger, Oliver, Williams, & Evans, 2003).

As people leave the hospital or treatment setting and return to their familiar pre-injury activities they begin to form a better understanding of changes in their abilities and how these affect their everyday functioning (Turner, Fleming, Ownsworth & Cornwell, 2011). People often experience activity restrictions (e.g., driving, work, alcohol consumption and sports), increased dependency on family, changes in social roles and relationships, and financial strain (Karlovits & McColl, 1999;

Turner et al., 2009). At the time of the injury, a young adult is typically in the process of establishing an independent lifestyle and career path. Conversely, an older adult may have been looking forward to retiring with financial security and plans to pursue new interests. Aptly stated by Evans (2011), brain injury 'throws people off the life-course they had anticipated' (p. 117).

Due to the long-term nature of brain injury and its consequences, people are faced with chronic stressors and periods of heightened stress due to various transitions, such as leaving hospital, moving to a more (or less) independent living situation, and efforts to return to work. People vary considerably in their psychological reactions to these stressors, with some experiencing depression, anxiety or anger regarding their situation (Ownsworth et al., 2011; Turner et al., 2011), and others showing remarkable resilience and optimism despite significant losses. Some of these contrasting reactions are depicted in Figure 4.1, as reported in our research by family members and people with brain injury.

Family members' perspectives

I did not really expect the depression and … the agitation that has happened…He just, you know, he just will not get off that chair half the time (Turner et al., 2011, p. 81)

He [person with brain injury] was hitting things, screaming, yelling, swearing with a lot of aggression in the voice (Turner et al., 2011, p. 82)

He's always been a very positive optimistic person anyway … He's the most resilient person I know…and so I think it's that bounceability that he can see the positive side in everything (Turner et al., 2011, p. 83)

Perspectives of people with brain injury

It's just more frustration you know the things that you took for granted that I can't do now. I can't play with the children the same, I can't do my own hair, I can't just make the bed and do the housework (Turner et al., 2011, p. 83)

I was in shock for weeks just going, what's this?...The biggest thing I've found through the whole thing was acceptance, just to accept what's happened and I don't fight it (Turner et al., 2011, p. 84)

[I] asked if I could volunteer, just help them out, just anything to kill the time, to feel useful... That is the main thing; I have never been this useless (Turner et al., 2009, p. 617)

I appreciate a lot of things that I probably took for granted you know, getting up every morning. I'm just happy to get up and have a shower and be able to go to work (Turner et al., 2011, p. 85)

I am an extremely lucky man. I have a wife that cares about me and I've managed to find the right people to fit with my idea of what's necessary to get this where it's going (Turner et al., 2011, p. 81)

Figure 4.1 Perspectives on the impact of brain injury during the first few months post-discharge

Reported rates of psychological distress differ in the literature. For depression, rates have been found to vary between 15–61 per cent following TBI (Fleminger et al., 2003; Kim et al., 2007) and 16–39 per cent following brain tumour (see Ownsworth et al., 2009). Based on an analysis of 51 studies, Hackett, Yapa, Parag and Anderson (2005) reported a pooled estimate of 33 per cent for post-stroke depression at different time points. The prevalence of anxiety after TBI ranges from 18 to 60 per cent across studies (Hibbard, Uysal, Kepler, Bogdany & Silver, 1998), with a meta-analysis of 12 studies reporting an overall prevalence of 29 per cent for anxiety disorders following TBI (Epstein & Ursano, 1994). Anxiety appears to be particularly prevalent following a diagnosis of brain tumour with rates ranging from 30 to 58 per cent (Ownsworth et al., 2009). Anxiety is also common following stroke; for example, Barker-Collo (2007) reported that 39 per cent of their sample displayed anxiety levels in the clinical range, and 21 per cent were in the moderate to severe range. Co-morbidity rates for depression and anxiety have been reported to be as high as 65 per cent (Moore, Terryberry-Spohr, & Hope, 2006). Overall, rates of emotional distress are likely to vary due to sampling issues (e.g., inpatient versus community-based samples) and different approaches to measurement and classification. A clear finding from the literature is that many people adjust to the effects of brain injury without experiencing significant or prolonged emotional distress.

Similar to the grieving process, adjustment to brain injury does not follow a linear course or a set of defined stages. Rather, identity transition has been described as a dynamic and cyclical process, characterised by 'contraction, expansion and tentative balance' (Muenchberger, Kendall & Neal, 2008). Others have referred to 'recurrent psychological reorganisation' that is required to adapt to ongoing stressors and new challenges (Cantor et al., 2005). Gelech and Desjardins (2011) proposed that there are many aspects of self involved in reconstruction of personhood, which include continuity, negotiation, resistance, transcendence and moral growth. Despite this complexity, adjustment can be broadly summarised to entail developing awareness of changes in one's functioning and lifestyle (self-awareness), making sense of changes to self (sense-making appraisals) and learning to cope with or manage these changes (coping and adaptation).

Figure 4.2 provides a framework of the psychological adjustment processes which contribute to people's working model of self after brain injury. This framework depicts the influence of premorbid characteristics, neuropsychological functioning and social context on the process of updating sense of self. Empirical support for different components of this framework will now be reviewed.

Self-awareness of changes in functioning

The adjustment process generally begins when people start to notice changes in their physical, cognitive or behavioural functioning or life situation (e.g., receiving a diagnosis or being hospitalised). This may occur quite suddenly, for example, noticing weakness down one side of the body and changes in speech during a stroke, or more gradually due to a slow growing tumour or deterioration in health due to a viral

58 *Psychological adjustment and self-identity changes*

Premorbid personality and coping style

Social context

Diagnosis and assessment: Access to information about brain injury and effects on functioning

Feedback on changes to self and reactions of support network

Opportunities to learn about self and develop coping strategies through activities and social interaction

Personal appraisals and reactions

Self-awareness
Awareness of changes in self, functioning and lifestyle

Sense-making appraisals
Meaning derived from the injury: Sense of threat, controllability and positive gains

Coping efforts
Reactions to changes in self and lifestyle and ways of managing stressors

Neuropsychological processes and neural networks

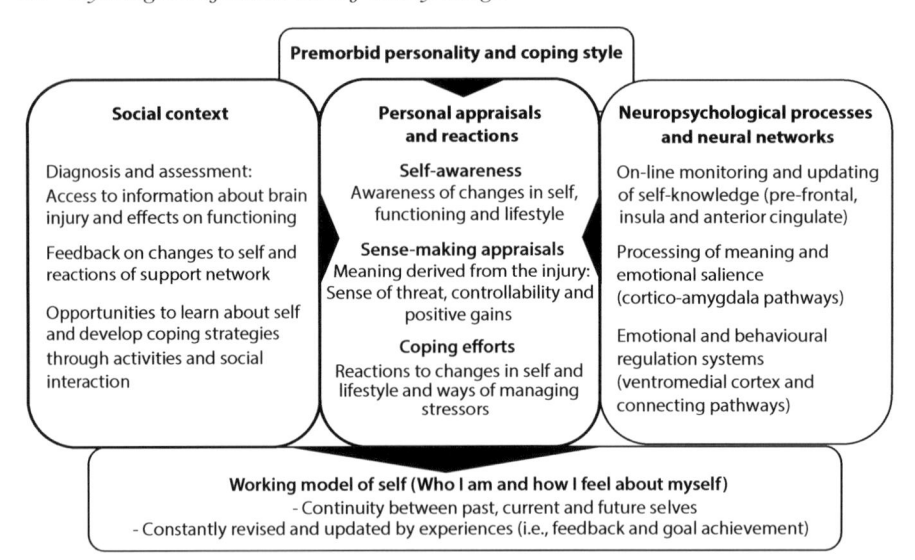

On-line monitoring and updating of self-knowledge (pre-frontal, insula and anterior cingulate)

Processing of meaning and emotional salience (cortico-amygdala pathways)

Emotional and behavioural regulation systems (ventromedial cortex and connecting pathways)

Working model of self (Who I am and how I feel about myself)
- Continuity between past, current and future selves
- Constantly revised and updated by experiences (i.e., feedback and goal achievement)

Figure 4.2 Biopsychosocial framework of the inter-related processes of self-awareness, sense-making and coping that contribute to self-identity after brain injury (adapted from Douglas, 2012; Gracey & Ownsworth, 2012)

infection. In the case of the latter, gradually worsening or sporadic symptoms may be misattributed to other more benign causes (e.g., headaches and nausea to 'the flu') (Ownsworth, Chambers, Hawkes, Walker & Shum, 2011). Following TBI, a person may not initially recall that they have had a brain injury or recognise the effects of the injury due to their acute neurological status (e.g., confusion, disorientation and rapid forgetting during post-traumatic amnesia).

Although lack of awareness of the brain injury and related impairments may initially protect individuals from emotional distress, it can complicate adjustment by delaying the start of medical investigations or impeding treatment and rehabilitation efforts. Salander, Bergenheim, Hamberg, and Henriksson (1999) found that delays in diagnosis of brain tumour were related to a combination of factors, including the person's own reactions (e.g., denial or avoidance of medical contact), their family (e.g., dismissive or passive reactions to symptoms) and medical professionals (e.g., belief in alternative diagnoses), thus complicating adjustment to the illness. The process of registering changes in one's functioning can be perplexing and confronting, as exemplified by the following case illustration.

Graham, a 65-year-old taxi driver who developed mild weakness down his left side, delayed seeking medical help for 10 days after his stroke. He explained that he could still drive and was able to 'drag' his leg in and out of the car each day. When Graham was asked why he did not seek help earlier, he acknowledged that he initially thought the numbness and heaviness in his leg was due to his usual cramping and circulation problems. He later recognised the persistence of the symptoms and realised it was more serious, although he still delayed seeking medical attention: 'Looking back ... I guess I wanted to stay in the dark as long as I could, and keep driving'.

Awareness impairments can be neurologically-based (i.e., disruption to neural circuitry underlying awareness and self-reflective capacity), reflect psychological mechanisms for coping with threats to one's self-image, independence and lifestyle, or arise from a complex interplay of these factors (Ownsworth, Clare & Morris, 2006). Premorbid personality traits related to denial include high levels of defensiveness, conscientiousness and perfectionism (Ownsworth, 2005; Ownsworth, McFarland & Young, 2002; Weinstein & Kahn, 1955). The social environment can also influence the extent to which people perceive changes in self, through having access to objective information about their brain injury and post-injury impairments. People may also underreport their difficulties because they are concerned about the consequences of disclosing their impairments, including negative reactions from others or the loss of certain resources or entitlements (e.g., a driver's licence, the ability to manage one's own finances) (Ownsworth, Clare et al., 2006).

Krefting (1989) referred to the use of concealment as a 'recasting strategy' which reflects a conscious effort to reduce the visibility of one's deficits to assist the person to appear normal to others. Therefore, although some people appear to lack awareness of post-injury changes, concealment of problems may reflect a strategy to protect their self-image and social persona (Ownsworth, 2005). For example, Janelle, a woman who was very independent and valued her privacy before her injury, would become highly anxious in situations where her actions (and potential mistakes) could be observed by others. She explained 'I can't bear for people to see me like this' and avoided having visitors to her home to help maintain the impression that she was coping fine. Similar strategies for controlling information about self and managing self-presentation style in social situations were described by Nochi (1998).

Prigatano (1999) highlighted how the deficits arising from brain injury can be emotionally threatening and difficult to make sense of, and that individuals with 'partial awareness' may employ defensive coping strategies such as denial or avoidance to protect against emotional distress. Consistent with this view, we found in our research (Ownsworth et al., 2002) that individuals with a highly defensive personality style appeared to perceive their impairments on some conscious level, and thus could still develop compensatory strategies, but were reluctant to disclose their difficulties to others. Even people with a non-defensive personality or coping style may continue to behave as though everything is normal in the face of obvious problems, and use rationalisation or find alternative explanations to preserve their self-image (Prigatano, 1999). This may be particularly common for individuals with neurologically-based awareness deficits who may not recognise their errors or difficulties on tasks, or are unable to recall these experiences accurately in order to update their self-knowledge (Ownsworth, Clare et al., 2006).

As an illustration of this phenomenon, the father of a man with unilateral neglect and severe awareness deficits following right fronto-parietal brain injury recalled the following experience with his son Peter at the gym. While his father was talking to another gym member, Peter loaded weights onto only the right side of the bar before using the bench press. When he went to lift the bar he instantly became unbalanced and fell off the bench. Peter's initial reaction was shock and bewilderment at his own mistake. However, later that day he recalled the situation differently and made the indignant remark, 'People should really tell you if they are going to borrow your weights so you don't fall over and hurt yourself'.

Empirical research supports that awareness impairments for specific sensory-perceptual or motor domains (e.g., anosognosia for hemiplegia) are most common following fronto-parietal lesions, particularly in the right hemisphere (Pia, Neppi-Modona, Ricci, & Berti, 2004). A more in-depth discussion of the neurological basis of domain-specific impairments is provided by Prigatano (2010) and Feinberg (2011b). The precise neuroanatomical site/s underlying more generalised awareness deficits (i.e., lack of awareness extending across multiple functional domains) is less well established, although Feinberg (2011b) noted that disturbances in awareness of self in relation to the environment are most common following damage to the prefrontal cortex and insula and anterior cingulate regions. Consistent with this view, generalised awareness deficits are found to be related to impaired online monitoring and self-regulation (e.g., rule following, set shifting) (Ciurli et al., 2010; Ownsworth, Fleming, Strong, Radel, Chan & Clare, 2007).

The development of self-awareness is facilitated by aspects of people's social environment, including participation in familiar activities, receiving feedback and having the opportunity to learn about post-injury changes in a supportive context (Fleming & Ownsworth, 2006). For example, feedback from a neuropsychological assessment may pose a threat to one's self-image, or validate and support understanding of one's impairments. The impact of feedback is likely to depend on the person's receptiveness to this information, the therapeutic relationship and the manner in which feedback is delivered, as follows:

> I've got a smart psychologist, one who is a real person and actually told me the meaning of some of these things that were happening ... if you understand what's happening, you can then take steps to do something about it.
> (Turner et al., 2011, p. 81)

Kristensen (2004) found that prior to rehabilitation individuals strived to maintain 'the former self' whereas after the programme they demonstrated greater 'self-realisation' and adjustment to their current situation. In a longitudinal study of the first 12 months post-injury, Dirette, Plaisier and Jones (2008) found that people with TBI developed self-awareness through comparison of their current and pre-injury performance on occupational activities and the need to use compensatory strategies. O'Callaghan, Powell, and Oyebode (2006) identified that the emergence of awareness occurred through personal discovery and by observing other people's reactions, and was associated with fear, grief and loss. Rehabilitation supported individuals to make sense of these experiences by explaining and normalising the effects of brain injury and promoting acceptance.

Conversely, some authors have noted that high levels of support provided by family or professionals can help to ensure that individuals largely experience success on tasks and protect them from a sense of failure (Ownsworth, Fleming et al., 2006; Ylvisaker et al., 1998). Peter from the previous example regularly experienced high levels of support on tasks and positive feedback regardless of his performance. His mother closely supervised his completion of tasks in daily living and provided prompts and assistance to avert any errors (e.g., when he was helping with cooking or doing laundry). Similarly, his co-workers at a charity organisation constantly praised his efforts as a volunteer and would correct any mistakes (e.g., incorrect sorting of clothing) after his shift. From their perspective, they wanted to prevent him from feeling frustrated and being reminded of his injury. Such reactions undoubtedly contributed to Peter's emotional well-being and positive self-concept following severe TBI. He often spoke with pride about his ability to work and be independent. The potential disadvantages of this 'shielding' approach to support will be considered later in this chapter.

Krefting (1989) described the common tendency for individuals with brain injury and their family members to redefine the common social meanings of particular concepts (e.g., work and independence). She provided an example of the parents of a woman with brain injury referring to their daughter's volunteering position as 'work' because she was engaged in productive activities. This helped to retain the meaning of a valued concept and maintain a sense of normality despite her inability to participate in the competitive job market. Such mechanisms serve to enhance the social status of the person with brain injury and also assist family members to cope with the major changes to their loved one.

Efforts to downplay the impact of brain injury and constructively redefine people's participation in society are often motivated by the desire to protect an individual from the distressing reality of their post-injury circumstances. More generally, it is recognised that the development of self-awareness can have positive or negative effects on a person's adjustment to brain injury. Accurate self-appraisal of impairments can be adaptive when this contributes to more realistic expectations of recovery, greater motivation to participate in rehabilitation and the pursuit of achievable and satisfying goals. In support of this view, in a systematic review we identified that individuals with greater self-awareness from the outset of rehabilitation generally experienced better rehabilitation outcomes (Ownsworth & Clare, 2006). Further, using cluster analysis we found that people in the 'good self-awareness' subgroup had better psychosocial outcomes than people with awareness deficits related to executive function impairments (i.e., 'poor self-awareness' subgroup) (Ownsworth et al., 2007). The latter subgroup demonstrated poor self-knowledge and impaired error monitoring and self-regulation which, in combination, may have contributed to their poorer community re-integration outcomes.

However, it is also well established that the development of self-awareness can be associated with heightened emotional distress (Fleming, Strong & Ashton, 1998; Godfrey, Partridge, Knight & Bishara, 1993). Specifically, there is considerable evidence that people who perceive high levels of impairment or changes in their functioning are at greater risk of developing depression (Malec, Brown, Moessner, Stump & Monahan, 2010; Ownsworth, Fleming et al., 2011). In our cluster analysis study, we found that individuals in the 'high symptom reporting' subgroup reported higher levels of depression and anxiety and had poorer interpersonal functioning than those in the 'high defensiveness' subgroup who minimised their symptoms (Ownsworth et al., 2007). As noted by Malec et al. (2010), there are two dimensions of impaired awareness; namely, a lack of awareness of post-injury changes and the tendency to focus excessively on one's post-injury deficits. Overall, more accurate self-appraisal of one's strengths and limitations is likely to facilitate adaptive adjustment to brain injury (Gracey & Ownsworth, 2012). In particular, recognising changes in one's functioning stimulates sense-making processes that may better support people to negotiate their identity transition (Muenchberger et al. 2008).

Sense-making appraisals

When people begin to notice changes in their functioning or lifestyle they undergo a series of cognitive appraisals to make sense of these changes and determine what these mean for them. Various cognitive theories of stress, appraisal and adaptation (e.g., Lazarus & Folkman, 1984; Taylor, 1983) have been applied to understand adjustment and meaning-making processes after TBI (Godfrey et al., 1996; Moore & Stambrook, 1995; Kendall & Terry, 2009), stroke (Rochette, Bravo, Desrosiers, St-Cyr-Tribble, & Bourget, 2007; Thompson, 1991) and brain tumour (Ownsworth, Chambers et al., 2011; Strang & Strang, 2001). These theories broadly propose that when faced with a significant threat to one's life, functioning or personhood, people strive to make sense of their experiences and regain a sense of control over their lives to restore their self-esteem (Taylor, 1983). Initially, the personal significance of the stressor is appraised in terms of the degree of potential threat/harm or challenge/gains it poses. Individuals then evaluate how well they can cope with or manage the demands faced according to their personal and social resources (Lazarus & Folkman, 1984). In general, perceptions of high threat, low control and less adequate resources for coping are proposed to contribute to greater emotional distress.

These theoretical perspectives were supported by Kendall and Terry (2009) who found that early appraisals of threat influenced both short-term (1 month post-discharge) and long-term (9 months post-discharge) emotional well-being after TBI. Self-esteem was found to have a protective effect on emotional well-being in the short-term and family support had a significant direct effect on longer term emotional adjustment. Similarly, Rochette et al. (2007) found that lower perceptions of threat and increased controllability at 2 weeks post-stroke were associated with better emotional adjustment and participation at 6 months follow-up.

The concept of brain injury posing a threat to self was first described by Goldstein (1943, 1952) who recognised that a 'catastrophic reaction' of intense anxiety may be triggered when individuals experience difficulty on tasks that they had previously mastered or completed with ease. Consistent with self-comparison and self-discrepancy theories discussed in Chapter 2, Goldstein proposed that anxiety is elicited by the sense of threat that failure on a task poses to one's self-concept. In order to reduce anxiety and protect their self-concept, individuals avoid certain situations where failure is possible, and thus restrict their activity participation. Guided by Goldstein's ideas, Riley, Brennan and Powell (2004) investigated the relationship between threat appraisals, activity avoidance, and anxiety after brain injury. Their findings indicated that people's experience of failure or challenge in situations can trigger threat appraisals, heightened anxiety and associated avoidance of these situations. Threat appraisals were particularly common and related to avoidance for 'doing things' (i.e., performing activities that they used to do before their injury), suggesting that the experience of task difficulty or failure triggers comparisons between pre-injury and post-injury selves, or negative self-discrepancy (Riley et al. 2004). Threat appraisals and avoidance were also evident for 'dealing with people' (e.g., not fitting in, negative evaluations from others), 'awkward situations' (e.g. being reminded of the injury) and 'personal safety' (e.g. getting hurt or reinjured).

Taylor's (1983) theory of cognitive adaptation proposes that following adversity people have a natural tendency to try to find ways to feel good again and restore their self-esteem. Social withdrawal and avoidance of threatening situations may provide short-term relief from discomfort and reduce anxiety. However, for people to adjust well after a major life stressor and rebuild their self-confidence, it is important that they regain a sense of mastery and control over their lives. The loss of meaningful social interaction and activity participation can contribute to an ongoing cycle of maladaptive appraisals and coping reactions with detrimental effects on self-concept, as depicted in Figure 4.3. Moore and Stambrook (1995) similarly proposed that over time people with brain injury can develop self-limiting belief systems and overgeneralise the effects of their injury, which results in poor self-efficacy, avoidance and emotional distress.

As an illustration of this cycle, after sustaining a TBI three years ago, Janelle felt nervous about using public transport in case she took the wrong train and needed to ask others for help. One day she mustered the courage to catch a train in the hope of seeing a new art exhibit in the city. When the train passed the first station she realised that the train was going in the wrong direction and she became intensely anxious about her safety and appearing foolish to others. She managed to change trains and caught the train straight home. This experience reinforced a core belief ('I can't trust myself to function') that had developed in relation to her perceived failures (e.g., cooking, doing crosswords, holding normal conversation) since her injury, and she decided not to use public transport again. In doing so, she relieved her anxiety about facing the situation again, but also restricted herself from visiting friends and grandchildren and pursuing valued hobbies and interests. Janelle's avoidance strengthened her belief that she could not cope with basic activities in life, and she developed severe social anxiety and depression (see Ownsworth, 2005). Her experience highlights the interplay between the experience of task difficulty, cognitive appraisals, anxiety and avoidance, and the implications for self-concept. Janelle's cognitive-behavioural therapy programme is described in Chapter 6.

Although threat appraisals and development of maladaptive self-beliefs are common, the event of brain injury and its associated life changes can also act as

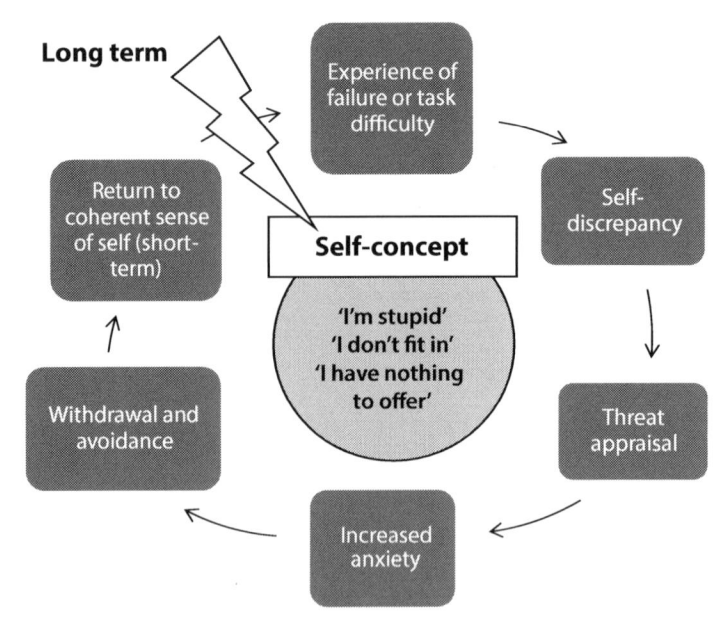

Figure 4.3 Cycle of appraisals, anxiety and avoidance and the impact on self-concept

a catalyst for personal growth (Ownsworth & Fleming, 2011). It has been found more generally that individuals can find positive meaning in their experiences of serious illness and trauma (Folkman, 1997). Various authors have proposed changes to traditional models of coping and adjustment to account for positive psychological effects of trauma, including post-traumatic growth and benefit finding (Collicutt McGrath & Linley, 2006; Folkman, 1997; Tedeschi & Calhoun, 1996). Post-traumatic growth refers to psychological developments that extend beyond pre-trauma functioning, and include recognition of new possibilities in life, increased personal strength, deepened spirituality, enhanced appreciation of life and closer relationships with others (Tedeschi & Calhoun, 1996).

Research on post-traumatic growth in the brain injury field is still in its infancy (Ownsworth & Fleming, 2011). Nonetheless, preliminary findings indicate that post-traumatic growth increases over time (Powell, Ekin-Wood, & Collin, 2007), is related to greater use of particular coping styles (e.g., cognitive restructuring and downward social comparison) (Gangstad, Norman & Barton, 2009) and is inversely associated with depression and anxiety (Collicutt McGrath & Linley, 2006; Hawley & Joseph, 2008). Studies have also indicated that post-traumatic growth is facilitated by greater recognition of post-injury impairments (Silva, Ownsworth, Shields, & Fleming, 2011) and early emotional distress (Collicutt McGrath & Linley, 2006; Kangas, Williams & Smee, 2011). Such findings suggest that post-traumatic growth requires individuals to initially perceive that the brain injury has consequences for their functioning or lifestyle, and experience a sense of threat that challenges their assumptions about themselves and the world (e.g., sense of safety and control). Further, heightened emotion is important to stimulate the meaning-making processes (e.g., rumination, self-disclosure) that contribute to changes in self-schema (Wright & Telford, 1996).

Qualitative research by Nochi (2000) highlighted positive themes in adjustment to TBI, which were referred to as 'reconstructed self-narratives' or ways in which people had revised their own personal stories in relation to the past and future. Five main types of self-narrative included: the recovering self, the self better than others, the grown self, the protesting self and the self living here and now. Particular narratives supported individuals to view themselves in a positive light 'in spite of' or because of their TBI. They did this by making favourable comparisons with what could have been (e.g., 'I've survived, things could be worse'), focusing on remaining strengths, and recognising the positive outcomes of TBI on their lives. For some individuals, the TBI increased their appreciation of life and other people, helped them to form character strengths or prompted them to make better life decisions. Their self-narratives indicated schema-level changes and alteration of life values. It is noteworthy that the participants in this study had sustained their TBI 3–28 years prior, and thus reflect more long-term perspectives on adjustment and adaptation to brain injury.

Coping and adaptation

The process of making sense of brain injury is closely related to coping, or the ongoing thoughts and behaviours an individual employs to manage stressful events in their lives (Glanz, Rimer & Lewis, 2002). Emotion-focused coping refers to ways of regulating emotional distress, including the usually adaptive approach of trying to understand one's own feelings and expressing these, and the less adaptive approaches of denial and avoidance (Stanton, Danoff-Burg, Cameron, & Ellis, 1994). Problem-focused coping involves active efforts to solve or manage the problem and includes seeking information and support, anticipation and planning ahead, and developing strategies to cope with the effects, such as the use of compensatory aids (e.g., for memory problems). Meaning-based or appraisal-focused coping refers to efforts to maintain well-being through reappraisal and benefit finding, or searching for the 'silver lining' of a situation (Glanz et al. 2002). In relation to the latter, Taylor (1983) referred to the positive function of 'illusions' or viewing the facts of a situation from a certain angle. This approach to coping may serve to increase a person's sense of control over an otherwise uncontrollable situation. After brain injury, this may be demonstrated by efforts to avoid dwelling on one's impairments and to focus more on personal abilities and success in recovery, as follows.

> I know how bad it could've been and being in rehab, like there's many different levels you know? ... I felt lucky that I wasn't as bad as some people.
> (Turner et al., 2011, p. 85)

However, in a more extreme form, illusions may reflect 'blind spots' or strong beliefs about one's functioning that are contrary to the facts of the situation

(Krefting, 1989). As an example, a person may insist that he or she is a safe driver despite being shown mistakes on a hazard perception test. Blind spots can reflect a temporary strategy that allows people time to cope with the otherwise overwhelming reality of their situation. Alternatively, blind spots may represent a dominant and enduring way of coping that implies a broader lack of acceptance of the brain injury. Individuals with this coping style are likely to make external attributions for undesired outcomes, such as the belief that restrictions are being placed on them by professionals or that they are being discriminated against in society (see also the 'protesting self'; Nochi, 2000). Blind spots may be a form of self-deception or defence mechanism employed to protect a person's ego (Krefting, 1989), and thus efforts to directly challenge these beliefs are often futile and potentially harmful.

The manner in which individuals cope with the effects of their injury is likely to be influenced by premorbid personality and coping style. In particular, some individuals show optimism from the outset of the injury and ongoing resilience (or 'bounceability', see Figure 4.1) despite setbacks and frustrations. Accordingly, Ramanathan, Wardecker, Slocomb and Hillary (2011) found that dispositional optimism was negatively associated with psychological distress following TBI. Interestingly, dispositional optimism was indirectly related to outcome through an association with improved psychological functioning, which in turn was predictive of better cognitive and functional outcomes (Ramanathan et al., 2011). People may draw on pre-existing coping resources including goal setting and persistence, for example:

> You set yourself a goal ... and it doesn't matter what it's for whether its mustering cattle or bloody building a new fence ... that way you just push yourself that little bit ... that's what I've always done in life, not just since the accident.
> (Turner et al., 2011, p. 82)

As discussed earlier, high levels of defensiveness also influence psychological adjustment after brain injury. Individuals who excessively try to present themselves in a favourable light have been found to underreport their brain injury symptoms and experience better long-term emotional adjustment and psychosocial functioning (Ownsworth et al., 2007). However, an overreliance on denial and impression management may place individuals at greater risk of psychological distress if confronted with situations where their problems are exposed or personal virtues are questioned. As an example, the repetitive assessments and close scrutiny of a person's functioning during a protracted medico-legal claim can be highly threatening to a person with high defensiveness (see Ownsworth, 2005). Goldstein (1952) proposed that people who consistently try to avoid thinking about their injury or withdraw from activities that expose their difficulties may experience poor psychological adjustment in the long term. Such reactions may reduce the opportunity to develop more effective ways of coping and regain mastery over their circumstances. Of greater concern, these maladaptive responses may contribute to deterioration in functioning over time through psychological decompensation

(Ownsworth, 2005). In support of this view, use of avoidant coping has been found to be associated with poorer psychological adjustment after brain injury (Anson & Ponsford, 2006a).

Curran, Ponsford and Crowe (2000) found that coping strategies that entailed rumination (e.g., worry and self-blame) and wishful thinking were associated with higher levels of depression and anxiety. In contrast, problem-focused strategies and meaning-based coping (i.e., focusing on the positives) were associated with lower anxiety. The ability to flexibly apply a range of strategies as needed in different situations is generally viewed as more adaptive than overreliance on a particular coping approach (Carver, Scheier & Weintraub, 1989). However, neuropsychological deficits such as impaired planning, inhibition and cognitive flexibility may comprise people's ability to drawn upon effective coping strategies as needed in situations. Krpan, Levine, Stuss and Dawson (2007) found that impaired executive function was related to greater use of emotion-focused coping (e.g., denial and avoidance) and lower use of problem-focused coping. Damage to the prefrontal cortex is likely to produce more emotion-driven or threat-based responses due to disruption of top-down control processes that support cognitive reappraisal and regulation of emotions (Etkin, Egner & Kalisch, 2011). Therefore, although individuals may plan to use particular coping strategies in stressful situations (e.g., use of deep breathing to calm down before overreacting in an argument), their ability to implement these strategies may be compromised by damage to areas underlying emotional and behavioural self-regulation (Stuss, 2007).

The associations among self-awareness, self-appraisals and coping were empirically supported in a cluster analytic study by Medley, Powell, Worthington, Chohan and Jones (2010). They identified that the 'low control/ambivalence' cluster had low perceived control, poor self-awareness, a lack of understanding of their injury and a tendency to employ more avoidant coping strategies. This subgroup contrasted with the 'high salience' cluster which had a high level of perceived control and good self-awareness, and reported more varied use of coping strategies (especially problem-focused strategies). The third cluster, referred to as 'high optimism', reported high perceived control and low use of avoidant coping in the context of poor self-awareness. This group was proposed to reflect individuals with neurologically-based awareness deficits; however, the potential role of premorbid coping style was not investigated.

A major source of stress after brain injury relates to changes in functioning, which often produce a discrepancy or 'mismatch' between a person's abilities, the environment and expectations of performance. The principles of compensation framework (Bäckman & Dixon, 1992) and the selective optimisation with compensation model (Baltes, 1987) were developed to explain the processes by which people adapt to loss of function due to the ageing process or disability. Both theories have been applied to brain injury to account for the different ways in which people adapt to physical, language, cognitive and behavioural impairments (Broomfield et al., 2010; Wilson & Watson, 1996). According to Baltes (1987), *selection* refers to adjustment of one's goals and expectations and channelling personal efforts towards a typically smaller number of achievable goals. *Optimisation* involves engaging in behaviours that capitalise on preserved skills and resources to maximise the outcomes of valued activities and goals. *Compensation* entails efforts to bypass or make up for a loss or reduction in skills below the level required for adequate functioning.

Bäckman and Dixon (1992) proposed the following four mechanisms of compensation:

- *Remediation:* greater investment of time and effort through training and repeated practice to relearn and improve one's skill level (e.g., speech therapy exercises to improve articulation);
- *Substitution:* development of new skills or making the most of preserved skills to take over and adjust for impaired abilities (e.g., learning to use assistive technology for communication deficits);
- *Accommodation*: adjustment of personal goals and expectations to address the gap between the demands of a situation and the person's skills (e.g., focusing on part-time work in a less demanding position than one's pre-injury role);
- *Assimilation:* modification of the environment and/or changing expectations of other people (e.g., selecting supportive work environments and educating employers).

Individuals typically employ a combination of these mechanisms after brain injury, which varies according to the phase of recovery, nature of their impairments, personality style and aspects of the social environment. Similar to coping, excessive use or overreliance on a particular mode of compensation may be detrimental. This was exemplified in Chapter 3 by Jasmine's intense time investment in her studies and resistance to considering different career options. As discussed earlier in this chapter, Peter's social support network helped to compensate for the effects of his injury by altering their expectations of his performance and averting or correcting his errors on tasks in the home and community. Because Peter was unaware of the mismatch between his skill level and the environment, he had not developed his own strategies for coping with cognitive impairments (e.g., his mother kept his diary for him). Despite this, he was very conscious that life was not going in the direction he wanted. His goals were to resume his pre-injury work as an engineer and regain his independent lifestyle, which included driving and living alone. The positive feedback from family and co-workers on Peter's performance in daily living served to reinforce his belief that these achievements were realistic. Consequently, he regularly contacted his previous employer to ask when they would have a position for him.

In summary, the processes of developing awareness, making sense of changes to self and learning to cope with the effects are closely related after brain injury. These adjustment processes feed into and support people's working model of self or self-identity.

Research on changes in self-identity after brain injury

In comparison to psychological adjustment, the literature focusing specifically on self-concept and identity after brain injury is relatively sparse. However, a growing body of studies demonstrates that brain injury can have a negative impact on self-concept (e.g., Cooper-Evans, Alderman, Knight & Oddy, 2008; Gracey et al., 2008; Howes, Edwards & Benton, 2005; Nochi, 1998; Tyerman & Humphrey, 1984). Changes to self after brain injury have been investigated using quantitative tools (i.e., questionnaires and rating scales) and qualitative methods such as life history, narrative and ethnographic approaches (e.g., Gelech & Desjardins, 2011; Krefting, 1989; Muenchberger et al., 2008; Nochi, 1997; 1998; 2000). A meta-synthesis of 23 qualitative studies by Levack, Kayes and Fadyl (2010) identified that six of eight core themes depicting the enduring experience of TBI were related to disconnection with self (i.e., mind/body, pre-injury identity, social world) and reconstructing one's self-identity, place in the world and personhood. The self and social disconnection was attributed to complex changes in people's functioning and life situation. To illustrate this perspective, the impact of physical changes and memory, language and socio-emotional impairments will be considered before examining the broader literature on self-concept and identity changes.

Changes in physical appearance, such as scarring and weight changes, have been found to contribute to poor self-concept after brain injury due to perceived or actual negative reactions from the public (Morris et al., 2005). Altered body image has been found to reduce the self-esteem of younger adults with stroke (Keppel & Crowe, 2000) and people with brain injury (Howes et al., 2005). In one study, people with TBI described their body as 'an enemy' due to the experience of physical symptoms (e.g., pain, fatigue and medication side-effects), which reduced their sense of control and normalcy (Jumisko, Lexell & Soderberg, 2005). Tyerman and Humphrey (1984) found that 30–40 per cent of their TBI sample experienced changes in physical self-concept, as follows: 'no longer a whole person', 'people only have pity for me', and 'everyone stares at me' (p. 16). Yet, 80 per cent endorsed the view that 'physically disabled can live normal lives just like everyone else' (p. 16).

The impact of physical impairments and loss of mobility on sense of self has received most attention in the stroke literature. Ellis-Hill, Payne and Ward (2000) identified the notion of 'self–body split' within the first year after stroke. Individuals perceived their body as a separate, precarious and perplexing entity in hospital and continued to perceive their bodies as unreliable at one year post-stroke. Clarke and Black (2005) found that to cope with physical impairments people with stroke reordered their priorities and modified normal activities to maintain participation on tasks that were closely tied to their identity. Barker, Reid and Cott (2004) found that older adults with stroke viewed their use of a wheelchair in one of three ways: 1) a necessity that was reluctantly accepted; 2) a useful aid to mobility that was gratefully accepted; or 3) 'a part of me', reflecting internal acceptance of the wheelchair as a substitute for declining physical abilities. Acceptance was related to the extent to which people felt that the wheelchair supported their continuity in life, such that it not only increased their mobility, but also their strength, self-confidence and security. Barriers in the person's physical and social environment further influenced acceptance of the wheelchair.

Brain injury can also alter how people experience and express their sexuality. People can experience reduced or increased sex drive and problems with sexual functioning (e.g., erectile dysfunction, impotence, pain or inability to orgasm) and behaviour (Giaquinto, Buzzelli, Di Francesco & Nolfe, 2003; Korpelainen, Nieminen & Myllylä, 1999; Ponsford, 2003). Sexual changes impact on people's ability to establish and maintain relationships, enjoy intimacy and their self-confidence. A combination of physical, psychological and social factors (e.g., reduced opportunity) appears to contribute to sexual difficulties (Ponsford, 2003). There is currently a lack of research investigating the impact of sexual changes on self-identity after brain injury. Although this is important for people in long-term relationships, sexuality is a significant issue for adolescents and young adults in forming their identity.

Memory impairments have received considerable focus in research examining disturbances in consciousness and self (Feinberg, 2011b; Wilson, Kopelman & Kapur, 2008). The subjective experiences of people with amnesia offer insight into the impact of loss of autobiographical memory on self. HM provided the following reflection on his experience of severe amnesia after surgery for intractable seizures.

> Every day is alone, whatever enjoyment I've had, whatever sorrow I've had ... Right now, I am wondering, have I done or said anything amiss? You see, at this moment everything looks clear to me, but what happened just before? That's what worries me. It's like waking from a dream.
>
> (Milner, 1970, p. 37)

Qualitative research by Nochi (1997, 1998) referred to blank periods of memory loss as a 'void' which disrupted people's understanding of their past and present and threatened their sense of agency. The term void also referred to the sense of unknown and difficulty making sense of their injury, particularly during the early recovery phase. People typically 'filled the void' by seeking information from family and professionals about past events. Cloute, Mitchell and Yates (2008) similarly identified how loss of consciousness, post-traumatic amnesia and ongoing memory problems affected people's ability to offer their own personal account of their brain injury, thus contributing to their 'passive positioning' within the medical system and society. Participants used conversational strategies (e.g., humour and well-learnt descriptions from significant others) to cope with gaps in memory about their brain injury. As described in Chapter 3, Dan recorded his daily experiences in a journal to compensate for episodic memory loss and support his continuity of self.

Self-identity has been closely linked to personal narrative, or people's own account of their experiences as represented through words, metaphors and other symbols. Nochi (1997) emphasised that such personal accounts often differed from the 'objective truth' or facts about their brain injury. Lorenz (2010) described how the combined use of photographs and conversation assisted a woman with brain tumour to form a 'visual illness narrative' and discover her new identity after brain injury. If telling one's own story is central to understanding self after brain injury, this raises the question of how communication impairments impact on self-identity.

This issue has received considerable attention in research investigating adjustment to aphasia (Shadden, 2005; Shadden & Koski, 2007; Silverman, 2011). Silverman (2011) identified that people's perceived control over their social environment or 'communication power' influenced their ability to participate in life with aphasia. Shadden and Koski (2007) observed that people with aphasia often found it difficult to reconstruct their sense of self, due to the loss of opportunity for social interaction. Supportive interactions (e.g., an aphasia communication group) were perceived to help overcome barriers associated with language impairments and facilitate the social reconstruction of self. Renegotiating self-identity in the context of aphasia depends largely on how successfully people with aphasia and their significant others adapt to their communication difficulties (Shadden, 2005).

Some of the most perplexing and distressing changes to self after brain injury include social perception and emotion-regulation deficits, such as loss of empathy and perspective-taking skills, lack of emotional responsiveness, reduced tolerance to stress and poor anger control. Jumisko et al. (2005) identified that people with TBI had a sense that they had 'lost something of themselves', but were often unable to clearly define this fundamental change. It was observed that they had difficulty understanding their own feelings as well as reading the emotions of others. As previously described in Chapter 3, the complex and often less visible changes in social cognition particularly interfere with adolescents' ability to establish and maintain relationships and pursue vocational goals. Other authors have similarly identified how changes in social skills and emotional regulation contribute to loss of relationships and diminished social networks for adults with brain injury (Douglas, 2012; McDonald & Flanagan, 2004).

Overall, changes in physical, cognitive and socio-emotional functioning can alter the 'experience of self in the world' (Gracey et al., 2008, p. 639). More specifically, these impairments can reduce people's sense of agency, independence and participation in society. The subjective meaning of these impairments and people's capacity to maintain valued activities and life roles is paramount to preserving or rebuilding one's sense of self.

The broader research on self-identity after brain injury has mainly focused on self-concept or self-esteem, because these related constructs are more amenable to measurement than self-identity. Studies that used a validated interview schedule or questionnaire to assess self-esteem, self-concept or sense of identity after brain injury are summarised in Table 4.1. A consistent finding in this literature is that poor self-concept after brain injury is associated with lower ratings of quality of life and emotional well-being (Cantor et al., 2005; Cooper-Evans et al., 2008; Doering, Conrad, Rief & Exner, 2011; Vickery, Gontkovsky & Caroselli, 2005).

The earliest study to systematically assess changes in self-concept was conducted by Tyerman and Humphrey (1984), who used a semantic differential rating scale (i.e., a list of personality and behavioural attributes) on which people with severe head injury rated their present self, past or premorbid self, future self, a typical person and a typical head-injured person. Present self was viewed as vastly different from past self, with

Table 4.1 Summary of studies investigating changes to self and identity after brain injury

Studies	Participants and design	Assessment of self-concept	Main findings
Tyerman & Humphrey (1984)	25 people with severe head injury (2–15 months post-injury); cross-sectional study	Semantic Differential Scale, anxiety, depression	Present self was viewed as vastly different from past self, although a return to past self was predicted within the year. Present self was viewed less positively than a typical person, but more positively than a typical head-injured person.
Wright & Telford (1996)	50 people with mainly mild TBI at 6 months and 21 followed up at 3 years post-injury	Head Injury Semantic Differential Scale (HISD)	Participants rated their present self more negatively than their pre-injury self and anticipated a return to past self in the future. Greater past/present and past/future self-discrepancies were related to more severe psychological distress.
Ellis-Hill & Horn (2000)	26 people with first-time stroke and 26 controls; cross-sectional study with within-group (current and 6 months pre-stroke) and between-group comparisons	HISD II (updated version)	Stroke participants perceived their current self-concept as significantly poorer than pre-injury (e.g., less capable, independent and in control). Self-concept was not significantly related to physical disability (mobility).
Vickery, Gontkovsky & Caroselli (2005)	19 individuals with ABI; cross-sectional study	Self-concept (Tennessee Self-Concept Scale 2; HISD)	Ratings of self-concept were positively correlated with quality of life.
Cantor et al. (2005)	21 individuals with TBI (2–33 years) or mild to severe severity; cross-sectional study	Selves Interview and Selves Adjective Checklist	Significant association between emotional distress and self-discrepancy on the checklist ($\rho > .80$), but not on the interview.
Secrest & Zeller (2007)	51 individuals with stroke; repeated measures (1, 3 and 6 months post-stroke); 33 completed the study	Continuity/Discontinuity of Self Scale	Continuity/self, continuity/other and discontinuity was significantly related to depression and quality of life. Sense of continuity and discontinuity did not change over time.
Cooper-Evans, Alderman, Knight & Oddy (2008)	22 individuals with brain injury; within-subjects design (re-assessment after 2 weeks), chronicity 16–348 months (average: 122 months)	Rosenberg Self-Esteem Scale (RSES)	Ratings of self-esteem were stable over a 2-week period and were negatively associated with anxiety and depression. Higher ratings of self-esteem were associated with poorer cognitive and executive functioning and lower self-awareness.
Carroll & Coetzer (2011)	29 individuals with TBI, chronicity: 2.3–40 years (average: 11.2 years); cross-sectional study	HISD-III, RSES, Brain Injury Grief Inventory	Negative changes in identity were related to greater emotional distress and poorer self-esteem. Poorer self-awareness was associated with higher self-esteem.
Doering, Conrad, Rief & Exner (2011)	35 participants with mixed brain injury in post-acute rehabilitation (chronicity: at least 3 months, range not specified); cross-sectional study	Frankfurt Self-Concept Scale	Participants rated their self-concept more negatively than normative data on most indices. Self-concept was related to subjective cognitive complaints but not cognitive test scores. Self-concept for achievement mediated the relationship between subjective cognitive complaints and subjective well-being.
Jones, Haslam, Jetten, Williams, Morris & Saroyan (2011)	630 individuals with brain injury (chronicity unknown) recruited through a brain injury support network; cross-sectional study	Trauma and Recovery Experiences Tool, assessing aspects of identity, stigma, discrimination, social support and well-being	Injury severity was positively associated with life satisfaction, identity strength and social changes. Identity strength was the strongest mediator of the relationship between injury severity and life satisfaction.

negative changes (e.g., more bitter, dependent and irritable) most commonly reported, although some changes were positive (e.g., more mature and appreciative). Despite the major differences perceived between present self and past self, participants with brain injury anticipated a return to past self within the year. Present self was viewed less positively than a typical person, but more positively than a typical head-injured person. Therefore, despite recognising the effects of brain injury on their current functioning, people held optimistic and unrealistic expectations of recovery and used downward social comparison (i.e., others are worse off than me) to cope with changes to self.

Consistent with Tyerman and Humphrey's (1984) findings, Wright and Telford (1996) found that individuals with predominantly mild brain injury rated their present self more negatively than their pre-injury self, and anticipated a return to past self in the future. Greater discrepancies between past and present self and past and future self were related to more severe psychological distress. No changes in self-concept were evident between the assessments at 6 months post-injury and 3-year follow-up, suggesting that self-discrepancies persist over time.

Guided by Self-Discrepancy Theory (Higgins, 1987; see Chapter 2), Cantor and colleagues (2005) examined self-discrepancies as a potential mechanism underlying emotional distress after TBI. Self-discrepancies were assessed using two approaches: 1) Selves Interview, an open-ended interview involving descriptions and ratings of actual (pre-injury and current), ideal and ought selves; and 2) Selves Adjective Checklist (SAC). Interestingly, scores on the two measures were not significantly related, and greater self-discrepancies on the SAC only were associated with increased depression and anxiety (see Chapter 5 for further details).

Self-discrepancies and changes in self-concept are also evident following stroke. Ellis-Hill and Horn (2000) found that people experienced a significant reduction in their overall self-concept, and viewed themselves as less capable, independent and in control, as well as feeling less satisfied, interested, active, confident, and of less value since their stroke. Self-concept changes were not found to be related to physical status (i.e., mobility). Furthermore, Secrest and Zeller (2007) reported that after stroke people's sense of continuity (i.e., experience of oneself as continuous with 'who I was') and discontinuity (i.e., loss of aspects of self, sense of control, independence and connection with others) remained relatively stable between one and six months post-stroke. Therefore, despite improvements in their functional status, individuals' sense of continuity and discontinuity with their pre-stroke selves was unchanged. Levels of continuity/discontinuity were related to depression and quality of life at both time points. At 6-months follow-up individuals who perceived greater discontinuity had poorer functional status, which suggests that level of disability contributed to their sense of disconnection with pre-stroke selves.

In addition to documenting changes in sense of self, a number of studies have examined cognitive and metacognitive factors related to self-concept after brain injury. The findings are consistent with those previously reported for children with brain injury (see Chapter 3) in one important respect. Specifically, Carroll and Coetzer (2011) and Cooper-Evans et al. (2008) reported significant positive associations between awareness deficits and self-esteem, indicating that lack of awareness may protect individuals' self-esteem after brain injury. Cooper-Evans et al. (2008) also found that individuals with lower general cognitive ability (IQ) and poorer executive functioning reported higher self-esteem.

However, Doering et al. (2011) found that self-reported cognitive deficits were more closely related to self-concept than objective cognitive performance. Self-concept relating to achievement mediated the relationship between subjective cognitive complaints and subjective well-being. Specifically, individuals who perceived greater cognitive difficulties were less confident in their ability to achieve personal goals, make decisions and solve problems, which in turn lowered their mood state and life satisfaction. Due to lack of collateral ratings it is not possible to determine whether their perceived impairments were accurate (i.e., consistent with significant others) or reflected an overestimation of their deficits, which typically co-exists with depressive symptoms (Ownsworth et al., 2007).

The key influence of subjective perspectives of change on well-being was emphasised in a large survey study ($n = 630$) by Jones, Haslam, Jetten, Williams, Morris and Saroyan (2011), who reported a 'counterintuitive positive relationship' between injury severity and life satisfaction. This relationship was mediated by personal identity strength and social changes, whereby individuals with more severe injuries were more likely to perceive themselves as stronger because of the injury and perceive positive changes in their relationships and support. Identity strength, or agreeing with the statement 'Having had a brain injury has made me a stronger person' (p. 358), was the strongest individual mediator. The identity strength and social change variables largely explained why people with more severe injuries reported greater life satisfaction.

Changes in group membership and social identity after brain injury have been reported by many authors (Douglas, 2012; Douglas & Spellacy, 2000; Gracey et al., 2008; Haslam et al., 2008). People can feel misunderstood and stigmatised, and experience a 'loss of self in the eyes of others' (Nochi, 1998). Relatives can inadvertently reinforce this message with comments such as 'he [or she] is no longer the person I married', which may reflect a complex grief reaction to the loss of a person who still living (Krefting, 1989). A number of studies have emphasised the importance of social groups and activity participation for maintaining self-worth after brain injury.

For example, Gracey et al. (2008) used structured group exercises to elicit personal constructs of individuals with acquired brain injury based on comparison of pre-injury, current, and ideal selves. One of the major themes, namely, 'experience of self in the world' related to people's experience of themselves in social and activity contexts. Self-descriptions within this theme included 'feeling part of things vs. do not fit in, (or) belong'; 'doing things that reinforce who I am vs. loss of key activities, not doing personally important things'; and 'struggle to be part of a group, a burden vs. feel useful and able to contribute'. The findings highlighted that sense of self after brain injury is influenced by the meaning derived from social interaction and activity participation.

Guided by social identity theory (see Chapter 2), Haslam and colleagues (2008) found that belonging to multiple social groups prior to stroke and maintaining these group memberships was predictive of life satisfaction. Specifically, stronger pre-existing social networks increased the likelihood of maintaining some social connections after the stroke. Subjective cognitive impairment influenced life satisfaction by impacting on people's ability to maintain their group memberships. Haun and Rittman (2008) also identified that levels of social connectedness and isolation influenced people's experiences of recovery during the first year post-discharge after stroke. Approximately half of their sample initially experienced isolation, while many re-adjusted and were able to reconnect with their social networks.

Strong-tie expressive support has been found to be the dimension of social support most closely related to well-being of people with brain injury and their family members (Douglas & Spellacy, 2000). This aspect of support involves being able to share one's feelings, problems and dreams with someone close, and to feel accepted and empathised with (Douglas, 2012). However, people with brain injury find it especially difficult to develop and maintain close and reciprocal relationships. In the absence of these social ties, they may require considerable support to re-establish their sense of connectedness and social identity. In Douglas's (2012) account of 'Michael' his mother made a specific link between lack of social connection and loss of self: 'he (Michael) feels lost because he doesn't interact with others … we have to find a way he can be Michael' (p. 237).

Qualitative research by Douglas (2012; 2013) identified two interrelated self-concept themes, namely, 'Who I am' (knowledge of personal attributes and goals) and 'How I feel about myself' (evaluation of self and one's achievements). Self-concept was conceptualised as a dynamic process of appraising the outcomes of self-defined goals. This is similar to James's (1890) notion that self-esteem 'depends entirely on what we back ourselves to be and do' (p. 310), as discussed in Chapter 2. In describing personal attributes participants typically did not make reference to their brain injury, thus indicating that they did not view the injury as a core aspect of themselves. As a third theme arising from the analysis, Douglas (2012) identified 'facilitators' that supported people's sense of connection with society, including family, friends, carers, pets, and 'social snacks'. The latter term refers to tangible reminders of social bonds such as photos, cards and certificates that represent relationships and shared experiences (Douglas, 2012).

Overall, it is well supported that social resources can act a buffer for the losses associated with brain injury. More supportive social interactions (e.g., empathic responses and reminders of personal achievements and social bonds) and opportunities to engage in meaningful activities tied to one's identity are likely to enhance psychological adjustment. As covered in more detail in Chapters 7, group and community-based activities that enhance people's social participation can facilitate the identity reconstruction process.

Summary and theoretical integration

As summarised in Table 4.1, the literature indicates that poor self-concept after brain injury is more likely to be experienced by individuals with less severe cognitive and executive deficits, and by those who perceive greater functional impairments. Conversely, those with severe cognitive deficits and poor self-awareness appear less likely to experience self-discrepancies, or make unfavourable comparisons between their current and pre-injury selves. There is also some evidence that people with more severe brain injury can experience a greater sense of survivorship, which in turn is associated with increased life satisfaction (Jones et al., 2011). However, some caution is needed in drawing firm conclusions from these studies due to various methodological issues.

Firstly, with the exception of research by Secrest and Zeller (2007) and Wright and Telford (1996), most studies examining changes in self-concept or self-discrepancies after brain injury have been cross-sectional and involved small and relatively chronic samples (i.e., > 2 years post-injury). Although research by Secrest and Zeller (2007) and Cooper-Evans and colleagues (2008) indicates that sense of self is relatively stable after brain injury, prospective longitudinal research with a large and representative cohort is needed to depict the identity transition process. Qualitative research by Turner et al. (2011) indicated that self-discrepancies were not usually evident at discharge or one month post-discharge, but began to emerge at 3 months post-discharge, as reflected by self-descriptions (see Figure 4.1). Secondly, in the study by Jones et al. (2011) single-item scales were used to assess identity strength and life satisfaction, and participants were asked to estimate their length of coma as an index of injury severity. A further methodological issue is that different measures of self-concept have been employed across studies, often with conflicting findings (see Cantor et al., 2005). These assessment issues will be considered in more depth in Chapter 5.

Overall, relatively few studies have examined factors influencing self-concept and identity changes after brain injury. The findings of the study by Doering et al. (2011) indicated that self-perceived consequences of the injury are more closely related to self-concept than objective indices of impairment. Hence, people with more severe injuries or more extensive functional impairments do not necessarily experience greater changes to sense of self. In fact, some research suggests that those with poorer neurocognitive status report better self-esteem (Cooper-Evans et al., 2008; Jones et al., 2011). To make sense of these somewhat paradoxical findings, it is helpful to consider Gracey and Ownsworth's (2012) model of neuropsychological and social processes influencing adjustment after brain injury.

Our model proposes that level of engagement in occupational activities and social groups provide the input for experiences that may challenge or reinforce sense of self after brain injury. Meaning derived from day-to-day interactions provides feedback that can affirm or disconfirm one's abilities, foster a sense of belonging or exclusion, and influence the extent to which a person feels understood and supported. Information about self is initially processed rapidly via lower order sensory-perceptual, cognitive and emotional systems (mapping onto the somatosensory cortex, thalamus, parietal lobe and amygdala) to guide responses in a situation, for example, a person's immediate response to feedback (LeDoux, 1996). Self-relevant information is also processed at a deeper level through monitoring and reflecting upon one's experiences across many situations. This process entails drawing on stored self-representations in autobiographical memory and abstracting meaning in relation to one's goals and self-schemas. Through these higher order processes (supported by fronto-temporal circuitry) people compare their pre-injury and post-injury abilities and update their self-knowledge and beliefs. As previously described in Chapter 2, effortful cognitive processes are required to resolve self-discrepancies and assimilate feedback about self (Eisenstadt et al., 2002). If feedback is accepted that is in line with one's rejected or feared self, this is likely to alter self-schemas in a detrimental manner (e.g., 'People don't want to spend time with me, no-one cares about me').

Gracey and Ownsworth's (2012) model can explain why people with more severe injuries and cognitive impairments sometimes maintain a more positive self-concept after brain injury. Specifically, damage to brain systems subserving neuropsychological processes (e.g., memory, metacognitive and executive functioning) may restrict people's ability to monitor and evaluate their task performance and compare their pre-injury and post-injury selves as needed to update their self-knowledge. Impairments in memory, self-awareness and executive function can therefore serve to maintain existing self-schemas (Agnew & Morris, 1998; Carroll & Coetzer, 2011; Cooper-Evans et al., 2008). Conversely, individuals with greater metacognitive and executive abilities are better able to compare their current abilities with their premorbid performance and update their self-knowledge. The self-discrepancies that arise from this self-comparison can be emotionally threatening (Cantor et al., 2005; Nochi, 1998) and lead to threat appraisals, avoidance of activities and social withdrawal (Riley et al. 2004). Lack of opportunity to adapt to one's impairments and regain a sense of mastery over one's environment is likely to contribute to poor self-concept and depression (Nochi, 1998; Ownsworth, 2005).

The first main implication of this account is that loss of meaningful activities and experience of social exclusion can contribute to self-discrepancies, a sense of threat and unhelpful coping reactions which impede people's ability to develop an adaptive post-injury identity (Gracey & Ownsworth, 2012). Therefore, assessing changes to self after brain injury is essential to guide support interventions, as discussed in Chapter 5. The second key implication is that rehabilitation approaches that focus on maintaining or re-establishing a person's activity and social participation are key to facilitating identity reconstruction. Individual, group and community-based interventions are reviewed in Chapters 6 and 7.

Overall, psychological adjustment to brain injury is highly individualised and successful adjustment is not reflected by one particular way of viewing one's circumstances or coping. For some, positive long-term adjustment may be evident from realistic and balanced self-appraisals, use of strategies to participate in valued activities and a sense of survivorship linked to their injury (Nochi, 1998; 2000). Others may feel they have acknowledged and dealt with the brain injury to the extent that it no longer influences their sense of self, as reflected by the following email from 'Ted' who sustained a severe TBI in 1996.

> I have done so much with my life since having the brain injury. It will always be an important chapter in my life, but I have moved past it. It rarely comes up in conversation with my family, and you'll note that I no longer refer to my brain

injury on my website. Surviving a brain injury is one of the many things I have achieved in my life, but it no longer defines me.

Conclusions

This chapter has highlighted that psychological adjustment to brain injury is a complex process influenced by people's pre-injury personality, neuropsychological status, social reactions and opportunities to re-engage in meaning activities and roles. Research suggests that heightened awareness of impairments and negative self-appraisals can lead to activity avoidance and social withdrawal which, in turn, contributes to poor self-concept. Optimistic yet realistic perceptions of one's capabilities motivate people to find ways to maintain participation in valued activities and social roles. In doing so, they can regain a sense of mastery and purpose in life. More generally, people's daily experiences need to provide meaning and reinforce their notions of who they are. In the following chapter, approaches for assessing psychological adjustment and changes to sense of self are reviewed.

5 Approaches for assessing changes to self after brain injury

A main objective of psychological assessment after brain injury is to determine how individuals perceive, make sense of and cope with changes in their functioning and lifestyle. This chapter describes approaches used in clinical practice and research to assess self-perceptions and changes to self and self-identity after brain injury. Based on the framework presented in Chapter 4, approaches for assessing self-awareness, sense-making appraisals, coping and adaptation are initially reviewed. Following this, measures assessing self-concept and changes in self and identity after brain injury are appraised according to their theory-base, psychometric properties, research applications and clinical utility. Although the chapter mainly focuses on assessments used with adults, approaches are also considered for children and adolescents based on existing literature and a discussion of tools developed for other paediatric populations that have potential utility for brain injury.

Issues surrounding the measurement of self and identity

Perceptions of one's own distinctiveness and sameness over time are central to definitions of self and identity. Hence, the self is a personal construction that cannot be directly observed or verified by another person (Damon & Hart, 1982). Authors have long questioned the legitimacy of attempts to capture the essence of self in an objective manner (Hume, 1738; cited in Hume, 2003). As noted in Chapter 2, experimental studies of self-referential processing pose various conceptual and methodological quandaries for neuroscience; yet, the field has advanced by developing a set of common assumptions and clear caveats regarding these assumptions (Northoff et al., 2011). Although the view that the self cannot be directly observed or verified is acknowledged (see Hume, 2003), endeavours to measure sense of self are important in research and clinical practice for many disorders where disturbances in self are a core feature, including autism, brain injury, dementia, psychosis and personality disorder. Such measurement can provide valuable insight into people's experience of their illness or condition and guide effective management and treatment.

The focus of this chapter is on approaches for assessing the subjective impact of brain injury and changes to sense of self. To assist this review it is useful to briefly consider broad approaches for measuring the concept of self. Brinthaupt and Erwin (1992) described three main ways of 'getting to know someone' or finding out what a person is really like. One approach is to observe someone closely when they are unaware they are being observed, in order to capture their naturalistic tendencies. A second approach is to ask people very close to the person to share their knowledge and observations. The third and most direct approach is to interact with the person and ask questions that cover a broad range of personal characteristics (e.g., demographics, preferences, values and attributes). Brinthaupt and Erwin (1992) distinguished between 'reactive' self-report methods that involve providing a list of specific items on a questionnaire or interview and 'spontaneous' methods that entail open-ended approaches, such as the Who Are You (WAY) technique and the related Twenty Statements Test (Bugental & Zelen, 1950; Kuhn & McPartland, 1954).

In considering the relevance of these three broad approaches to brain injury, the first approach of covert observation is problematic from an ethical perspective. However, the use of naturalistic observation in real-life settings with people's consent can provide valuable insight into their characteristic self-perceptions and coping reactions (e.g., Krefting, 1989). The second approach of assessing an individual's characteristics by proxy may have utility in certain contexts. The use of significant others' reports to assist in measuring aspects of self will be considered later in this chapter. The third approach of self-report via interviews and questionnaires is the most frequently used and practical method for measuring the constructs of self and identity (Brinthaupt & Erwin, 1992). The use of an interview guide to elicit self-narrative is a common qualitative approach for exploring changes to self and identity after brain injury (Levack et al., 2010). This approach is based on the view that self-identity is a language constructed phenomenon, and we are the stories we tell about ourselves (Freeman, 1992).

There are many practical advantages to using self-report methods for studying the self. These typically brief measures require individuals to describe, rate or endorse particular personal characteristics or tendencies. A broad range of cognitive, developmental, psychological and socio-cultural factors influence the information gained through self-report (for an in-depth review see Brinthaupt & Erwin, 1992). Of particular relevance to brain injury, reporting about the self relies upon access to and organisation of self-knowledge and schemas, which in turn is influenced by cognitive processes such as working memory, autobiographical memory and the filtering and abstraction from personal experiences. The ability to recall recent experiences and update self-knowledge based on feedback and perceptions of task success and failure is often compromised by brain injury (Ownsworth, Clare et al., 2006). Disrupted access to or selective recall of self-relevant information may produce biased self-reports that resemble one's pre-injury self and overestimate current abilities. Developmental issues influence the content of self-reports, whereby younger children find it easier to report concrete physical and behavioural characteristics than psychological traits. Due to their more advanced reasoning skills, older children and adolescents are better able to identify more abstract and generalised characteristics and psychological traits (Brinthaupt & Erwin, 1992; Harter, 2012).

Psychological factors also influence the nature of self-reported information. In particular, a conscious or unconscious desire to protect one's self-image (i.e., self-deception) and impression management (i.e., social desirability) may contribute to underreporting of unfavourable information about self or personal shortcomings. Information-processing biases (e.g., self-enhancement or self-depreciation) influence the filtering of self-relevant information and affect people's self-presentation style. A common tendency is to report information that is more consistent with the ideal self (or ought-other self) than the actual self. Various contextual factors, including people's affective state, motivation, recent life experiences and demand characteristics of the situation influence self-reported information (Brinthaupt & Erwin, 1992). Further, the assessment format (e.g., open or closed questions) influences the type and specificity of responses. The self has been described as a working personal construction for which components are selectively activated in a given setting (Markus & Nurius, 1986).

Due to the interactive influence of these factors, Brinthaupt and Erwin (1992) advise that there will always be information about self that is not reported. This may be because it is not consciously perceived or accessible to the person, or because he or she is unwilling to disclose this information in a specific assessment context. Additionally, the approach employed may not effectively elicit such information due to the particular wording or format of questions.

Assessment of self-awareness, sense making and coping strategies

Following brain injury, people's compromised language and cognitive capacity and lack of insight have been identified as issues that influence the accuracy of information obtained from interviews and questionnaires (see Paterson & Scott-Findlay, 2002; Fleming, Strong & Ashton, 1996). Self-reports are still considered the most appropriate source of information about changes in self and identity, bearing in mind two main points. First, the approach to measurement inevitably influences the information gained and may not be comparable or consistent with that gained from other sources. Second, accessing multiple sources of information about the person with brain injury (e.g., self-reports, collateral information from significant others and behavioural observation) is ideal and can be valuable for examining degree of consistency and areas of discrepancy.

Self-perceptions after brain injury have been investigated using a range of quantitative methods (i.e., questionnaires, rating scales and structured interviews; see Tate, 2010) and qualitative approaches that include open-ended interviews (e.g., Nochi, 1997; 1998; 2000) and eliciting self-perceptions and reactions in social and activity contexts (Gracey et al., 2008; Krefting, 1989; Ownsworth, Turpin et al., 2008). For an in-depth review of the methodology of qualitative studies exploring people's experience of TBI, readers are referred to a meta-synthesis by Levack and colleagues (2010). The following sections provide a review of assessment tools that are in common use in brain injury research, as well as novel approaches that have potential clinical utility but require further psychometric evaluation. Based on the framework presented in Chapter 4, approaches are initially reviewed for assessing self-awareness, sense-making appraisals and coping strategies. A summary of measures commonly used to assess these constructs is presented in Table 5.1.

Table 5.1 Summary of measures assessing self-awareness, sense-making appraisals and coping after brain injury

Construct and measure	Description of measure	Example of content	Research applications
Self-awareness Patient Competency Rating Scale (PCRS; Prigatano et al., 1986)	30 items rated on a 5-point Likert scale ('Can't do' to 'Can do with ease'), focusing on degree of difficulty or current competency. Items sample four domains (Prigatano & Leathem, 1993). A modified 13-item version (PCRS for neurorehabilitation) is available for assessing self-awareness in inpatient rehabilitation (Borgaro & Prigatano, 2003).	• Activities of daily living (preparing meals, dressing) • Cognitions (remembering names and daily schedule) • Interpersonal function (handling arguments, accepting criticism) • Emotional behaviour (controlling crying, temper and depression).	Used extensively in research: e.g., distinguishing between people who overestimate or underestimate deficits (Prigatano & Altman, 1990), assessing development of awareness of deficits over time (Fleming et al., 1996), investigating cross-cultural differences (Prigatano & Leathem, 1993), and evaluating the efficacy of rehabilitation (Ownsworth, Fleming et al., 2008).
Awareness Questionnaire (AQ; Sherer Bergloff, Boake, High, & Levin, 1998a)	17-item measure assessing perceived changes in functioning from pre-injury status. Items are rated on a 5-point rating scale (1 = much worse, 3 = about the same, 5 = much better). Factor analysis supports three components or subscales: cognitive, behavioural/affective and motor/sensory (Sherer et al., 1998a).	• Cognitive (concentration, memory for recent events) • Behavioural/affective (get along with people, keep feelings in control) • Motor/sensory (able to see, hear, move arms and legs).	Used to investigate development of awareness between the acute recovery phase and 12 months follow-up (Hart, Seignourel & Sherer, 2009), neuroanatomical basis of awareness deficits (Sherer et al., 2005), relationship between awareness deficits and functional outcomes (Sherer et al., 1998b) and efficacy of awareness interventions (Schmidt et al., 2013).
Self-Awareness of Deficits Interview (SADI; Fleming et al., 1996)	A semi-structured interview with open questions and prompts for three sections: (1) awareness of deficits, (2) awareness of the functional implications of deficits and (3) ability to set goals. A checklist with corresponding items is completed by a significant other (relative/close friend or therapist) and scoring involves comparing the responses of the person with brain injury with a significant other. Administration time is approximately 20–30 minutes.	• Section 1: 'Are you any different now compared to what you were like before your accident?' • Section 2: 'Does your head injury have any effect on your everyday life?' • Section 3: 'What do you hope to achieve in the next 6 months?' (Tate, 2010, p. 269).	Most commonly used interview schedule to monitor emergence of self-awareness during hospital transition (Fleming et al., 1998), investigate the aetiology of awareness deficits (Ownsworth et al., 2002), and evaluate the efficacy of awareness training (Cheng & Man, 2006).

Sense making Stress Appraisal Measure (SAM; Peacock & Wong, 1990)	28 items assessing primary appraisals related to anticipatory stress (threat, challenge and centrality), secondary appraisals focusing on perceptions of control (controllable-by-self, controllable-by-others and uncontrollable-by-anyone) and overall stressfulness. Items on the seven SAM scales are rated on a 5-point Likert scale (1 = not at all, to 5 = extremely).	• Threat (potential for harm/loss) • Challenge (potential for gain) • Centrality (importance for one's well-being) • Controllable-by-self (skills to overcome problem) • Controllable-by-others (support or help available) • Uncontrollable (problem can't be resolved by anyone).	Rochette et al. (2007) reported that higher appraisals of threat and centrality and lower appraisals of challenge at 2 weeks post-stroke were associated with an increase in depressive symptoms 6 months later. Ownsworth, Hoffmann et al. (2011) also found that early cognitive appraisals (at hospital discharge) were associated with psychological adjustment at 5–6 months post-discharge after stroke.
Appraisal of Threat and Avoidance Questionnaire (ATAQ; Riley et al., 2004)	36-item measure of threat appraisals and related avoidance behaviours after TBI. Each item is rated yes (= 1) or no (= 0) across three categories. Scoring includes a threat appraisal score and avoidance score for each category and overall threat appraisals and avoidance scores.	• Personal safety (e.g., worry about falling or injuring self) • Dealing with people (e.g., worry that people think I'm stupid) • Doing things (e.g., get upset or frustrated if do things wrong).	Initial research by Riley et al. (2004) found that 100% of TBI participants (n = 50) identified at least one threat appraisal and 74% identified ≥ 10. 74% reported at least one avoidance behaviour and 32% reported ≥ 10. Subsequent research found that the relationship between threat appraisals and avoidance was moderated by coping resources and self-esteem (Riley et al., 2010).
Coping strategies Coping Scale for Adults (CSA; Frydenberg & Lewis, 2012)	74 items that assess 18 distinct coping strategies and reflect four dimensions of coping: 'Dealing with the problem', 'Nonproductive coping', 'Optimism' and 'Sharing'. The CSA has short and full versions of both general concerns and specific concerns.	• Dealing with the problem (e.g., tackling a problem systematically) • Sharing (e.g., enlisting support of others) • Non-productive (e.g., self-blame and worry) • Optimism (focusing on positive outcomes).	Coping styles on the CSA have been found to correlate with emotional adjustment and self-esteem (Anson & Ponsford, 2006a; Spitz et al., 2013). The CSA was sensitive to detecting change in adaptive coping after a coping skills intervention (Anson & Ponsford, 2006b).
Ways of Coping Questionnaire – Revised (WCQ; Folkman & Lazarus, 1985)	66-item measure of problem-focused coping and emotion-focused coping based on the Transactional Theory of Stress and Coping. Various shortened or revised versions of the WCQ exist, with items ranging from 28 (Rochette & Desrosiers, 2002) to 40 (King et al., 2002).	• Confrontive coping • Distancing • Self-controlling • Seeking social support • Accepting responsibility • Escape-avoidance • Planful problem solving • Positive reappraisal.	Most commonly used coping measure in stroke and TBI research. Findings generally indicate that greater use of problem-focused coping and less use of emotion-focused coping (e.g., avoidance, and wishful thinking) is related to better psychosocial function (Kendall & Terry, 2008; Medley et al., 2010; Rochette & Desrosiers, 2002).

Self-awareness: Self-knowledge of abilities and impairments

In the context of brain injury, self-awareness refers to an individual's capacity to recognise changes in personal abilities and understand the implications for everyday functioning and future goals (Fleming et al., 1996). This section focuses on measures of self-awareness that broadly span physical, cognitive, emotional and behavioural functioning (for a review of domain-specific awareness disorders see Prigatano, 2010). Subjective perceptions of impairment or symptoms following brain injury can be assessed using an infinite number of formal and informal measures, rating scales and checklists. However, particular measures have been specifically designed and validated to assess self-awareness.

The most common approach to measuring awareness of deficits is to compare ratings of the presence, frequency or severity of functional problems by the person with brain injury and a significant other (e.g., a therapist or family member) to yield a discrepancy index. Some authors have used generic measures of well-being or disability developed for other clinical populations, such as the Sickness Impact Profile, and compared self-ratings and significant other ratings (Pagulayan, Temkin, Machamer & Dikmen, 2007). Other measures were specifically designed to broadly assess the sequelae of brain injury and include both self-report and informant versions, thus enabling a discrepancy-based awareness index to be calculated. These include the Mayo-Portland Adaptability Inventory, European Brain Injury Questionnaire and Neurobehavioural Functioning Inventory.

Some self-report measures focus on awareness of behavioural difficulties, such as the Patient Competency Rating Scale (PCRS), Dysexecutive Questionnaire (DEX) and Head Injury Behaviour Rating Scale (HIBS). Other scales assess changes in behaviour or functioning since the brain injury, including the Key Behaviors Change Inventory, and Awareness Questionnaire (AQ). The PCRS and AQ have been used extensively and validated in brain injury research (see Table 5.1). Self-report measures are practical and brief to administer and provide multiple indices that enable a comparison between individuals' self-perceived functional difficulties (e.g., PCRS, HIBS) or perceived change from premorbid functioning (e.g., AQ) and one or more significant others' ratings. Informant versions are available for a family member or clinician to complete. A particular advantage of these questionnaires is that both positive and negative discrepancies are clinically meaningful to identify because some individuals may overestimate their functional abilities while others underestimate their functional abilities (Ownsworth et al., 2007). The PCRS and AQ are available in Tate's (2010) compendium and on the Centre for Outcome Measurement in Brain Injury website (http://www.tbims.org/combi), as part of an extensive collection of online resources, which include the rating forms and psychometric properties.

Although there are many advantages of questionnaire-based measures of awareness, a potential shortcoming of tools such as the PCRS, AQ, DEX and HIBS is that scoring and interpretation relies upon the veracity of ratings provided by significant others. It is well recognised that family members' and clinicians' ratings of the person's functioning are prone to bias and inaccuracy due to a range of factors. For example, therapists are typically unfamiliar with the person before the injury and may not have the opportunity to observe the person's functioning in a range of settings. Relatives may not be aware of how the person has changed during the early hospitalisation period, and their own mood state and personality style may contribute to a tendency to report excessively high or low levels of impairment for the person with brain injury. Another option is to compare individuals' self-ratings with more objective indices of functioning such as neuropsychological tests (see Allen & Ruff, 1990; Anderson & Tranel, 1989). However, neuropsychological tests cannot sample the broad range of functions for which awareness may be compromised (e.g., interpersonal skills and emotional regulation). Due to these limitations, some authors have advocated the need for more in-depth assessment of awareness using interview schedules (Fleming et al., 1996; Simmond & Fleming, 2003).

The Self-Awareness of Deficits Interview (SADI; Fleming et al., 1996) is a validated semi-structured interview designed to assess self-awareness in three areas: (1) awareness of deficits (e.g., physical, cognitive, emotional and social); (2) awareness of the functional implications of deficits (e.g., independent living, work, family, relationships and leisure); and (3) ability to set goals (e.g., goals for the next six months and future expectations of recovery). As presented in Tate's compendium (2010), the initial broad questions for Section 1 are: 'Are you any different now compared to what you were like before your accident? In what way? Do you feel that anything about you, or your abilities has changed?' (Fleming et al., 1996, p. 14). These questions are followed by further questions and prompts that enable an in-depth exploration of individuals' awareness of their deficits, understanding of the functional implications and future impact on goals and functioning.

A key advantage of the SADI involves the flexible format for phrasing questions and follow-up prompts to elicit information, rather than asking the person to rate their abilities on a constrained set of questionnaire items. Similar to the AQ and PCRS, scoring requires collateral information from significant others (therapist or family member), who complete the SADI checklist. However, clinical judgement is also exercised based on the researcher's or therapist's own observations and knowledge of the effects of brain injury. The three sections of the SADI are scored on a 4-point scale (0 = no disorder of awareness to 3 = severe disorder of awareness), with a total score ranging from 0 (accurate knowledge, good understanding of functional implications and realistic goals) to 9 (inaccurate knowledge of deficits, poor awareness of functional implications and unrealistic goals). The SADI has strong psychometric properties, including inter-rater reliability, test-retest reliability and construct validity (see Tate, 2010), and has been used extensively in research (see Table 5.1).

Some potential limitations of questionnaires and interview-based measures of awareness are that such approaches rely upon verbal skills and accurate recall of past experiences, and are influenced by cultural issues (e.g., the extent to which items are phrased in a culturally appropriate manner). Therefore, for some individuals awareness of deficits may be more validly assessed by observing their behaviour on naturalistic tasks. Many researchers have combined behaviour observation with self-rating scales to more broadly assess people's metacognitive skills, including self-knowledge of impairments prior to task performance and the ability to anticipate or predict problems with future task performance (i.e., self-predictions), correct errors and use strategies during performance (i.e., on-line awareness), and self-evaluate performance after the activity (Abreu, Seale, Scheibel, Huddleston, Zhang, & Ottenbacher, 2001; Hart, Giovannetti, Montgomery & Schwartz, 1998; Ownsworth et al., 2006; Schmidt et al., 2013). Overall, multidimensional approaches to assessing self-awareness that combine interviews, validated questionnaires and observation of behaviours reflecting awareness during task performance are optimal.

Sense-making appraisals

As discussed in Chapter 4, as people begin to recognise the impact of the brain injury on their functioning they typically start to process what the injury means for their well-being, lifestyle and the future. This subjective appraisal process has significant implications for emotional adjustment and self-concept. Therefore, efforts to understand people's sense-making regarding their brain injury are important in clinical practice. Qualitative approaches that focus on understanding individuals' phenomenological experience can provide valuable insight into meaning-making processes (e.g., Nochi, 1998; 2000; Ownsworth et al., 2011; Strang & Strang, 2001). However, questionnaires represent the most practical approach to assessing sense-making appraisals in clinical practice and research. Questionnaires specifically developed or modified for use with people with brain injury will now be reviewed.

A common sense-making appraisal examined is self-efficacy, or the extent to which a person perceives that they can cope with or manage stressors related to the brain injury (Rutterford & Wood, 2006). Self-efficacy researchers recommend that measures be tailored according to the specific domain of functioning or situation for which self-perceptions are being assessed (Bandura, 1989; Lorig, Stewart, Ritter, González, Laurent, & Lynch, 1996). Accordingly, measures of self-efficacy have been developed or modified for use in TBI or stroke. For example, Robinson-Smith, Johnston and Allen (2000) developed a modified version of the Strategies Used by People to Promote Health (SUPPH) for use in stroke. The SUPPH was originally developed for people with cancer (Lev & Owen, 1996) and focuses on self-care self-efficacy. A 23-item version was used in stroke research which retained three subscales assessing people's degree of confidence (1 = very little confidence to 5 = extremely confident) in using coping strategies, reducing stress and enjoying life. Robinson-Smith et al. (2000) reported excellent internal consistency (α = .95) for the tool and found that self-care self-efficacy was significantly related to quality of life and depression at 1-month and 6-months post-stroke.

The Self-Efficacy for Symptom Management Scale (Cicerone & Azulay, 2007) is a 13-item scale developed to assess people's ability to manage common challenges associated with TBI. Adapted from a tool developed by Lorig et al. (1996), the scale requires people to rate their degree of confidence (1 = not at all confident to 10 = totally confident) in being able to access help or support and manage their physical, cognitive and emotional difficulties in everyday life. For example, one item requires people to rate their degree of confidence in being able to compensate for any cognitive difficulties related to the injury such that problems do not interfere with what the person wants to do. The measure has good internal consistency for the total scale (.93) and three subscales (Self-efficacy social [SEsoc] = .76, Self-efficacy cognitive [SEcog] = .93 and Self-efficacy emotional [SEemot] = .92). The construct validity of the measure was supported by factor analysis and significant correlations with measures assessing related constructs (Cicerone & Azulay, 2007). Further, the authors found that perceived self-efficacy was the best predictor of global life satisfaction, and mediated the relationship between community integration and global life satisfaction.

Also developed for use in TBI, the Perceived Control Scale for Brain Injury (PCS-BI; Malec, 2012) assesses self-efficacy regarding advocacy for individuals with brain injury. An example item includes: 'I can influence decisions that affect people with brain injury in my community', with ratings made on a 4-point scale (Strongly agree to Strongly disagree). This measure is available on the Centre for Outcome Measurement in Brain Injury website (http://www.tbims.org/combi). The tool has sound psychometric properties, based on Rasch analysis (Person Reliability = .78; Item Reliability = .99) and additional analyses of concurrent and construct validity (see Malec, 2012).

Another assessment option is to capture different types of cognitive appraisal using the same instrument. Based on Cognitive-Relational Theory (Lazarus, 1966), the Stress-Appraisal Measure (SAM; Peacock & Wong, 1990) assesses primary and secondary appraisals relevant to stress and coping (see Table 5.1). Applied in the context of stroke (Ownsworth, Hoffmann et al., 2011; Rochette et al., 2007), items on the SAM reflect the anticipated impact of the stroke (i.e., perceived harm/loss, gain/growth and importance for one's well-being) and perceived controllability of stressors associated with stroke. Rochette et al. (2007) used the SAM to assess the relationship between cognitive appraisals and depression symptoms following stroke; however, they did not conduct any psychometric analysis on the SAM. Ownsworth, Hoffmann et al. (2011) also used the SAM in stroke research and found that internal consistency was generally acceptable across the subscales, with alphas ranging from .61 (Centrality) to .79 (Controllable-by-others). The main advantages of the SAM include its sound theoretical underpinnings and brief assessment of different primary and secondary stress appraisals. Further research examining the SAM's psychometric properties for the brain injury population is needed.

Similar to the SAM, the Illness Perceptions Questionnaire-Revised (IPQ-R; Moss-Morris, Weinman, Petrie, Horne, Cameron & Buick, 2002) assesses different cognitive appraisal processes. However, unlike the SAM, these appraisals specifically relate to illness representations and are based on Leventhal's Self-Regulatory Model (Leventhal et al., 1997). The IPQ-R is comprised of three sections: identity, beliefs and causal attributions. In the illness identity section, the presence of 18 symptoms and their perceived association with the illness are assessed using a yes/no format. In the beliefs section, illness representations are rated on a 5-point scale (strongly disagree to strongly agree). The factor-derived dimensions and sample items from Moss-Morris et al. (2002, pp. 5–6) include: consequences (e.g., 'My illness is a serious condition', timeline acute/chronic (e.g., 'My illness will last a short time'), timeline cyclical (e.g., 'My symptoms come and go in cycles'), personal control (e.g., 'I have the power to influence my illness'), treatment control (e.g., 'My treatment can control my illness'), illness coherence (e.g., 'I don't understand my illness') and emotional representations (e.g., 'My illness makes me feel angry'). The third section assesses causal attributions on the same 5-point scale, and includes psychological attributions (e.g., 'My personality), risk factors (e.g., 'My own behaviour'), immunity (e.g., 'A germ or virus') and accident or chance (e.g., 'Chance or bad luck').

Moss-Morris et al. (2002) examined the reliability and validity of the IPQ-R in a large mixed chronic disease sample. The authors note that the applicability of subscale content is likely to vary for different illness populations. Accordingly, a modified version of the IPQ-R was investigated for mild TBI by Snell, Siegert, Hay-Smith and Surgenor (2010). They reported satisfactory internal consistency for the Identity Scale ($\alpha = .79$), and factor analysis of the Beliefs Scale yielded eight factors (each containing 3–7 items) that were largely consistent with the original factor solution, with the exception of the personal control and treatment control items which loaded onto the same factor. The Causal Attributions Scale loaded onto three factors, including psychological (8 items), environmental/biological (8 items) and risk behaviour (2 items). Internal consistency was satisfactory for all belief and causal attribution subscales with three or more items (.71–.90). Overall, despite the rich information gained from the IPQ-R and the evidence of sound psychometric properties for use with mild TBI, the large number of items (71 items across three scales) may affect the utility of the measure in some contexts. Nevertheless, the importance of assessing sense-making appraisals was highlighted by Whittaker, Kemp and House (2007), who found that early illness beliefs (consequences) best predicted functional outcome at 3-months follow-up after mild head injury.

Based on Goldstein's (1952) account of threat-related anxiety and avoidance, Riley et al. (2004) developed an approach for assessing common threat appraisals and associated avoidance behaviours after TBI. Stage one of development entailed conducting interviews and focus groups to identify a large number of specific activities that people with TBI avoided and the nature of related threat appraisals or 'implicit or explicit anticipation of negative consequences' (p. 874). Following a thematic analysis, stage two involved developing the Appraisal of Threat and Avoidance Questionnaire (ATAQ; 41 items) and the Specific Activities and Avoidance Questionnaire (SAAQ; 26 items). Details of the content and example items of the ATAQ are provided in Table 5.1. The SAAQ lists specific activities (e.g., paid work, filling in forms, driving, being in a crowd) for which people respond Yes/No to four questions: a) 'Did you do this before your injury?' (p. 875); b) 'Do you feel less confident about it now, compared to how you felt before your injury?' (p. 875); c) 'Do you do it less often now?' (p. 875); and d) 'Is your lack of confidence one of the reasons why you do it less often?' (p. 875).

Riley et al. (2004) reported that internal consistency was satisfactory for the overall threat appraisals and avoidance subscales ($\alpha = .92–.94$) and the following categories: personal safety ($\alpha = .73–.79$), dealing with people ($\alpha = .86–.92$) and doing things ($\alpha = .87–.92$). However, internal consistency was inadequate for awkward situations ($\alpha = .30–.35$), and hence the authors excluded these five items from the ATAQ in their subsequent research (Riley et al., 2010). Internal consistency for the SAAQ was satisfactory for Questions b), c), and d) ($\alpha = .81–.84$), but not for Question a) ($\alpha = .56$).

The 36-item ATAQ was used to investigate the role of coping and self-esteem as moderators of the relationship between threat appraisals and avoidance behaviours (Riley et al., 2010). There was further support for the internal consistency of the ATAQ ($\alpha = .89–.91$) and concurrent validity was demonstrated with measures of self-esteem and coping. Although further psychometric investigation of the ATAQ and SAAQ is warranted, these tools enable researchers and clinicians to examine the link between threat appraisals and reduced activity and role participation, which may guide intervention efforts.

Coping strategies

The influence of coping strategies on adjustment to brain injury has been examined using diverse approaches, including self-report measures (e.g., Curran et al., 2000; Kendall & Terry, 2008; King et al. 2002; Rochette & Desrosiers, 2002), contextualised assessment (Kendall, Shum, Lack, Bull & Fee, 2001; Krpan, Stuss & Anderson, 2011), and interview schedules in qualitative research (Karlovits & McColl, 1999; Krefting, 1989). Donnellan, Hevey, Hickey and O'Neill (2006) reviewed the conceptual basis, domains and psychometric properties of self-report measures of coping after stroke and identified ten main tools employed in research. As described in Table 5.1, the Ways of Coping Questionnaire Revised (WCQ-Revised; Folkman & Lazarus, 1985) was the most frequently employed, followed by the Freiburg Questionnaire on Coping with Illness (35 items) and the Coping Orientation for Problem Experience (COPE, 19–52 item versions). Some researchers have employed a modified version of the WCQ-Revised (66 items), reducing the number of items to 28 or 40 items (King et al. 2002; Rochette & Desrosiers, 2002). Two stroke-specific measures of coping include the Mental Adjustment to Stroke Scale (40 items; Eccles, House & Knapp, 1999) and the Ways of Coping – Cardiovascular Accident (31 items; Johnson & Pearson, 2000), however, the utility of these measures is uncertain due to lack of psychometric evaluation.

Psychometric analysis of the WCQ-Revised in brain injury samples has indicated that Cronbach's alpha is generally adequate for the coping domains ($\alpha = .63–.73$) (De Sepulveda & Chang, 1994), but is variable across the strategies ($\alpha = .59–.90$) for the shortened or revised versions (King et al. 2002; Rochette & Desrosiers, 2002). Moore and Stambrook (1994) identified ten distinct factors on the WCQ-Revised for their TBI sample, with main coping themes including resignation, planning, escape and denial. Kendall and Terry (2008) obtained the common three-factor solution (i.e., emotion-focused, perception-focused and problem-focused coping) in their TBI sample, although the number of items included in their modified version of the WCQ was not stated.

The Coping Scale for Adults (Frydenberg & Lewis, 2012) has been employed in many TBI studies (Anson & Ponsford, 2006a; 2006b; Curran et al., 2000; Spitz et al., 2013). Anson and Ponsford (2006a) used the CSA to identify coping strategies related to poorer emotional function (i.e., avoidance, worry, wishful thinking and self-blame) and higher self-esteem (i.e., working on the problem, use of humour and engaging in enjoyable activities) and to evaluate the effectiveness of coping skills training (Anson & Ponsford, 2006b). Internal consistency was acceptable for the non-productive coping subscale ($\alpha = .73$), lower than satisfactory for the adaptive coping subscale ($\alpha = .65$) and poor for the optimism and sharing subscales ($\alpha = .42-.45$). Nonetheless, there was evidence of validity based on theory-consistent associations between coping styles on the CSA and emotional adjustment and self-esteem following TBI (Anson & Ponsford, 2006a), and sensitivity to change in response to a coping skills intervention (Anson & Ponsford, 2006b).

A main advantage of self-report measures of coping is that these provide a structured format for identifying the use of a broad range of coping strategies, and an approach to stimulate self-reflection and discussion in therapy. For scoring purposes, the strategies are often clustered together to reflect adaptive versus maladaptive coping or productive versus non-productive coping efforts. The basis for this distinction is sometimes unclear and may vary according to the nature and chronicity of the stressor (Kendall et al., 2001). For example, use of denial or efforts to mentally distance oneself from the impact of brain injury may be helpful strategies in the short-term to protect from an overwhelming sense of loss, whilst in the longer term these strategies are typically less adaptive (Ownsworth, 2005). Therefore, it is important to take into account the context in which the person is employing a particular strategy and the function it may serve in supporting adjustment. As discussed in Chapter 4, flexible use of varied coping strategies is likely to be most adaptive for managing different stressors experienced after brain injury.

The length of administration for self-report measures of coping appears to be a key issue in brain injury research and clinical practice, given the need to minimise the burden of assessment on participants or clients of a service. However, shortened versions with fewer items on each scale or domain can compromise the reliability of the measure (e.g., the Brief Cope has two items per subscale). Efforts have been made to revise or adapt the WCQ, with recognition that types of coping behaviour employed to manage stressful situations after brain injury are likely to differ from the general population, as are the nature of situations considered stressful (e.g., King et al., 2002; Riley et al., 2010). As noted by Donnellan et al. (2006) the use of revised versions can be problematic because psychometric evaluation is typically not conducted prior to use and different adaptations of the same measure are often employed across studies. A common methodological issue identified for self-report measures of coping is that people's responses may be influenced by demand characteristics of the situation and self-deception or denial. The validity of responses is also influenced by a person's ability to recall stressful situations and their awareness of how they typically appraise and react to these (Krpan et al., 2011).

As an alternative to self-report measures of coping, some authors have developed performance-based measures or contextualised assessment in relation to particular problems or stressors (e.g., Kendall et al., 2001; Krpan et al., 2011). Kendall et al. (2001) developed four video-based vignettes of stressful situations (1.5–2 minutes duration each) to assess perceived stress (10-point rating scale) and coping strategies. The scenarios included stressful situations that people with TBI may face, namely, the inability to gain a driver's licence, discrimination at a job interview, unsuccessful social interaction and memory problems. After each vignette, participants were asked to describe how they would cope, or how they did cope if they had actually experienced this or a similar situation, with prompts used to identify all types of coping response within the person's repertoire. Coping responses were coded and classified according to whether the strategies were active or passive, emotion- or problem-focused, and the flexibility of coping style (i.e., constant or varied use of coping styles across the scenarios). The merits of using four common stressful scenarios to stimulate discussion include the increased specificity and immediacy of the situation and the ability to derive both qualitative and quantitative data. One possible limitation is that individuals may provide socially acceptable responses concerning what they should do, rather than what they are actually likely to do in the situation, although Kendall et al. noted that participants often described socially undesirable responses (e.g., punching a wall).

A further performance-based assessment of coping behaviour that could help to overcome this issue is the Baycrest Psychosocial Stress Test (BPST) developed by Krpan et al. (2011). The BPST is based on the Trier Social Stress Test (Kirschbaum, Pirke, & Hellhammer, 1993) and aims to simulate real-world stress in order to observe coping behaviour. Specifically, participants receive the verbal instructions that they will need to deliver a 5-minute speech to an expert in communications (a confederate) while being video-taped. Individuals' coping behaviours and physiological responses are recorded for the 10-minute anticipation/preparation period leading up to the stressor and during the task itself. In addition to the speech, they are asked to perform mental arithmetic (subtracting 13 from 1,022) as quickly and accurately as possible, with errors requiring them to start again. Participants were interviewed after the task to gain further insight into their strategy use. Coping behaviours were coded and categorised by three independent raters, and yielded excellent inter-rater reliability and Cronbach's alpha for planful behaviour (ICC = .98, α = .98) and avoidant behaviour (ICC = .95, α = .95). Support for the validity of the BPST was evident, with people with moderate to severe TBI engaging in more avoidant behaviour than planful behaviour than matched controls. Interestingly, control participants' performance was significantly related to their self-report of coping styles on the WCQ, whereas this was not the case for the TBI sample. There were no differences in state anxiety or physiological responses between TBI and control participants. Both groups demonstrated a stress response according to heart rate and skin conductance recordings and reported increased anxiety in relation to the task.

Overall, the BPST provides an innovative approach to assessing actual coping behaviours employed in a stressful situation. As noted by the authors, participants' background and the perceived threat associated with the task may influence their stress response and coping behaviours. Further research on the psychometric properties of the BPST would enhance its clinical utility.

Assessing the impact of brain injury on sense of self

A number of measures developed for the general population have been used to assess self-esteem and self-concept after brain injury. As summarised in Table 5.2, the Rosenberg Self-Esteem Scale (RSES; Rosenberg, 1965) has been most

Table 5.2 Overview of approaches for assessing self-concept and identity change after brain injury

Measure	Reliability and validity for brain injury	Research applications	Clinical considerations
Tennessee Self-Concept Scale-2 (TSCS-2; Fitts & Warren, 1996); 82 items	TSCS-2 scores were significantly correlated with the Head Injury Semantic Differential Scale ($p = .72$) and measures of depression and quality of life (Vickery et al., 2005). Evidence of convergent validity with the RSES (Keppel & Crowe, 2000) and sensitivity to change after intervention (Helffenstein & Wechsler, 1982).	Helffenstein & Wechsler (1982); Keppel & Crowe (2000); Vickery et al. (2005)	A comprehensive standardised measure that assesses self-concept across multiple domains and incorporates validity scores (e.g., inconsistency, faking good, self-criticism). Reliability analyses have not been conducted for the brain injury population.
Rosenberg Self-Esteem Scale (RSES; Rosenberg, 1965); 10 items	Ratings of self-esteem were stable over a 2-week period ($r = .86$) and were negatively associated with anxiety and depression (Cooper-Evans et al., 2008). High internal consistency (.89) and convergent validity with the HISD III has been reported (Carroll & Coetzer, 2011; Cooper-Evans et al., 2008).	Anson & Ponsford (2006a; 2006b); Carroll & Coetzer (2011); Cooper-Evans et al. (2008); Kelly, Ponsford & Couchman (2013); Kendall et al. (2001); Keppel & Crowe (2000); Riley et al. (2010); Vickery et al. (2005)	A brief measure of global or trait self-esteem. Utility for TBI and stroke population is supported by extensive use in research. Sensitivity to change in the context of intervention is not evident (e.g, Anson & Ponsford, 2006b; Kelly et al., 2013; Simpson, Tate, Whiting & Cotter, 2011).
Robson Self-Concept Questionnaire (Robson, 1989); 30 items	Factor analysis with a brain injury sample identified four factors: perceived self-worth, likeability, resilience and confidence. Self-concept was associated with depression and anxiety (Longworth, Deakins, Rose & Gracey, 2012). Sensitivity to change in the context of therapy was supported by a case study (Ashworth, Gracey & Gilbert, 2011).	Ashworth et al. (2011); Longworth et al. (2012)	A brief multi-dimensional measure of self-esteem with some preliminary psychometric support for use with brain injury.
Coopersmith Self-Esteem Inventory (CSEI; Coopersmith, 1989), multi-forms: adult form – 25 items; School form – 50 items	Adequate split-half reliabilities of .71–.74 and test-retest reliabilities of .80–.82 over a 5-week period were reported for the general population (Bedian, Teague & Zmud, 1977). The CSEI was associated with overall psychosocial outcome (Tate & Broe, 1999). Sensitivity to change has not been demonstrated (Medd & Tate, 2000).	Tate & Broe (1999); Medd & Tate (2000); Hawley (2012)	Brief measure of self-esteem that reflects attitudes towards self in social, academic, family and personal areas. Psychometric data are yet to be reported for the brain injury population.

Measure	Psychometric properties	References	Comments
Head Injury Semantic Differential Scale (I, II, III); Tyerman (1987, personal communication), 18 items on the HISD III	HISD and HISD II: Internal consistency (.88–.93) and split-half (.87–.93), factor analysis, sensitivity to effects of severe TBI, change in response to rehabilitation and group therapy, stability over time. Convergent validity with the Frankfurt Self-Concept Scale. Theory-consistent associations between self-discrepancies with mood symptomatology. HISD III: internal consistency (.92–.93) and convergent validity with the RSES and Brain Injury Grief Inventory (BIGI) (Carroll & Coetzer, 2011).	TBI: Tyerman & Humphrey (1984); Wright & Telford (1996); Carroll & Coetzer (2011); Stroke or mixed brain injury: Ellis-Hill & Horn (2000); Vickery et al. (2006); Doering et al. (2011)	A theory-guided, brief and easy to administer measure. Ratings are likely to be influenced by language ability and retrospective recall (past self). Reliability and validity supported by extensive research applications in TBI, stroke and mixed brain injury samples.
Selves Interview (Strauman, 1990; Tangney, Niedenthal, Covert & Barlow, 1998) and Selves Adjective Checklist (SAC; Cantor et al., 2005), 38 items	Interview: Adequate reliability in general population (3 year test–retest reliability = .56; interrater reliability = .86). The SAC has only been used in TBI research. There was no significant association between the interview and SAC. Significant associations between emotional distress and self-discrepancies on the SAC, but not the interview.	TBI: Cantor et al. (2005)	Sound theoretical and empirical basis for general population; the Selves Interview was expanded and modified for TBI (prompts and cues added); option of using open-ended interview or forced choice checklist, however, different information is yielded. Psychometric properties are yet to be reported for the brain injury population.
Continuity/Discontinuity of Self Scale (Secrest & Zeller, 2003), 24 items	Two subscales derived from factor-analysis; Continuity of self (α = .87) and Discontinuity of self (α = .87). Three factors emerged from a further factor analysis; Continuity/self, Continuity/other and Discontinuity. Scores were stable over a 6-month follow-up interval.	Secrest & Zeller (2003; 2006; 2007)	Sound theoretical and empirical basis; brief and easy to administer. Research applications with stroke samples.
Brain Injury Grief Inventory (Coetzer, Vaughan & Ruddle, 2003), 20 items	Internal consistency is better for the Loss scale (α = .84) than Adjustment scale (α = .65) and test–retest reliability is good for Loss (r = .89) but low for Adjustment (r = .58). A negative association was reported between the scales (r = −.75). No factor analysis conducted to date, although there is evidence of convergent validity with the HISD III.	Carroll & Coetzer (2011); Ruddle, Coetzer & Vaughan (2005)	Theory-guided tool; brief and easy to administer. The Loss scale has greater relevance to self-identity and better psychometric properties than the Adjustment scale. The tool requires further psychometric analysis to support clinical application.

commonly used in TBI and stroke research, with findings consistently indicating a negative association between self-esteem and emotional distress (Anson & Ponsford, 2006a; Carroll & Coetzer, 2011; Cooper-Evans et al., 2008; Kendall et al., 2001; Keppel & Crowe, 2000; Riley et al. 2010; Vickery et al., 2005). Research supports the psychometric properties of the RSES as a measure of global self-esteem for the brain injury population (Carroll & Coetzer, 2011; Cooper-Evans et al., 2008). The Coopersmith Self-Esteem Inventory (Coopersmith, 1989) was employed in research by Tate and Broe (1999) and Medd and Tate (2000); however, no psychometric properties were reported for their TBI samples. Other tools that appear to have utility as multi-dimensional measures of self-concept include the Robson Self-Concept Questionnaire and the Tennessee Self-Concept Scale–2 (see Table 5.2), although further psychometric analysis is required for the brain injury population.

A review of the literature identified five tools that have been specifically developed to assess changes to self and identity after brain injury. As presented in Table 5.2, these tools include the Head Injury Semantic Differential Scale (Tyerman & Humphrey, 1984), Selves Interview, Selves Adjective Checklist (Cantor et al., 2005), Continuity/Discontinuity of Self Scale (Secrest & Zeller, 2003) and Brain Injury Grief Inventory (Coetzer et al., 2003). The following provides a review of the development, theoretical basis, psychometric evaluation and research applications of each measure.

Head Injury Semantic Differential Scale (HISD)

Development and theoretical basis

The HISD was developed by Tyerman and Humphrey (1984) to assess changes in self-concept after brain injury for research and clinical purposes. The measure arose from an identified need to capture the subjective impairments or changes to self as experienced by the person with brain injury. The original HISD consisted of 20 bipolar adjective pairs rated on a 7-point scale from 1 (negative pole) to 7 (positive pole). The approach is based on the semantic differential rating method of Osgood, Suci and Tannenbaum (1957) for measuring the meaning of concepts, including attitudes and personality descriptors. The 20 items are rated according to Past Self (6 months prior to injury), Present Self (over the last few days) and Future Self (expectation for one year into the future). Total scores on the HISD ranged from 20 to 140 to enable comparisons between past, present and future selves. Further ratings may be obtained for Ideal Self, 'Typical person of their own age and sex' and 'Typical head injured person' (Tyerman & Humphrey, 1984), although these ratings have been less frequently used in research. The two revised versions of the HISD will be described in the next section.

Psychometric evaluation

Psychometric properties of the original HISD were examined in a sample of 60 individuals receiving rehabilitation after severe TBI (Tyerman, 1987). The HISD demonstrated good internal consistency (Cronbach's alpha = .88) and split half reliability (Guttman's = .87), concurrent validity with a measure of emotional distress (Leeds scale), and theory-consistent differences based on comparison between people with TBI and orthopaedic controls. Further, the responsiveness of the HISD was examined through repeated measurements on the HISD between rehabilitation admission and discharge (improved self-concept) and discharge and follow-up (decline in self-concept). Factor analysis identified six factors that together accounted for 70 per cent of the variance. These factors and example items included: Self-esteem (e.g., Worthless–Of Value), Boredom (e.g., Bored–Interested), Sociability (e.g., Unfriendly–Friendly), Positive expectation (e.g., Despondent–Hopeful), Negative affect (e.g., Emotional–Stable) and Caring/Unfeeling (single item).

Two revised versions of the HISD (HISD II and HISD III) have subsequently been developed, based on longstanding routine use of the HISD as an outcome measure at the Community Head Injury Service in Aylesbury, UK (Tyerman, personal communication). The most recent version (HISD III) is provided in Appendix A. In 1992 the HISD was revised (HISD II) with modification of five items; specifically, the skill-related items of Forgetful–Mindful and Stupid–Clever were replaced by two items more related to personality (Aggressive–Unaggressive and Impatient–Patient) and the wording of three other items was modified. Further psychometric analysis on a sample of 42 individuals with very severe brain injury was conducted which provided strong support for the tool's reliability (Cronbach's alpha = .93, Guttman's = .93). Five factors emerged from factor analysis, including Contentment (9 items), Aggression (3 items), Loss of belief (5 items), Sociability (5 items) and Boredom (3 items). However, due to overlap between the factors Tyerman cautioned against using subscale scores, and identified the need for further research (Tyerman, personal communication). As further evidence of validity, Ellis-Hill and Horn (2000) found that there were significant differences between Past self and Present self on the HISD II for stroke participants but not for matched controls.

Further revisions were made to the scale in 1997 (i.e., HISD III), which involved excluding the Caring–Unfeeling and Cooperative–Uncooperative items based on clinical observations of the inappropriateness of these items for self-report. The Impatient–Patient item was reversed to provide a balance between the order of positive–negative items (see Appendix A). A significant new development entailed the creation of a relative's version (HISD-R) which includes 17 items of the HISD III (note: the Cooperative–Uncooperative item was retained for this version), but excludes two items (Attractive–Unattractive and Of Value–Worthless) and substitutes the Sensitive–Insensitive item for the original Caring–Unfeeling item. Therefore, the differences between the 18-item versions of the HISD III-R and HISD III relate to items 9 and 10, with Sensitive–Insensitive and Cooperative–Uncooperative used only for the relative's version and Attractive–Unattractive and Of Value–Worthless included only in the version for the person with brain injury.

To administer the HISD III, the person with brain injury (or relative) is informed that the measure assesses changes in how the person sees him- or herself (or how the relative views the person) after the injury. The scale may be administered orally or completed in writing, with the clinician or researcher present to assist and provide any necessary clarification and support. The first item of Bored–Interested is used an example, although it is also calculated in the total score, to ensure that respondents understand the instructions, which involve placing an 'X' on the appropriate line between the adjectives to indicate how they viewed themselves in the past (or present or future). Initially, the person or relative rates the set of 18 adjectives on the Past scale, and then rates the same adjectives on the Present scale, followed by the Future scale. To score the self-rated and relative-rated versions of the HISD III, the scores for each item (rated 1–7) are summed to produce a total score of 18–126 (Tyerman, personal communication). When re-administering the measure in the context of rehabilitation, only the Present and Future scales are completed. Graphical representation of the 18 items can be useful to present feedback on changes in self-concept over time or, when appropriate, on the differences between the perspectives of the person with brain injury and his or her relative. Such graphical representation is commonly used in research to depict group-level data (see Ellis-Hill & Horn, 2000; Tyerman & Humphrey, 1984).

Carroll and Coetzer (2011) reported high Cronbach's alphas for both past self (.93) and present self (.92) on the HISD III and found that ratings were significantly associated with sense of loss ($r = .53$) and adjustment ($r = -.35$) scales on the Brain Injury Grief Inventory.

Research applications

In Tyerman and Humphrey's (1984) original study of changes in self-concept after severe TBI, present self on the HISD was viewed as vastly different from past self, whilst participants anticipated a return to past self within the year (see Chapter 4 for further discussion). Wright and Telford (1996) used the original HISD to examine changes in self-concept after TBI at 6 months post-injury with a sample described as having 'predominantly minor' injuries. Similar to Tyerman and Humphrey, they found that present self was rated more negatively than pre-injury self and that participants anticipated a return to past self in the future. Data for a subgroup at 3 years post-injury follow-up revealed no significant changes on the HISD, suggesting that self-discrepancies were stable over time. Wright and Telford found that self-discrepancies (present vs. past self and past vs. future self) were significantly associated with psychological distress.

Vickery et al. (2005) used the original HISD to evaluate a 6-week self-concept group intervention for 18 people with brain injury (72 per cent TBI). Their post-intervention evaluation indicated a significant overall improvement in self-concept (present self), with significant changes evident for five of the 20 items. Although caution is needed when interpreting this outcome due to the lack of control group, such findings indicate that the HISD is responsive to change in the context of rehabilitation. In the context of stroke, Ellis-Hill and Horn (2000) found a significant reduction in overall self-concept on the HISD II, although differences were only significant for eight items. Specifically, participants viewed themselves as less capable, independent and in control, and felt less satisfied, interested, active, confident, and of less value since their stroke.

To date, the HISD III has been used in one study by Carroll and Coetzer (2011), who examined the associations among grief, self-awareness and identity for a long-term TBI sample (mean time since injury of 11 years). Consistent with other studies, the authors reported that individuals perceived their current self in a more negative light than their pre-injury self. Greater changes in self-identity on the HISD III were significantly related to lower self-esteem and increased grief and depression.

Overall, the benefits of using the HISD extensively in clinical practice to inform revisions are evident, with the authors taking considerable care to improve the wording of the HISD as a client-centred instrument. Further psychometric analysis is required for the HISD III and HISD III-R, including investigations of temporal stability and sensitivity to change in the context of intervention.

Selves Interview and Selves Adjective Checklist

Development and theoretical basis

The development of the Selves Interview (Strauman, 1990) and Selves Adjective Checklist (Tangney et al., 1998) was guided by Self-Discrepancy Theory (Higgins, 1987), which proposes that discrepancy between one's actual self and ideal self contributes to depression whilst discrepancy between one's actual self and ought self underlies anxiety. Based on this theory, Cantor and colleagues (2005) adapted the Selves Interview from the original Selves Questionnaire, and developed the Selves Adjective Checklist to examine self-discrepancies as a potential mechanism underlying emotional distress after TBI.

The Selves Interview is an open-ended interview involving descriptions and ratings of three *current* selves, namely, actual, ideal and ought selves, as well as *pre-injury* actual self. Respondents are asked to generate at least six descriptors for each self and rate the degree of applicability (1 = slightly true of me, to 5 = extremely true of me). The descriptors given for the ideal, ought and pre-injury selves are compared with those given for the actual current self using a thesaurus, yielding four codes: a) *matches* (synonymous descriptors used and a difference of ≤ 1 rating point for applicability), b) *mismatch of degree* (synonymous descriptors used, but > 1 rating point difference in applicability), c) *mismatches of descriptors* (descriptors antonymous to current actual self), and d) *nonmatches* (descriptors were not synonymous or antonymous). Discrepancy scores are calculated for the three different discrepancy indices (i.e., current actual self versus pre-injury self, current actual self versus ideal self, current actual self versus ought self) by summing the number of mismatches (degree and descriptors) and subtracting the number of matches (note: nonmatches are not included in the scoring). Higher positive scores indicate a greater degree of self-discrepancy.

The Selves Adjective Checklist (SAC) requires respondents to select from a list of 38 forced-choice bipolar adjectives (e.g., 'easy-going/irritable') for each of the four selves, with the option of stating 'not applicable' for any adjective pair. Using this approach, respondents indicate which adjective is most descriptive of each self, with one descriptor of each pair viewed as more desirable than the other. Three codes are derived, including: a) *matches*, whereby the same descriptor is selected for the two selves being compared; b) *negative mismatches*, whereby the antonym descriptor is selected and is less desirable for current actual self than another self; and c) *positive mismatches*, in which the antonym descriptor is selected and is more desirable for current actual self than another self. Using the same subtraction approach as the Selves Interview, self-discrepancy indices for the SAC are calculated for the current actual self versus pre-injury self, current actual self versus ideal self, current actual self versus ought self.

Although the list of adjective pairs contains attributes that are typically viewed as desirable or undesirable, this is not straightforward for certain adjective pairs (e.g., 'ambitious/not ambitious', 'working/not working', 'interested in sex/not interested in sex'). However, this is taken into account in the scoring by considering the person's ideal selves, which represent qualities considered desirable from his or her perspective. Consistent with the Selves Interview, larger positive discrepancies for each index indicate greater self-discrepancy. One advantage of the SAC is that this approach also enables identification of positive changes in self-concept (i.e., positive mismatches) following TBI.

Psychometric evaluation

Considerable detail is provided by Cantor et al. concerning the selection of these tools and their development or modifications for use with people with cognitive impairment. However, to date, there has been limited psychometric evaluation of the Selves Interview and SAC for use with brain injury. Cantor et al. found that scores on the two measures were not significantly related for their small sample ($n = 21$). Higher levels of self-discrepancy on the SAC, but not the Selves Interview, were associated with depression and anxiety, and these associations were large for each discrepancy index ($r > .50$). It was noteworthy that there was a larger degree of variability on the SAC than the Selves Interview. The open-ended format and complexity of scoring procedures used for the Selves Interview may have also contributed to the non-significant findings. In particular, the validity of the interview approach may be compromised by participants' cognitive deficits and their ability to generate relevant self-descriptors. Furthermore, the reliability of scoring procedures, which involve the use of a thesaurus to calculate distance between adjectives, is uncertain. Overall, the reliability and validity of both measures is yet to be determined.

Research applications

Cantor et al. (2005) used the SAC and Selves Interview in a pilot study to investigate the role of self-discrepancy in understanding anxiety and depression. As previously described, there were significant positive associations between each discrepancy index on the SAC and level of anxiety and depressive symptoms. As noted by the authors, the direction of these associations is unclear, as individuals with greater anxiety and depression may have had a negative response bias when completing the SAC. Although no known research has subsequently employed the Selves Interview or SAC, the related approach of Gracey et al. (2008) is noteworthy. As discussed previously in Chapter 4, in small groups (i.e., two groups with 18 and 14 participants respectively) people with brain injury were asked to consider how they saw themselves before the injury, how they see themselves now and how they would like to be. With prompting and support from the facilitator, group members collaboratively generated bipolar personal constructs. A thematic analysis identified key themes relating to current, pre-injury and ideal selves. The constructs were commonly stated as phrases and related to physical and psychological attributes and activity and social contexts; for example:

- 'Good social life vs being lonely' (Gracey et al., 2008, p. 648)
- 'Not having confidence in relationships' vs 'feeling confident, able to trust' (p. 648)
- 'Having a plan for the future' vs 'being uncertain about the future' (p. 648)
- 'Engaged, doing things that reinforce who I am' vs 'loss of key activities, not doing personally important things' (p. 649).

Given the inductive process employed, the constructs generated may be more meaningful to people with brain injury than the SAC adjective pairs. Further research is needed to examine the broader relevance of these constructs for people with brain injury, which in turn may guide modification of the Selves Interview and SAC.

Continuity/Discontinuity of Self Scale (CDSS)

Development and theoretical basis

The CDSS (Secrest & Zeller, 2003) assesses the extent to which people feel connected to or continuous with their previous self and lifestyle, as well as their sense of discontinuity, or loss of aspects of self, perceived control, independence and connection with others. Items are rated on a three-point scale (agree, neutral/don't know, disagree) according to people's agreement with statements such as: 'I feel as though I have lost part of myself' (Secrest & Zeller, 2003, p. 246). A particular strength of this tool is that items were derived from an existential-phenomenological study of people with stroke (Secrest & Thomas, 1999), which identified that people experience both continuity and discontinuity in their experience of self with respect to sense of control, independence and connection with others (Secrest & Zeller, 2003). Therefore, the CDSS has a strong conceptual basis, guided by theories of identity and research investigating the subjective experiences of people with stroke.

Psychometric evaluation

The CDSS was originally developed as a 45-item scale for assessing the meaning of recovery after stroke in terms of people's sense of continuity and discontinuity (Secrest & Zeller, 2003). Using a stroke sample ($n = 55$, 1–260 weeks post-stroke), an initial principal components analysis identified two defined factors with 10 items loading onto each factor, labelled as Continuity (e.g., 'I have control of my life') and

Discontinuity (e.g., 'I sometimes give up on something because it is too much trouble') (p. 246). The 20-item CDSS displayed good internal consistency (α = .87 for each subscale), with the subscales showing a modest inverse association ($r = -.29$, $p < .05$). The Continuity subscale was positively associated with functional independence and quality of life, and Discontinuity subscale was negatively associated with quality of life.

In a replication study, Secrest and Zeller (2006) conducted a factor analysis on the 45 items with a larger sample ($n = 105$) that included the previous sample. Although the two-factor solution was robust across the two smaller independent samples, a three-factor solution emerged from the analysis with the combined sample. Specifically, the solution supported the Discontinuity subscale (10 item), but identified two dimensions within Continuity, namely Continuity/self (7 items relating to control and independence) and Continuity/other (7 items relating to connection with others).

Research applications

To date, the CDSS has only been used in research with stroke samples by the authors. Longitudinal research by Secrest and Zeller (2007) examined the relationship between levels of continuity and discontinuity and depression, functional ability and quality of life. They found that individuals' sense of continuity and discontinuity remained relatively stable over the 1 to 6-month follow-up despite improvements in functioning. Levels of continuity/discontinuity were related to depression and quality of life at both time points. At 6-months follow-up individuals who perceived greater discontinuity had poorer functional ability, thus suggesting that level of disability contributed to their sense of loss or disconnection with the past.

Brain Injury Grief Inventory (BIGI)

Development and theoretical basis

The BIGI (Coetzer et al., 2003; Ruddle, Coetzer & Vaughan, 2005) was developed as a measure of grief and adjustment following TBI. The items and format were based on existing measures of grief, and guided by theoretical literature on grief and loss as well as the authors' clinical experiences in brain injury rehabilitation. The questionnaire was initially piloted with clinical psychologists and people with brain injury, who provided feedback to improve the tool's face validity and clarity. The BIGI is a 22-item measure comprised of two scales; the Loss scale (Factor 1, e.g., 'I have found myself longing for the time before my brain injury'; Carroll & Coetzer, 2011, p. 296) and the Adjustment scale (Factor 2, e.g., 'I have stopped comparing how things were before my injury'; p. 296). Items are rated on a 3-point scale (0 = never, 1 = sometimes, 2 = mostly). Together, these scales examine the extent to which people focus on the losses associated with brain injury and are able to make sense of and come to terms with their injury.

Psychometric evaluation

Internal consistency of the BIGI was found to be acceptable for the Loss scale ($\alpha = .84$), although was somewhat low for the Adjustment scale ($\alpha = .62$) (Carroll & Coetzer, 2011). Cronbach's alpha improved to .65 for the adjustment scale with removal of two items (see the 20-item version of the BIGI in Appendix B). Test–retest reliability was found to be good for the Loss scale ($r = .89$) and low for the Adjustment scale ($r = .58$) (Ruddle et al., 2005). A large negative association was reported between the two scales ($r = -.75$). Although there has been no factor analysis conducted on the BIGI to date, the Loss and Adjustment scales have shown evidence of convergent validity with the HISD III discrepancy score ($r = .53$ and $-.35$ respectively) and Rosenberg Self-Esteem Scale ($r = -.59$ and $.56$ respectively) (Carroll & Coetzer, 2011). A factor analysis would be helpful to examine the scale structure of the BIGI.

Research applications

Ruddle et al. (2005) examined the influence of age, gender and marital status on the BIGI scores, and found that younger people with TBI reported more positive adjustment than older people. Females reported a greater sense of loss than males and, interestingly, married people with TBI reported less positive adjustment than single people. Coetzer, Ruddle and Mulla (2006) found that the BIGI scales were significantly associated with emotional status. Specifically, the Loss scale was positively associated with anxiety ($r = .40$) and the Adjustment scale was negatively associated with depression ($r = -.48$). Carroll and Coetzer (2011) reported significant associations between the BIGI scales and measure of depression, self-esteem and identity change. The BIGI has recently been translated into French (Coetzer, personal communication).

Summary

A number of measures developed for the general population have been used to assess self-esteem or self-concept after brain injury. There are five main tools that were specifically developed to assess changes in self or identity after brain injury. Overall, the different versions of the HISD have been most commonly used in empirical research and demonstrated the most evidence of reliability and validity.

Assessment of self-concept for children and adolescents with brain injury

Investigation of changes to sense of self after paediatric brain injury has been largely overlooked in research. This may be due in part to the lack of tools specifically validated for this purpose, with most existing studies using measures developed for the general paediatric population or non-validated approaches. For example, self-awareness has been measured using questionnaires that assess quality of life and behavioural functioning, with self-ratings compared with parent ratings (Stancin et al., 2002; Wilson et al., 2011) and by comparing self-ratings prior to test performance with actual cognitive performance (Hanten et al., 2000). Qualitative research by Jacobs (1993) supported the utility of semi-structured interviews for exploring children's understanding of brain injury and changes in their functioning. However, for clinical and research applications, standardised measures of self-awareness with a validated scoring protocol are required.

Beardmore et al. (1999) developed the first purpose-built questionnaire and interview for assessing self-awareness in children with brain injury. Based on Jacob's qualitative findings, the Knowledge Interview for Children (KIC) is a semi-structured interview that assesses: a) knowledge of TBI spanning 12 areas (story of the accident, hospitalisation, brain injury, coma and long-term effects of TBI); and b) awareness of deficits with 10 possible problem areas after TBI (e.g., memory, language and behaviour). The KIC is scored using information from the child's medical file and an interview with parents. The KIC yields the following indices: knowledge of TBI score, spontaneous problems reported by the child and parent, a discrepancy index from the two later scores, and number of problems endorsed on the checklist. Items on the Knowledge of TBI index are scored on a 2-point scale (0 = do not know or incorrect answer, 1 = partial or vague answer, 2 = adequate answer) to yield a total possible score of 24. The Awareness Discrepancy Index is calculated as the difference between the number of problems endorsed by the parents and the child's self-endorsed problems.

The clinical utility of the KIC is supported by its reasonable administration length (20 minutes) and preliminary psychometric properties. Specifically, Beardmore et al. (1999) reported excellent inter-rater reliability ($r = .96$) between two raters and acceptable internal consistency ($\alpha = .75$). Children with TBI were found to report significantly fewer problems on the Awareness of Deficits index than their parents, thus supporting the checklist's construct validity. The Knowledge of TBI score was not significantly related to the Awareness Discrepancy Index, suggesting the indices assess different aspects of self-knowledge, although the small sample size ($n = 21$) may have contributed to this finding. Nonetheless, the two KIC indices showed different patterns of association with other measures, namely, the Knowledge of TBI score was significantly correlated with memory performance ($r = .52$), whilst the Awareness Discrepancy Index was significantly associated with self-esteem ($r = .48$). The KIC was used to evaluate the efficacy of a single-session educational intervention (i.e., injury information) as compared with a control intervention (i.e., school study information) for children with TBI. The findings indicated an overall improvement in scores on the KIC (Knowledge of TBI); however, this improvement did not vary between groups. In general, the psychometric properties of the KIC, including sensitivity to change, require further investigation.

Children's self-concept after brain injury has been assessed using measures developed for the general paediatric population. Beardmore et al. (1999) used the Piers-Harris Children's Self-Concept Scale (CSCS; Piers, 1984), which is an 80-item scale that assesses six domains of self-concept and produces a total self-concept score. The more recent version of the scale, the Piers-Harris Children's Self-Concept Scale, 2nd Edition (Piers & Herzberg, 2002) has fewer items (60 items) and an administration time of approximately 10–15 minutes. The tool is appropriate for children and adolescents (7–18 years), and uses a Yes/No format that requires endorsement of personal strengths and weaknesses (e.g., 'I am smart', 'I am well behaved in school'). Scoring yields a global self-concept total score, six domain self-concept scores (i.e., Physical appearance and attributes, Intellectual and school status, Happiness and satisfaction, Freedom from anxiety, Behavioural adjustment, and Popularity), and validity indices (inconsistent responding and response bias). The Piers-Harris 2 Self-concept Scale (SCS) has been found to be the most commonly used measure of children's self-concept over the last 20 years (Butler & Gasson, 2005). The tool has good internal consistency for the total score ($\alpha = .90$) and each subscale ($\alpha = .71–.81$), adequate test–retest reliability ($r = .75$ over 10 weeks) and shows convergent validity with other self-concept measures, including the Coopersmith Self-Esteem Inventory (CSEI; Coopersmith, 1989) (Butler & Gasson, 2005).

As previously discussed, the CSEI has multiple forms and has been used with adults with TBI (Tate & Broe, 1999; Medd & Tate, 2000). The School form (ages 8–15) has sound reliability and validity and has been widely used in educational research. The 50 items assess general self-esteem and four sub-scales measure general self (20 items); social self (8 items); home–parents (8 items), and school–academic (8 items). There is an 8-item validity scale which measures defensiveness or socially desirable ratings. The scale has a maximum score of 100 and a minimum score of 0, with higher scores indicating higher self-esteem (Coopersmith, 1989). The CSEI was used by Hawley (2012) to assess self-esteem in children with TBI, who were on average two years post-injury. She found that children with TBI reported significantly poorer self-esteem than a peer control group and normative data and that lower self-esteem was significantly associated with greater symptoms of anxiety and depression.

Measures with potential utility for paediatric brain injury

The Social-Emotional Questionnaire for Children (SEQ-C; Wall, Williams, Morris & Bramham, 2011) was developed to assess socio-emotional difficulties and awareness of deficits of adolescents with brain injury. The original adult version of the SEQ was developed to assess social and emotional difficulties which commonly occur after damage to the prefrontal cortex (Bramham, Morris, Hornak, Bullock & Polkey, 2009). The SEQ-C includes a 30-item self-report version and parent/guardian version, with the discrepancy score between the two providing an index of self-awareness. A copy of each version of the SEQ-C is provided by Wall et al. (2011). In a preliminary study involving 109 typically developing adolescents (aged 11–14), a principal components analysis identified the following three factors for the self-report version: Emotion Recognition and Empathy (9 items; e.g. 'I notice when other people are happy'), Prosocial Behaviour (3 items; e.g., 'I am impatient with other people'), and Sociability (5 items; e.g., 'I have difficulties making and keeping close relationships'). Internal consistency was acceptable for the Emotion Recognition and Empathy ($\alpha = .87$), Social Conformity ($\alpha = .77$) and Prosocial Behaviour ($\alpha = .69$) subscales. There was evidence of convergent validity with the Dysexecutive Questionnaire for Children (DEX-C) and Strengths and Difficulties Questionnaire

(SDQ). A subgroup of adolescents ($n = 18$) with a history of concussion or mild head injury scored significantly lower on the Emotion Recognition and Empathy subscale than adolescents with no neurological history. There were no differences in scores between the adolescent and parent/guardian SEQ-C versions. Discrepancy scores did not vary according to age, gender or head injury status.

Overall, the SEQ-C shows promise as a new measure specifically designed for use in paediatric brain injury rehabilitation. Although the questionnaire measures functions assessed by existing tools (e.g., DEX-C, SDQ), the SEQ-C more specifically focuses on self–other perceptions and the social and emotional difficulties that can develop in the context of brain injury. However, the SEQ-C requires a more comprehensive psychometric evaluation in an adolescent brain injury sample prior to clinical use.

The Self-Understanding Interview (Damon & Hart, 1988) is based on a substantive body of theoretical and empirical literature concerning developmental changes in self-understanding from early childhood to adolescence. The general approach of the interview is to ask children to describe themselves, and then a content coding procedure is applied to score their responses. The Self-Understanding Interview is comprised of seven dimensions and related questions, including *self-definition* (e.g., what you are like as a person), *self-evaluation* (e.g., what you are proud of or like most about yourself), *self in past and future* (e.g., how you perceive you will be – the same or different in 5 years, and changes from 5 years ago), *self-interest* (e.g., what you hope for and want to be like), *continuity* (e.g., how you feel you change and stay the same each year), *agency* (e.g., how you feel you became the person you are) and *distinctiveness* (e.g., what makes you different from other people) (Damon & Hart, 1988).

Administration time is typically 30–60 minutes and wording is varied according to the child's comprehension needs, with probe questions used to facilitate self-descriptions. Interview responses are coded according to four self-as-object categories (i.e., physical, active, social and psychological aspects of the self) and three self-as-subject categories (i.e., continuity, distinctness and agency). Interviews are transcribed and divided into units or 'chunks' for scoring of self-statements according to Damon and Hart's (1988) coding scheme and scoring criteria.

Reliability investigations have indicated a high level of inter-rater agreement for modal-level score (84 per cent; $k = .75$), satisfactory internal consistency ($\alpha = .70-.83$), and acceptable 1-month test–retest reliability ($r = .49$) for a developmental measure (Damon & Hart, 1988). The interview has demonstrated theory-consistent differences in self-understanding of typically developing children and those with high functioning autism (Lee & Hobson, 1998; Yoshii & Yoshimatsu, 2003). With further validation, the Self-Understanding Interview may offer an in-depth approach for investigating emerging sense of self for children and adolescents after brain injury. In particular, the interview may help to identify the extent to which brain injury influences children's self-definition and their perceptions of continuity versus changes to self, personal strengths and difficulties, achievements and goals and hopes for the future. However, children's ability to convey their self-perceptions relies upon their verbal skills and understanding of abstract concepts such as time orientation.

Given the potential limitations of using interview schedules with young children, behavioural based measures of parent–child interaction may have promising applications. In their investigation of parenting style and child behavioural outcomes after brain injury, Wade et al. (2011) videotaped the parent–child dyad during 10 minutes of unstructured free play. They developed a coding system to rate caregiver and child verbalisations and behaviour. Parents' behaviour was rated on a 5-point rating scale according to dimensions of warmth, contingent responsiveness and negativity. Children's behaviour regulation or socially appropriate behaviour was also rated on a 5-point scale. A high level of inter-rater reliability was found for each dimension (ICC > .80). They formed two composite scales of warm responsiveness (warm and contingent responsiveness) and parent negativity, which were found to be significantly related to child behavioural problems (negative and positive associations, respectively) after severe TBI. The association between parenting style and internalising problems (e.g., anxiety, depression, withdrawal) is noteworthy due to the likely implications for self-concept. Overall, validated naturalistic observation may provide valuable insight into children's affect regulation and how they perceive themselves in relation to their social environment.

Conclusions

Assessment of changes to self and identity after brain injury requires broader consideration of individuals' psychological adjustment. Therefore, measures of self-awareness, sense-making appraisals and coping strategies are important to administer along with measures of self-concept and identity change. This chapter provided a review of the development, psychometric properties, clinical utility and research applications of key assessment approaches for understanding the impact of brain injury on sense of self. Further development and evaluation of measures for assessing developing sense of self after paediatric brain injury is particularly warranted. Access to validated measures is essential to evaluate the efficacy of intervention approaches, as covered in the next three chapters.

6 Individual psychotherapy and neurorehabilitation approaches

Identity-orientated therapy incorporates psychotherapy and neurorehabilitation approaches for supporting continuity of self and reconstruction of identity after brain injury. This chapter reviews individual interventions for adults, while group and community-based interventions (Chapter 7) and child and family interventions (Chapter 8) are discussed in separate chapters. Strategies for establishing a good working alliance and enhancing engagement in therapy are initially described. A diversity of therapy frameworks and strategies, including psychoeducation and feedback, goal-directed interventions, cognitive behavioural therapy, third-wave cognitive and behavioural therapies and project-based learning are presented with a review of empirical evidence to support their efficacy. The potential utility of technological aids to support sense of self is considered in the final section.

The therapeutic relationship and engagement in therapy

A collaborative and supportive therapeutic relationship is viewed as the backbone to successful engagement and change in therapy after brain injury (Judd & Wilson, 2005; Klonoff, 2010). Client-centred therapy entails the therapist and client working together to achieve mutually agreed upon goals, with the therapist providing guidance and encouraging the client's active participation in therapy. In the broader psychotherapy literature, it is well supported that 'common factors' influence treatment outcome regardless of the therapeutic paradigm and associated treatment techniques. For example, up to 85 per cent of variance in treatment outcome has been attributed to client, therapist and therapeutic relationship factors (Lambert, 1992). In a systematic review by Keijsers, Schaap and Hoogduin (2000) therapists' capacity for empathy, warmth, unconditional positive regard, and genuineness were the most reliable predictors of cognitive-behavioural therapy outcomes for different client groups. Such qualities enhance the working alliance or partnership formed, whereby the therapist is attuned to the 'client's theory of change' (see Robinson, 2009), and provides guidance to address the problems that he or she wants to address in therapy.

Many authors have recognised the importance of the therapeutic relationship and change processes in psychotherapy for people with brain injury (e.g., Ben-Yishay & Diller, 2011; Cicerone, 1989; Coetzer, 2007; Gracey et al., 2009; Judd & Wilson,

2005; Klonoff, 2010; Prigatano, 1999; Schönberger, Humle & Teasdale, 2006; Wilson et al., 2009). A good working alliance fosters trust in the therapist and the therapeutic process, thus creating emotional safety to explore the subjective meaning of the brain injury (Gracey et al., 2009). In contrast, a poor working alliance and use of techniques that elicit distress (e.g., confrontation and critical feedback) may activate threat-based coping reactions including denial, defensiveness and avoidance (Langer & Padrone, 1992). Various psychotherapy models have been developed to guide clinical practice in brain injury (Coetzer, 2007; Gracey et al., 2009; Klonoff, 2010).

Applying the Generic Model of Psychotherapy developed by Orlinsky and Howard (1987), Coetzer (2007) identified the following six common facets of psychotherapy with clients with brain injury:

- *Therapeutic contract*: clarifying the role of the client and therapist and practical aspects of therapy, including session length, duration and type of treatment;
- *Therapeutic operations*: assessment processes that support a shared understanding and collaborative approach to treatment planning;
- *Therapeutic bond*: characteristics of the client–therapist relationship, including establishing rapport and a mutual understanding of respective roles;
- *Self-relatedness:* clients' capacity to respond to themselves during interaction with other people and their environment (e.g., response to feedback);
- *In-session impacts*: clients' immediate experiences of psychotherapy (e.g., realisation and relief) as clients make sense of issues they have been grappling with and learn how to manage the consequences;
- *Phases of treatment*: the sequence of events across sessions that contribute to psychotherapy outcomes (e.g., developments in self-awareness, meaning-making, coping and acceptance, and psychological adjustment).

The Collaborative Model of Psychotherapy after Brain Injury by Klonoff (2010) has features in common with the generic psychotherapy model. These models share the view that the main goal of psychotherapy is to improve self-awareness, foster acceptance and realism and support people to derive meaning from their experiences after brain injury. Klonoff described the therapist as the facilitator of change with the client and therapist collaboration viewed as integral to this process. However, unlike the generic model, Klonoff's framework also incorporates the person's family and community connections. People's support networks facilitate and reinforce their 'renewed sense of identity, hope and meaning' (p. 2), as covered in more detail in Chapters 7 and 8. In Klonoff's multifactorial model, client factors (e.g., pre-injury personality, nature and extent of brain injury, cognition, emotion and behaviour) interact with therapeutic factors (e.g., working alliance, theoretical frameworks and techniques) and their family or social milieu (e.g., history, culture and environment) to influence the outcomes of psychotherapy, including self-awareness, coping and adjustment.

The 'Y-shaped' model by Gracey et al. (2009) depicts the relationship between processes of change and outcomes in rehabilitation (including psychotherapy), in order to understand *how* interventions work. The top of the 'Y' in the model represents initial social and psychological discrepancies that are identified and targeted in rehabilitation to promote the process of adaptation and social re-integration. As discussed in Chapter 4, a person may experience *personal discrepancies* between their current self (e.g., abilities) and aspired-to self (i.e., pre-injury or ideal self), *social discrepancies* (e.g., loss of relationships and social roles) or *interpersonal discrepancies* (e.g., a client and family member having different opinions regarding post-injury problems and support needs). These discrepancies create inner tension and pose threats to self, and often result in unhelpful coping reactions (e.g., avoidance and substance use) and emotional distress.

According to Gracey et al. (2009), psychotherapy supports people to resolve self-discrepancies, as reflected in the model by convergence at the centre of the 'Y'. This occurs through developing a safe environment and the therapist and client engaging in cyclical processes that include setting goals, making predictions, planning and performing activities, reflecting on their outcomes and developing shared formulations. The use of behavioural experiments and experiential learning serves to promote more adaptive and realistic self-representations and ways of coping. By reducing the threat posed by self-discrepancies, individuals are better able to explore the meaning of their brain injury and develop an adaptive post-injury identity (signified by the vertical trunk of the 'Y'). Such psychological growth involves 'updating' one's identity by recognising both continuity with and discontinuity from pre-injury self, and 'consolidating' the new identity through meaningful social and activity participation (Gracey et al., 2009). The focus on promoting psychological well-being and improving functionality is consistent with positive psychology perspectives on brain injury rehabilitation (see Evans, 2011; Feeney & Capo, 2010; Ownsworth & Fleming, 2011; Ylvisaker et al., 1998).

In summary, models of psychotherapy provide useful frameworks within which clinicians can plan their approach to therapy and select appropriate techniques. As recognised by each model, the initial process of engaging clients in psychotherapy is integral to its effectiveness.

Strategies to enhance engagement in psychotherapy

There are many potential barriers or challenges to engaging people with brain injury in therapy. These barriers relate to the person with brain injury, therapist and therapeutic relationship (Judd & Wilson, 2005). Although barriers related to the client are of primary focus here, it is important to recognise that the therapist's background (e.g., training and experience), values and attitudes (e.g., expectation of a positive outcome) can greatly influence the working alliance and therapy outcomes. There may also be constraints placed on therapists by their organisation and funding arrangements, such as specific referral criteria and session limits, which influence their capacity to offer psychotherapy to a client. The belief that a client should be insightful and motivated to change from the outset of therapy to derive benefits may prevent therapists from offering a programme, or affect their persistence when challenges arise. Judd and Wilson (2005) noted that a longstanding and still prevalent view is that people with brain injury are less likely to benefit from psychotherapy than other client groups due to their complex cognitive and behavioural impairments.

Conducting psychotherapy with people with brain injury can certainly be challenging, but very worthwhile. Some of my most rewarding experiences and positive client outcomes involved working with people who were excluded from other services due to poor insight, cognitive deficits, lack of motivation or other behavioural issues. When deciding whether to provide a psychotherapy intervention or not, it is important for therapists to be mindful of their own limitations and the constraints of their clinical setting. This involves considering their scope to provide an intervention of sufficient duration and intensity with follow-up support, and the need for appropriate training and supervision (Ownsworth & Clare, 2006). Judd and Wilson (2005) emphasised the importance of therapists having a high level of self-awareness and self-reflective skills to manage negative emotions (i.e., most commonly, frustration and anxiety) that can be experienced when working in this area of practice.

Various client characteristics influence the suitability of psychotherapy after brain injury. Some clients present with issues that may contraindicate psychotherapy at that time point, including poor physical health and an unstable medical condition, behavioural disturbance (e.g., severe aggression or apathy), psychotic symptoms and major substance abuse issues. In these circumstances other treatment and rehabilitation approaches may be warranted and prioritised from a funding perspective, including pharmacotherapy and environmental interventions such as family-based support and support worker training.

Judd and Wilson (2005) surveyed UK psychotherapy practitioners working with people with brain injury to identify the main challenges to forming the working alliance and their strategies or practice modifications. Common challenges included the client's lack of insight, disinhibition, emotional lability and impairments in memory, cognitive flexibility, attention and language. A related issue impacting the therapeutic relationship was different views or expectations held by the client and therapist with regards to goals and outcomes of therapy. Based on Judd and Wilson's findings, Table 6.1 summarises some key challenges to forming the working alliance and strategies to facilitate a collaborative understanding and enhance participation.

Although the strategies in Table 6.1 are likely to be useful in a general sense, their use relies on clients agreeing to attend psychotherapy. In some instances, clients will resist attending the first session or leave therapy early because they do not perceive any need or benefit, or even feel concerned about negative consequences of therapy. Issues that can contribute to these perceptions include lack of insight, anger and frustration, severe anxiety and sense of hopelessness. Table 6.2 presents four case vignettes to illustrate how these characteristics affected motivation for therapy and strategies that were helpful for building rapport in this context. Although not always the case, it can be more challenging to build rapport with clients referred by another person than those who self-identified the need for support and initiated contact with the therapist. Strategies for building rapport vary, but typically involve efforts to create a non-threatening and emotionally safe environment during initial contact. The general aim is to get a 'foot in the door' in the first session by fostering trust in the therapist and therapeutic process using the following approaches:

- Displaying warmth, empathy and a non-judgemental stance towards the client and his or her presenting concerns (e.g., validating distress or frustration);
- Asking the person about their preferences to increase their level of comfort in the therapy environment (e.g., use of a communication aid, presence of a family member, seating arrangements, note-taking, refreshments);
- Avoiding confrontational approaches (e.g., asking potentially intrusive questions, presenting challenging tasks that reveal deficits or providing critical feedback);
- Increasing people's sense of control over the therapy process by presenting options that people often find helpful and non-threatening (e.g., learning relaxation strategies, reading other people's stories and receiving general education about the brain);
- Reinforcing participation on any level (e.g., 'I really appreciated your feedback/ views on …') and, where appropriate, providing feedback on personal strengths;
- Motivational interviewing approaches (Miller & Rollnick, 2002), such as supporting clients to identify and explore the discrepancy between their current situation and their desired state (i.e., personal goals and how they want to feel and act) and to consider the possible benefits versus costs or risks of participating in therapy (see also Hsieh, Ponsford, Wong, Schönberger, McKay & Haines, 2012a).

Table 6.1 A summary of issues impacting the working alliance and strategies used by psychotherapists in brain injury (adapted from Judd & Wilson, 2005)

Issues impacting the working alliance and psychotherapy process	Strategies or modifications to practice
Impairments in memory, attention, language and executive function affecting people's capacity to attend to, understand and assimilate their therapy experiences	• Provide written summaries and use memory aids to record important details and assist learning • Involve significant others to reinforce information and strategy use at home • Shorten sessions and focus on one key issue at a time, and conduct therapy over a longer timeframe
Lack of insight into the effects of brain injury (impairments and abilities) and unrealistic goals and expectations of therapy outcomes	• Provide personalised education and information about brain injury and its effects • Use behavioural experiments to test the accuracy of client's self-perceptions and evidence of his/her impairments and skills • Support clients to reflect on their post-injury changes using guided discovery • Respect the client's right to hope • Identify short-term steps within broader goals and affirm the therapist's presence and support throughout the process
Behavioural/emotional problems (e.g., disinhibition and emotional lability)	• Develop a behaviour management programme • Reduce session length and involve significant others to reinforce strategies and support the client at home • Teach adaptive coping behaviours to enable participation in psychotherapy

Table 6.2 Case vignettes illustrating barriers to rapport and therapeutic strategies

Client characteristics	Barriers to rapport	Therapist's strategies during the initial session
Evan: referred by insurance company due to anger management problems. He displayed a lack of self-awareness and narcissistic features.	Evan was highly critical of all professionals and became verbally aggressive when asked about his injury or understanding of the reason for his referral. His view was: 'I don't need to see a head doctor – this is a [expletive] waste of time'.	• Validated Evan's frustration about feeling 'forced to attend' and avoided direct questions about his injury. • Invited Evan to provide feedback on a draft educational resource for people with brain injury. He was very critical of the resource, but acknowledged that some of it applied to him, and that he felt 'isolated and misunderstood'. • Encouraged Evan to reflect on the discrepancy between how he felt and how he wanted to feel and weigh up the possible 'pros' and 'cons' of attending therapy.
Amy: referred by case manager and mother due to aggressive behaviour on public transport and risk of losing her accommodation. She lacked self-awareness of the effects of her behaviour on others.	Amy was very angry with 'the system' and felt discriminated against in society. She felt a strong sense of injustice about her injury and believed that others were to blame. She also made many self-depreciating comments.	• Validated distress and frustration, taking care not to reinforce her views. • Encouraged Amy to identify her values and desired life situation, barriers to living the life she wants and aspects that were potentially within her control (including the choice to participate in therapy). • Provided positive feedback on her strengths (artwork, sense of humour and resourcefulness) and thanked her for openly sharing her views and experiences.
Janelle: referred by her lawyer due to severe social anxiety, defensiveness and unwillingness to attend medico-legal assessments.	Initially Janelle would not attend therapy in person or answer the telephone. She communicated through letters, expressing a concern that therapy would make her 'feel worse'. She wanted a guarantee that therapy would help.	• Validated concerns and distress regarding previous experiences with professionals (i.e., expecting they would help her). • Acknowledged that there was no guarantee that therapy would help, but also described common outcomes people achieved in collaboration with a therapist. • Presented Janelle with different options and asked to indicate her preferences to increase her sense of control. She expressed that she did not want to talk about the injury until she was ready.
Adam: referred by mother due to his suicidal ideation and hopelessness after losing his position in a law firm; lack of self-awareness of his emotion and behaviour regulation difficulties.	Adam believed that there was 'no point in therapy' because this could not help him get his former job back. Despite his sense of hopelessness, Adam stated he was 'not depressed'.	• Validated distress and recognised his efforts to 'get on with life' after his injury (active participation in rehabilitation and work trial). • Explored Adam's personal values to understand the meaning of his former work (i.e., his status and identity as a lawyer). • Encouraged Adam to weigh up the possible 'pros' and 'cons' of attending therapy. Cons included possibly feeling even worse and wasting his time; pros included the possibility of finding a way forward.

In addition to building the working alliance, it is important to monitor and maintain the alliance over time and be mindful of issues that can threaten or reduce the quality of the therapeutic relationship. For an in-depth discussion of the working alliance and process issues in psychotherapy for people with brain injury see Klonoff (2010). Overall, there is a lack of research investigating psychotherapy processes and the relationship between the working alliance and outcome in brain injury rehabilitation (Schönberger et al., 2006). Nevertheless, a growing body of literature supports the effectiveness of interventions that focus on self-awareness and client-centred goals to improve motivation and engagement in rehabilitation (see Doig, Fleming, Kuipers, Cornwell, & Khan, 2011; Doig, Fleming, Cornwell & Kuipers, 2010; McPherson, Kayes & Weatherall, 2009; Ownsworth et al., 2008; Ylvisaker, McPherson et al., 2008). An overview of these interventions and the evidence base will be presented in the next section.

Self-awareness and goal-directed interventions

Individuals' self-awareness of their post-injury impairments has been found to influence motivation, goal setting, strategy use and participation in rehabilitation (Fleming et al., 1998; Ownsworth & Clare, 2006; Ownsworth, McFarland & Young, 2000; Schönberger et al., 2006). A systematic review by Ownsworth and Clare (2006) identified that 10 out of 12 studies provided at least partial support for the view that greater self-awareness is associated with more favourable rehabilitation outcomes. Other researchers have found that people with awareness deficits can make meaningful gains in rehabilitation through task-specific learning and achieve positive community re-integration outcomes with appropriate environmental support (Malec, Buffington, Moessner, & Degiorgio, 2000; Sohlberg, Mateer, Penkman, Glang & Todis, 1998). Nonetheless, in the context of psychotherapy, more accurate self-appraisal is likely to support people to make sense of changes in their lifestyle (e.g., understand the reason why returning to a particular job is not feasible) and increase their use of self-management strategies.

Ownsworth and Clare (2006) proposed that interventions targeting awareness deficits may be beneficial in the following circumstances: a) lack of awareness represents a likely barrier to the person achieving his or her own valued goals; b) there is a concern for the person's safety that cannot otherwise be managed effectively, for example, through constant supervision; c) the perceived benefits of improving awareness outweigh the possible negative impact on the person's emotional state; and d) there is sufficient scope in the rehabilitation setting to employ evidence-based approaches to training awareness and support is available to buffer the psychological impact of increased self-awareness. The application of these guidelines has been illustrated in single-case studies (Ownsworth, Fleming et al., 2006; Ownsworth, Turpin et al., 2008).

The optimal timing of awareness interventions has been debated in the literature, with some authors cautioning the need to avoid confronting the person with their deficits or losses too early in rehabilitation (e.g., Langer & Padrone, 1992). However, awareness deficits can impede rehabilitation progress and interfere with the collaborative process of setting realistic goals (Judd & Wilson, 2005). Conversely, it has been found that the process of developing and working towards valued goals can enhance self-awareness and promote better psychological adjustment (Doig et al., 2010; 2011). In particular, after a brain injury people typically aim to resume their pre-injury activities and roles (e.g., return to the same occupation). These aspired-to outcomes can provide the impetus to participate in activities related to the attainment of this goal (e.g., vocational rehabilitation and work trials). Engaging in these activities provides people with the opportunity to receive feedback on their performance and to reflect on the meaning of these experiences. Through this process they can develop more accurate self-appraisals, become more realistic about the future and adjust their goals accordingly. The link between client goals and use of occupation to improve self-awareness is exemplified by the following case study (see Ownsworth, Turpin et al., 2008).

A case illustration: Craig

Craig was a 37-year-old man who sustained a right thalamic stroke four years prior. His main goals in community-based rehabilitation were to return to full-time work in his former vocation as an accountant and to increase his independence from his parents' support. Craig displayed a lack of awareness of his cognitive deficits (e.g., reduced processing speed, visuo-spatial and executive function impairments) and experienced regular periods of depression. Psychoeducation and feedback were identified as important components of a 12-session vocational rehabilitation intervention to increase his self-awareness, self-monitoring and use of compensatory strategies in daily living. Due to concerns about his emotional state and the possible negative impact of feedback, a bi-directional feedback approach was employed throughout the intervention. Specifically, the therapist provided feedback on Craig's performance during the session, while Craig's perspective on the value of different therapy exercises was sought during a 10–15 minute post-session debriefing (see Ownsworth, Turpin et al., 2008). This debriefing supported Craig to process the meaning of feedback he received and also helped the therapist to monitor the psychological impact of the intervention.

Craig's feedback indicated that he found psychoeducation about brain functioning and stroke 'very interesting'. However, asking him questions about the long-term effects of his stroke was not beneficial because this focus on his problems made him feel like 'a second class citizen'. In a self-estimation task he found it difficult to rate his cognitive abilities, because there was no 'benchmark' to compare himself against. During a role-reversal exercise the therapist overestimated her performance on cognitive tasks (e.g., list learning and line bisection) and Craig provided feedback on the accuracy of her self-estimation. After switching roles, Craig recognised the benefits of receiving immediate feedback on his performance, as follows: 'I think it's important to get it [feedback] early because you've got to know how you are measuring up against their standard … but it needs to be accurate feedback' (Ownsworth, Turpin et al., 2008, p. 703).

Craig received audiovisual and verbal feedback on his performance on real-life tasks (i.e., cooking, planning weekly activities and a work trial), and became increasingly more accurate at predicting and evaluating his own performance. Later sessions focused on Craig identifying both easy and difficult components of tasks and developing management strategies. He also received counselling to enhance his understanding of how cognitive deficits influenced the type of work he could achieve. After the final session, a work trial observation, Craig identified that the programme helped him to better understand his 'strengths and downfalls' and become 'realistic about the type of work you want to do' (p. 705). His modified goal was to work 2–3 days a week, 6 hours per day in one of a number of possible employment areas. Three weeks after the intervention Craig achieved part-time work (15 hours per week) as a retail assistant and maintained this position at long-term follow-up (6 and 9 months).

Psychoeducation and feedback

Craig's programme employed a number of theory-guided techniques for enhancing metacognitive skills, including psychoeducation, verbal and video-based feedback, role reversal and guided self-evaluation of performance prior to, during and after task performance (Fleming & Ownsworth, 2006; Toglia & Kirk, 2000). Because psychoeducation and feedback interventions are typically embedded in broader rehabilitation programmes, it can be difficult to evaluate their efficacy in isolation. It would also be pointless and potentially harmful to conduct interventions that focus solely on improving awareness of deficits (e.g., the ability to accurately report one's impairments). Rather, interventions need to focus on improving awareness as part of the process of achieving other clinically important outcomes such as improved self-regulation and emotional adjustment. Despite widespread use in brain injury rehabilitation, there has been little research investigating the efficacy of psychoeducation and feedback approaches. A systematic review by Schmidt, Lannin, Fleming, & Ownsworth (2011) identified 12 empirical studies evaluating self-awareness interventions with a feedback component. The main intervention strategies included:

- Direct verbal feedback from therapists (e.g., Cheng & Man, 2006);
- Comparing self-ratings of ability with therapist ratings and discussing discrepancies (e.g., Coetzer & Corney, 2001);
- Audiovisual feedback; a person observes his or her own task performance from an audiovisual recording (e.g., Ownsworth, Fleming et al., 2006; Ownsworth, Quinn et al., 2010);
- Experiential feedback or repeated practice in completing a functional task, usually incorporated into a broader intervention (e.g., Cheng & Man, 2006);
- Feedback during task performance, including the therapist's use of pause, prompt and praise to support the person to self-identify errors during an activity (e.g., Ownsworth, Fleming et al., 2006; Ownsworth, Quinn et al., 2010);
- Performance predictions prior to task completion, and post-task evaluation of strengths, limitations and strategy use by the person with brain injury and therapist (e.g., Goverover, Johnston, Toglia & DeLuca, 2007).

Most studies (i.e., 9 out of 12) employed single-case methodology with a pre-post design. A meta-analysis of three randomised controlled trials (RCT) (Cheng & Man,

2006; Goverover et al., 2007; Ownsworth, Fleming et al. 2008) that involved a total of 62 people with brain injury yielded a moderate effect size for improvement in self-awareness. Although this finding reinforces the clinical utility of feedback in rehabilitation, due to the diversity of feedback interventions employed within and between studies it was not possible to determine the most effective approach to feedback from the systematic review (Schmidt et al., 2011).

A subsequent RCT by Schmidt, Fleming, Ownsworth and Lannin (2013) investigated the relative efficacy of three feedback approaches for people with severe TBI (76 per cent were inpatients of a brain injury unit). The four-session interventions included combined video and verbal feedback ($n = 18$), verbal feedback ($n = 18$) and experiential feedback ($n = 18$). The combined video and verbal feedback intervention was associated with significantly greater gains in online awareness (i.e., error monitoring and correction) and intellectual awareness (i.e., AQ discrepancy) compared with the verbal feedback and experiential feedback interventions. Importantly, levels of depression, anxiety and stress did not change, and thus there was no negative impact on emotional status for any of the feedback interventions. The four main components of the combined video and verbal feedback intervention included:

1   The person with TBI performs a meal preparation task with the therapist using the pause, prompt and praise technique. This entails the therapist observing that an error has been made, delaying a response to create the opportunity for self-correction (e.g., 5–10 seconds) and then providing a non-specific prompt (e.g., 'Can I get you to stop and think about what you are doing'). If the error is not corrected a specific prompt is provided. Praise is consistently given for following the instructions accurately, using strategies effectively and self-correcting errors (see Ownsworth, Fleming et al., 2006).
2   The therapist and person with TBI independently complete the 'Meal Independence Rating Scale' (MIRS; Schmidt et al., 2013) to rate the amount of assistance required for task initiation, execution (organisation, sequencing, judgement and safety), and completion.
3   The person with TBI watches his or her videotaped performance with the therapist. The therapist encourages the person to recognise errors and areas of strength in task performance, and suggests future use of compensatory strategies.
4   The therapist and person with TBI verbally discuss any discrepancies in their ratings on the MIRS.

The experiential feedback intervention involved steps 1 and 2, whereas the verbal feedback entailed steps 1, 2, and 4. Interestingly, there were no differences in awareness outcomes between the verbal feedback and experiential feedback interventions, which suggests that improvements in online and intellectual awareness can largely be attributed to the video-based feedback component (i.e., step 3).

Due to the encouraging findings of the RCT, the authors developed guidelines for implementing the video and verbal feedback (Schmidt, Fleming, Ownsworth & Lannin, under review). Their guidelines for providing client-centred feedback (see Table 6.3) are most appropriate for clients with neuropsychologically-based awareness

Table 6.3 Guidelines for providing client-centred feedback in brain injury rehabilitation (adapted from Schmidt et al. 2013)

Client-centred feedback principles
1   Use a meaningful occupation (e.g., everyday tasks) as a medium to provide feedback, incorporate clients' choices and task preferences and focus on areas of occupational performance to improve rather than specific impairments.
2   Build therapeutic rapport to foster effective communication and trust in the therapist's feedback (i.e., explain the purpose and value of feedback).
3   Provide an opportunity for the client to independently self-recognise and correct errors using graded prompting (e.g., pause, prompt and praise).
4   Deliver feedback in a confidential and distraction-free environment and clarify how information will be used.
5   Use the 'sandwich approach' to providing feedback by describing the person's strengths before and after discussing areas of difficulty and suggested improvement.
6   Consider the timing of feedback in relation to task performance (i.e., soon after task completion to support recall of experiences) and the client's rehabilitation programme (i.e., provide feedback on occupational performance early in rehabilitation to facilitate awareness and adoption of compensatory strategies prior to discharge).
7   Monitor the client's emotional status and ensure adequate psychological support during and after feedback sessions, including the need for adjustment counselling.

deficits (i.e., executive dysfunction). Clients displaying defensive denial are more likely to benefit from non-confrontational approaches that focus more on building the therapeutic alliance and exploring the personal meaning of everyday difficulties (see Fleming & Ownsworth, 2006; Ownsworth, 2005), as exemplified by a case study later in this chapter. Similarly, clients at risk of developing significant emotional distress may require counselling in conjunction with a feedback intervention (see Ownsworth, Turpin et al., 2008).

Goal-directed interventions

As outlined in the previous section, clients' goals can support awareness interventions by helping to identify personally meaningful activities in which to update self-knowledge and develop self-regulation skills. However, goals have a more central role in identity-oriented therapy. Goals are closely linked to self-identity, particularly the notion of possible selves, or who a person might become in the future (Markus & Nurius, 1986). Therefore, goal setting and goal attainment is often a focus of intervention in brain injury rehabilitation (Doig et al., 2010; 2011; Evans, 2012; McPherson et al., 2009). However, the process of setting realistic and personally meaningful goals is not always straightforward for people with brain injury (Ylvisaker et al., 2008). A useful starting point is to support people to identify their values, or lifelong principles and beliefs that guide their actions.

Values are what matters most to us deep down, and what we believe that our lives stand for (i.e., how we want to relate to ourselves, others and the world) (Harris, 2009). Values are akin to the directions in which one travels, rather than destinations at which one arrives (i.e., goals). For example, a person may have a lifelong value of health and fitness, while actions congruent with that value (e.g., joining a gym and maintaining regular exercise, eating nutritious food) reflect personal goals. Values are freely chosen by an individual and in most cases reflect continuity with the past or aspects of self that have not changed despite the injury (Gelech & Desjardins, 2011). However, as discussed in Chapter 3, the experience of brain injury can alter people's priorities and directions in life, with new interests (e.g., becoming an advocate for others) sometimes superseding previous ones (e.g., achieving in one's former occupation). The physical, cognitive and behavioural consequences of brain injury can make it more difficult for people to live in accordance with their values (Evans, 2011). Therefore, exploring a person's values early in the therapy process can assist in setting personally meaningful goals and identifying obstacles or barriers to these goals. An example values worksheet is presented in Figure 6.1 for Bill, a 35-year-old man who experiences cognitive and behavioural difficulties in the context of brain tumour. The worksheet depicts the general steps of: identifying key values, developing value statements, exploring current levels of importance and success in living according to one's values, and identifying behaviours consistent with one's values, and obstacles or barriers (Harris, 2009).

As shown in Figure 6.1, there are a number of potential goals for Bill to increase his success in being a loving and caring partner to his girlfriend. These goals relate to managing his anger, completing household tasks and developing memory strategies. There is a growing body of literature that supports the efficacy of goal-directed interventions for improving outcomes in brain injury rehabilitation (Doig et al., 2010; 2011; Evans, 2012; Levine et al. 2000; McPherson et al., 2009; Jenkinson, Ownsworth & Shum, 2007). Techniques that support goal-directed programmes include use of SMART goals, Canadian Occupational Performance Measure, Goal Attainment Scaling and Metaphoric Identity Mapping.

SMART goal setting

Practical guidelines developed for goal setting in rehabilitation follow the SMART or SMARTER principles (see Bovend'Eert, Botell & Wade, 2009; Evans, 2012). There are variations to the wording associated with the acronym and some redundancy, as follows:

- S – Shared, specific, succinct and straightforward
- M – Monitored, measurable, meaningful and manageable
- A – Accessible, attainable, action-orientated and agreed upon
- R – Realistic, relevant and reasonable
- T – Timely, transparent, tangible and trackable
- E – Evolving (changing, as needed, with time)
- R – Relationship-centred.

These terms convey that goals should be personally valued by the person with brain injury and developed collaboratively in order to motivate behaviour change (Evans, 2012). Goals need to be realistic in the sense that change that is feasible within

118 *Individual psychotherapy and neurorehabilitation approaches*

\multicolumn{6}{c	}{**VALUES WORKSHEET**}
Name: Bill					Date: 12/3/13
Values	Value statements	Current importance (0–10)	Current success (0–10)	Behaviours consistent	Obstacles and barriers
Intimate relationship	*To be a loving and caring partner to my girlfriend*	*9/10*	*5/10*	*Keeping my cool when I'm frustrated, showing affection, helping out around the house, and completing tasks I've promised to do.*	*Anger management problems, loss of motivation, fatigue and memory difficulties*
Independence					
Health					
Family relations					
Recreation					
Work/career					
Friendships/ socialising					
Looking after or helping others					
Education/ training					
Community/ environment					
Spirituality					

Figure 6.1 Example values worksheet

a specified timeframe (i.e., short-, medium- or long-term) and clearly described in behavioural terms to enable measurement of progress. It is also optimal that goals reflect outcomes that are desired and supported by members of the person's support network including family, employers, support workers and rehabilitation professionals.

Canadian Occupational Performance Measure (COPM)

Based on the Canadian Model of Occupational Performance (see Law, Cooper, Strong, Stewart, Rigby & Letts, 1996), the COPM involves a semi-structured interview (approximately 30–45 minutes) that supports clients to identify problems experienced in the areas of self-care (i.e. personal care and functional mobility), productivity (e.g.

paid or unpaid work), and leisure and socialisation. Participants rate the importance of each activity (1 = not important at all; 10 = extremely important) to assist in prioritising areas to address. Typically, 3–5 activity areas are selected by the client, which form the basis of specific goals for the intervention. Self-ratings of current level of performance (1 = not able to perform; 10 = able to perform extremely well) and satisfaction with performance (1 = not satisfied at all; 10 = extremely satisfied) are obtained.

The COPM has been applied in various rehabilitation contexts, including inpatient neurological rehabilitation (e.g., Bodiam, 1999), outpatient rehabilitation (Trombly et al., 1998) and community-based rehabilitation (e.g., Jenkinson et al., 2007; Ownsworth, Fleming et al., 2008). The COPM has particular value for facilitating client-centred goal setting and increasing clients' participation in goal planning (Doig et al., 2010). Due to the focus on occupation, it is more straightforward to set activity-based goals (e.g., to improve meal preparation performance) than goals relating to emotional or cognitive functioning. However, SMARTER goal-setting guidelines can assist to identify behaviourally specific and action-oriented goals for impairment-based goals (e.g., managing depression or memory problems).

Research largely supports the COPM's responsiveness to intervention (e.g., Bodiam, 1999; Trombly et al., 1998; Jenkinson et al. 2007; Ownsworth, Fleming et al. 2008). However, satisfaction ratings can increase over time without intervention, which raises some concerns about stability in measurement (Jenkinson et al., 2007). A further potential limitation of the COPM is that awareness deficits may affect self-identification of problem areas and reliability of self-ratings, and hence the tool's capacity to detect change in response to intervention. For this reason, some researchers have obtained collateral ratings on the COPM. Interestingly, collateral ratings were generally found to be consistent with self-ratings (Jenkinson et al., 2007; Trombly et al. 1998), and COPM self-ratings were not significantly related to measures of awareness (PCRS) or cognitive function (Jenkinson et al., 2007). Nevertheless, due to perceived limitations of the COPM some researchers have used the COPM in combination with the more objective method of Goal Attainment Scaling (Doig et al., 2010; Trombly et al., 1998).

Goal Attainment Scaling (GAS)

GAS was developed as a measurement methodology to evaluate mental health programmes, but is now frequently used in brain injury rehabilitation (e.g., Bouwens, van Heugten & Verhey, 2009; Doig et al., 2010). GAS provides an objective approach to planning, monitoring progress and measuring goal attainment. The GAS framework supports formulation of individualised goals that are desirable to all (i.e., the client, therapists and family members). As outlined by Kiresuk, Smith and Cardillo (1994), the steps of GAS include:

1   Identifying specific goals for each problem area based on assessment (e.g., COPM or performance observation) and discussion with the client and significant others. Using Bill's example in Figure 6.1, a goal entailed reducing the frequency

of anger outbursts in order to increase positive and loving interactions with his girlfriend Clare.
2. Determining the methods for measuring goal performance, using an objective and clearly operationalised approach, e.g., Bill and Clare record the daily frequency of anger outbursts, defined from prior observation as instances in which Bill raises his voice excessively, swears, says something hurtful to Clare, and throws or hits objects.
3. Assessing current performance level, e.g., Bill has an average of two anger outbursts per day, with 13 recorded over a one-week baseline.
4. Setting expectations of performance. Bill and Clare identify that although the most desirable outcome is no anger outbursts, a reduction in the frequency of anger outbursts is more realistic and hence 5–6 anger outbursts per week is specified as the expected outcome of the intervention.
5. Completing the scaling of the GAS levels and corresponding behaviour. Scaling ranges from +2 (most favourable outcome) to –2 (least favourable outcome), e.g., see Table 6.4.
6. Reviewing the goal to ensure appropriate gaps between levels and monitoring performance over time.

The utility of GAS relies upon therapists having the knowledge and expertise to set accurate and realistic goal outcomes in collaboration with clients and their significant others (Evans, 2012). Where clients have multiple goals these can be weighted according to order of priority (e.g., of 4 goals, the most important is weighted as 4 and least important is weighted as 1) and overall progress can be assessed using a standard T score, as follows: > 50 = above expected performance, 50 = expected performance, and < 50 below expected performance. The process for calculating standard scores is outlined by Bovend'Eert et al. (2009). Quantitative measurement of goal attainment is beneficial for programme evaluation and research evaluating the efficacy of specific interventions (Doig et al., 2011). Using GAS to evaluate the efficacy of cognitive rehabilitation, Bouwens et al. (2009) found that setting at least three realistic goals for each client with brain injury was possible within a 30-minute period. GAS was considered less feasible for people with poor self-awareness or those with comorbidity or psychological problems. Despite many advantages in clinical practice, Evans (2012) raised some concerns about the use of GAS in RCTs due to low inter-rater reliability of goal attainment ratings.

Metaphoric identity mapping (MIM)

Ylvisaker and colleagues (Ylvisaker & Feeney, 2000; Ylvisaker et al., 2008) emphasise the importance of supporting people to re-establish an 'organised, compelling and reasonably realistic identity' (Ylvisaker et al., 2008, p. 715) after brain injury. Goals need to be linked to higher level self-representations (i.e., 'who I am' and 'who I want to be') to be personally meaningful and worth striving for. MIM is a theory-based set of procedures that facilitate goal setting and engagement in rehabilitation (see Ylvisaker et al., 2008). The approach entails supporting people to identify a

Table 6.4 GAS levels and corresponding behaviour for the example of Bill

GAS level	Outcome	Goal
+2	Much better than expected outcome	No anger outbursts over the week
+1	Somewhat better than expected outcome	1–4 anger outbursts over the week
0	Expected outcome	5–6 anger outbursts over the week
−1	Somewhat less than expected outcome	7–13 anger outbursts over the week (pre-intervention level)
−2	Much less than expected outcome	More than 13 anger outbursts over the week

personally meaningful metaphor (e.g., much-admired person, symbol, image or story) which is associated with positive thoughts, emotions and behaviour and supports the re-construction of an adaptive identity. Metaphors are concise internal representations (e.g., a lion depicting courage, strength and leadership) that resonate with an individual, serve to motivate and guide decisions and behaviour, and can be linked to meaningful tasks and action strategies. Visual representations of identity maps depict the person and his or her metaphor in the centre (e.g., Tony as a lion) and linked attributes (values, goals, feelings, action strategies and affiliations) in surrounding circles. As described by Ylvisaker et al. (2008), the main applications of MIM include:

- Forming the therapeutic alliance, and seeking to understand a person as he or she understands themselves. This process includes identifying values, interests and goals and current obstacles to achieving one's goals.
- Supporting individuals to set personally meaningful goals and action strategies for achieving these. Strategies include tying goals to positive metaphors and congruent actions.
- Developing strategies to overcome long-term obstacles for achieving goals, and practising and implementing these through task assignments and projects to foster a sense of accomplishment.
- Facilitating changes in identity and self-schema in the context of long-term psychotherapy.

MIM is often used in conjunction with or as part of formal psychotherapy and rehabilitation approaches such as project-based learning, as covered later in this chapter. An RCT by McPherson et al. (2009) compared the acceptability and clinical utility of Identity Oriented Goal Training (IOT) and Goal Management Training (GMT; see Levine et al., 2000) after TBI. Each intervention was conducted over 6–8 weeks and involved key workers engaging clients in goal setting and goal performance according to GMT or IOT. They used MIM as part of IOT to develop higher representations of what is important to the person to drive their goals. Based on a predominantly qualitative analysis (i.e., client and clinician interviews and focus groups), McPherson et al. (2009) identified that IOT and GMT were both acceptable to clients and clinicians. However, IOT was more useful for engaging clients in the goal-setting process while GMT provided a more structured framework to prevent errors when performing goal-related activities (e.g., preparing meals, shopping). There were no quantitative differences in goal attainment between GMT, IOT and usual care on the GAS, which may have been due to small sample size ($n = 32$).

In summary, self-awareness and goal-directed interventions are useful approaches for improving engagement in therapy and facilitating functional gains. These interventions are typically incorporated into broader psychotherapy and neurorehabilitation programmes. Individual psychotherapy approaches and their evidence for people with brain injury will now be reviewed.

Individual psychotherapy: Approaches and evidence

Many theoretical frameworks may be applied to individual psychotherapy with people with brain injury. These include psychoanalytic therapy, existential therapy, person-centred therapy, narrative therapy, behavioural therapy, cognitive-behavioural therapy, acceptance and commitment therapy and other third-wave behavioural therapies. A review of each framework and their applications in brain injury rehabilitation is beyond the scope of this chapter and can be found elsewhere (see Bowen, Yeates & Palmer, 2010; Coetzer, 2010; Klonoff, 2010; Kangas & McDonald, 2011; Lincoln, Kneebone, Macniven & Morris, 2012; Prigatano, 1999; Tyerman & King, 2008). In practice, individual psychotherapy is usually not conducted in isolation but rather is provided as part of a broader multi-disciplinary programme or within a holistic rehabilitation setting (see Klonoff, 2010; Wilson et al., 2009). The advantages of group and community-based interventions are discussed in Chapter 7.

The focus of this section is on reviewing the evidence base for individual psychotherapy approaches for people with brain injury and highlighting promising therapy advances. To date, controlled intervention studies on psychotherapy have primarily focused on mood or emotional adjustment outcomes, with very few studies assessing the impact on broader notions of self or self-identity (for exceptions, see Helffenstein & Wechsler, 1982; Medd & Tate, 2000; Thomas, Walker, Macniven, Haworth & Lincoln, 2013). Identity-oriented approaches do not just involve 'talking therapies' but incorporate functional approaches in neurorehabilitation to help people re-establish meaningful social and activity participation (Feeney & Capo, 2010; Ylvisaker et al., 2008). However, few intervention studies have evaluated the efficacy of psychotherapy combined with neurorehabilitation (e.g., Azulay, Smart, Mott & Cicerone, 2013; Dewar & Gracey, 2007; Tiersky et al., 2005). This approach is ideal for people with brain injury because the adjustment process involves both updating identity (i.e., through sense making and assimilation of the old and new self) and consolidating the new identity through everyday activities (Gracey et al., 2009; Klonoff, 2010). Wilson et al. (2009) similarly note that learning ideally occurs through interplay between experience and cognition, thus supporting changes in self at the implicational level. Creating regular opportunities for people to experience a sense of accomplishment and mastery can help overcome longstanding patterns of thinking and reacting that feed into negative self-concept (Ylvisaker & Feeney, 2000).

As well as describing approaches to psychotherapy, the evidence base for psychological treatment is essential to consider. According to the Oxford Centre for Evidence-based Medicine (OCEBM, 2011), systematic reviews of RCTs and n-of-1 trials constitute Level 1 evidence, the highest quality of evidence. An individual RCT or observational study with a very robust effect represents Level 2 evidence. Non-randomised controlled cohort or follow-up studies are rated as Level 3 evidence. A case-series, case-control studies or historical controls provide Level 4 evidence. Evidence-based mechanistic reasoning (or expert clinical opinion in this context) constitutes Level 5 evidence (OCEBM, 2011).

Table 6.5 summarises research that provides Level 1 or Level 2 evidence supporting the efficacy of individual psychotherapy or neurorehabilitation approaches for enhancing emotional adjustment to brain injury (for more in-depth reviews of psychotherapy and other behavioural approaches see Fann, Hart & Schomer, 2009; Tsaousides, Ashman & Gordon, 2013). Overall, there is evidence that psychotherapy is beneficial for reducing level of depression, anxiety and anger management problems after brain injury. For example, research supports the efficacy of CBT for reducing anxiety symptoms in people with clinical diagnoses of PTSD after mild to moderate TBI (Bryant et al., 2003) and other anxiety disorders after moderate to severe TBI (Hsieh, Ponsford, Wong, Schönberger, Taffe & McKay, 2012b).

A broader review of the psychotherapy literature indicates that the programme intensity and delivery format are important considerations. For example, brief mindfulness interventions (i.e., 1–5 sessions) failed to yield a significant improvement in emotional functioning for people with brain injury (McMillan, Robertson, Brock, & Chorlton, 2002; O'Neill & McMillan, 2012). However, an 8-week mindfulness-based cognitive therapy intervention by Bédard et al. (2012) was effective in reducing depressive symptoms, but not anxiety symptoms, for people with TBI ($n = 23$). Further, Azulay and colleagues (2013) found that 10 sessions of mindfulness-based stress reduction significantly improved quality of life, self-efficacy and working and attention skills for people with mild TBI ($n = 22$). Bombardier et al. (2009) demonstrated the efficacy of brief scheduled telephone-based counselling (i.e., up to seven sessions) for improving mood in the first 12 months after TBI (see Table 6.5). Yet, a subsequent larger multi-centre study of the same intervention approach failed to replicate these findings (Bell et al., 2011). Therefore, it is unclear whether telephone-based counselling is sufficient to enhance psychological adjustment during community re-integration after TBI.

Some preliminary research supports the efficacy of internet-delivered CBT. In a non-randomised group study, Topolovec-Vranic et al. (2010) evaluated the efficacy of six weekly sessions of internet-delivered CBT (MoodGym) for people with mild to moderate TBI who experienced depression ($n = 21$). They reported a significant reduction in depressive symptoms at post-intervention, which was maintained at 12-months follow-up. However, in addition to the lack of control group, their study had low retention rates (i.e., 64 per cent at post-interventions and 43 per cent at follow-up) and participants reported that concentration, memory and comprehension problems affected their participation in the internet-based sessions.

Table 6.5 Summary of Level 1 and Level 2 evidence supporting the effectiveness of psychotherapy for people with brain injury

Research evidence	Treatment focus	Study details	Psychological treatment approach	Overall findings
Level 1: Systematic reviews (note: results are reported separately where meta-analysis was not conducted)				
Hackett, Anderson, House and Halteh (2008) Cochrane review	Prevention of depression post-stroke*	Forster & Young (1996), $n = 240$, average of 8 sessions over 6 months	Specialist nursing intervention (problem-solving, goal setting and information provision). Control: usual care	Small but significant benefits for depression and psychological distress
		Goldberg, Segal, Berk, Schall & Gershkoff (1997), $n = 56$, weekly phone calls and monthly home visits for 12 months	Home-based multi-disciplinary psychosocial support (e.g., psychology; psychiatry; recreation therapy). Control: usual care	
		House (2000), $n = 450$, 1–10 (median of 5) fortnightly sessions	Treatment: Problem-solving therapy; Attention control: non-specific volunteer visits. Control: usual care, no visits	
		Watkins et al. (2007), $n = 411$, 4 weekly sessions	Treatment: motivational interviewing. Control: usual care	
Soo & Tate (2007) Cochrane review	Treatment of anxiety/PTSD after mild-moderate TBI	Bryant et al. (2003), $n = 24$, 5 × 90-minute weekly sessions	CBT: education, relaxation, exposure, cognitive restructuring; control: supportive counselling (education and problem-solving)	Significantly lower incidence of PTSD and level of PTSD and anxiety symptomatology
		Tiersky et al. (2005), $n = 20$, 3 × weekly for 11 weeks	50 mins of CBT and 50 mins of neurorehabilitation: stress management and coping skills training, and strategies for improving cognitive function. Control: wait list/attention control	Significant reduction in anxiety symptoms
		Helffenstein & Wechsler (1982), $n = 16$, 20 × 60-minute sessions	Interpersonal process recall therapy (video-taped interaction, reviewing video, feedback and skill development). Control: individual sessions with no feedback	Significant decrease in trait anxiety and improvement in self-concept, interpersonal and communication skills

Level 2: Individual RCTs

Study	Intervention	Participants	Description	Outcome
Medd & Tate (2000)	Cognitive behavioural intervention for anger management difficulties	16 participants with brain injury (mixed aetiology), 5–8 weekly sessions	CBT: stress inoculation training, self-awareness training and anger management strategies. Waitlist control: daily anger monitoring	A significant decrease in self-reported anger relative to waitlist. No differences in self-esteem, anxiety, depression or self-awareness
Powell, Heslin & Greenwood (2002)	Community-based multi-disciplinary rehabilitation	94 community-based participants with TBI. Outreach treatment for a mean of 2 sessions per week for 27 weeks	Individualised goal-planning and multi-disciplinary treatment in the home and community. Control: information provision on alternative resources	A higher proportion of individuals in the outreach intervention experienced improved psychological well-being compared with controls
Hodgson, McDonald, Tate & Gertler (2005)	CBT for social anxiety after ABI (mixed aetiology)	12 participants allocated to CBT (9–14 sessions) or the waitlist using a case-control procedure	CBT: relaxation, cognitive strategies, graduated exposure and training assertiveness skills. Control: waitlist	Improvements in general anxiety and depression, but not social anxiety or self-esteem, compared to waitlist
Bombardier et al. (2009)	Telephone-based support to reduce depressive symptoms in the first 12 months post-TBI	171 people with TBI discharged from an inpatient unit, up to 7 sessions over 9 months	Scheduled telephone intervention involving problem-solving and behavioural activation. Control: usual care.	Usual care participants developed more severe depressive symptoms in the first 12 months. Treatment group reported lower severity of depression symptoms
Hsieh et al. (2012b)	CBT and motivational interviewing for treating anxiety after moderate to severe TBI	27 participants with moderate-severe TBI, 12 weekly sessions	Motivational interviewing and CBT (MI+CBT), non-directive counselling (NDC) plus CBT and treatment as usual (TAU)	Both treatment groups displayed a greater reduction in anxiety than TAU. Those in the MI+CBT group displayed a significantly greater reduction in anxiety, stress and non-productive coping
Thomas et al. (2013)	CALM (communication and low mood) study of behavioural therapy for people with aphasia after stroke	105 people with stroke, therapy provided for up to 3 months (3–18 sessions)	Home-based behavioural therapy which combined supported communication, education, activity monitoring and scheduling and graded task assignments. Control: usual care	After controlling for baseline functioning, behavioural therapy was associated with significantly lower depression and higher self-esteem at post-intervention and 3-month follow-up

* A separate Cochrane review by Hackett, Anderson, House and Xia (2008) found no evidence to support the effectiveness of psychotherapy for treating people with a clinical diagnosis of depression post-stroke.

Ashman and Tsaousides (2012) compared the efficacy of 16 sessions of CBT ($n = 21$) and supportive psychotherapy (SPT, $n = 20$) for treating depressive disorders after TBI. The CBT programme focused on identifying and modifying unhelpful thoughts and behaviours to improve mood. It was adapted to address TBI-related cognitive deficits with compensatory strategies tailored to participants' needs. SPT was described as a client-centred programme designed to improve individuals' coping skills through problem-solving, education and positive behaviour support (see clinical trials NCT00211835). Within-group analyses indicated that remission rates of depression were significant for both interventions (i.e., 57 per cent for CBT and 40 per cent for supportive psychotherapy), but did not significantly differ between the groups, possibly because of inadequate power. It is noteworthy that effective principles of psychotherapy were incorporated in both interventions, and so it is likely that non-specific therapeutic factors (e.g., working alliance) contributed to the positive outcomes.

There are some mixed findings concerning the efficacy of psychotherapy for people with stroke. For example, although pilot findings of a CBT intervention for post-stroke depression were promising (Lincoln, Flannaghan, Sutcliffe & Rother, 1997), a subsequent RCT failed to support the efficacy of CBT for improving mood in individuals with post-stroke depression (Lincoln & Flannaghan, 2003). As summarised in Table 6.5, a systematic review by Hackett et al. (2008) found significant but small effects of motivational interviewing and problem-solving therapy for improving psychological adjustment after stroke. More recently, Watkins et al. (2011) investigated the longer-term effects of their early motivational interviewing intervention (Watkins et al., 2007). The 12-months follow-up revealed significant benefits of motivational interviewing over usual care for mood (48 per cent and 38 per cent normal mood respectively) and mortality (6.5 per cent and 13 per cent respectively). Such findings are based on a very large consecutive cohort ($n = 411$) who were not receiving other psychiatric or clinical psychology intervention at the time of recruitment. There is currently no Level 1 or Level 2 evidence to support the effectiveness of psychotherapy for treating people with a clinical diagnosis of depression after stroke (Hackett et al., 2008).

However, findings of the recent Communication and Low Mood (CALM) stroke study by Thomas and colleagues (2013) are very promising. A sample of 105 people with aphasia and 'low mood' (screened for using two brief self-report measures) were randomly allocated to behavioural therapy ($n = 51$) or usual care ($n = 51$). The behavioural therapy over three months (3–18 sessions) was home-based and combined supported communication, education, activity monitoring and scheduling and graded task assignments. After controlling for baseline functioning, behavioural therapy was associated with a significantly greater reduction in depression (self and observer rated) and higher self-esteem (Visual Analogue Self-Esteem Scale) at post-intervention and 3-months follow-up than usual care. The benefits of intervention did not extend to improvement in leisure participation or reduction in caregiver strain. It is noteworthy that the session content, intensity and duration of behavioural therapy varied considerably, as decided upon by the therapist, and therefore the mechanisms underlying improvement in psychological status need to be further investigated.

In addition to controlled group studies, the efficacy of CBT is supported by numerous case studies (Level 4 evidence). For example, Ownsworth (2005) described the successful application of CBT for treating social anxiety disorder and depression in a woman with severe TBI. Williams, Evans and Fleminger (2003) demonstrated the efficacy of combining neurorehabilitation and CBT to treat obsessive-compulsive disorder after TBI. Dewar and Gracey (2007) also combined CBT with neurorehabilitation strategies to treat anxiety and support identity reformation in a woman with herpes simplex viral encephalitis. Further, Gracey, Oldham and Kritzinger (2007) used CBT to treat seizure-related panic symptoms following stroke, and demonstrated positive changes in mood, coping and target cognitions.

In summary, there is a growing body of evidence that supports the efficacy of psychotherapy for people with brain injury, particularly approaches based on the CBT framework. The following sections provide an overview of CBT and ways of adapting therapy for people with brain injury.

CBT: An overview and applications in brain injury

CBT focuses on the role of cognitions in developing and maintaining emotional distress and maladaptive behaviours (Beck, 2005). A main premise of CBT is that psychological problems arise from the subjective interpretations that people give to their experiences, which are filtered through their core beliefs and assumptions (Bennett-Levy, Westbrook, Fennell, Cooper, Rouf, & Hackmann, 2004). The CBT framework broadly encompasses a range of therapy approaches including psychoeducation, collaborative goal setting, motivational interviewing, problem-solving, cognitive techniques (e.g., monitoring and restructuring thoughts) and behavioural therapy (e.g., exposure and behavioural activation). The general goals of CBT are to identify and modify biases in people's thinking, and develop and test new cognitions that give rise to more positive schemas about one's self and the world (Beck, 2005).

After building rapport, the initial focus of therapy is on examining how people process information about themselves and the world, and identifying common thinking patterns and the cognitive schemas these represent (Bennett-Levy et al., 2004). Interviews, self-report questionnaires and self-monitoring records are typically used for assessment. Self-monitoring of daily experiences using the ABC (i.e., Activating event, Beliefs and Consequences) framework provides information to guide the clinical formulation and psychoeducation regarding the role of cognitions in developing and maintaining psychological distress (i.e., the interaction between cognitions, physiology, behaviour and affect). The ABC exercise helps people to recognise their common cognitive distortions or unhelpful thought patterns (e.g., all-or-nothing thinking, catastrophising) (Fennell, 2000). The following case illustrates the use of the ABC exercise.

Janelle was a 45-year-old woman who developed severe social anxiety and depression following a TBI four year ago. She was taught to self-monitor distressing daily situations using the ABC framework and her diary entries were reviewed in therapy each week. Some example entries are presented in Figure 6.2 (see Ownsworth, 2005).

CBT involves a collaborative process of exploring, questioning and challenging underlying beliefs and unhelpful assumptions. Cognitive restructuring techniques include:

a. Guided discovery (or Socratic dialogue) using a series of questions to gradually uncover and challenge beliefs;
b. The three-questions technique to examine the evidence (e.g., What is the evidence for this belief? How else can you interpret this situation? If that was true, what would it mean for you?) to understand the basis for and meaning of self-defeating beliefs;
c. Thought challenging or counters concerning a belief (e.g., Is it accurate or realistic?) and weighing up the advantages and disadvantages of holding particular beliefs (e.g., Is it helpful to think this way?);
d. Cognitive rehearsal of an upcoming event and anticipating thoughts, emotions and behavioural reactions for both undesirable and desirable outcomes (Clark, & Beck, 1999; Fennell, 2000).

Behavioural techniques are an integral aspect of CBT, and include behavioural experiments (i.e., planned experiential activities designed to test the validity of beliefs and to develop and verify more adaptive ones), graded activity scheduling, systematic desensitisation, behavioural rehearsal or roleplay, relaxation exercises (e.g., deep breathing and progressive muscle relaxation), and social skills and coping skills training (e.g., assertiveness, problem-solving). Homework is an essential component of CBT, and may include self-monitoring, behavioural experiments, practising relaxation and cognitive restructuring exercises, and scheduled activities to promote generalisation and maintenance beyond therapy (Bennett-Levy et al., 2004; Fennell, 2000; Gracey et al., 2009).

Cognitive techniques used with Janelle included the downward-arrow technique (see Fennell, 2000), which entailed a series of probing questions regarding her beliefs from the recorded ABCs. Prompts included: 'If that was true, what would it mean to you?' and 'If so, why would that be so bad?' These questions led to the identification of general statements that reflected her core beliefs; '[It means] I don't have any control' and 'I'll never be a patch on who I was'. Her anxiety and avoidance in everyday situations appeared to represent deeper issues concerning perceived loss of control over her life and threats to her self-identity. Upon this realisation Janelle became quite distressed, and received emotional support from the therapist. She was very motivated to learn cognitive restructuring techniques and participate in behavioural experiments to test and modify her beliefs. Graded activity scheduling was used to develop opportunities for self-mastery and accomplishment (e.g., Tai Chi and craft). Janelle also participated in three group therapy sessions as part of an experiential learning exercise and to apply anxiety management skills. The final therapy sessions focused on goal setting and maintenance and generalisation of cognitive and behavioural strategies. After 13 therapy sessions Janelle's post-

A – activating event	B – beliefs (immediate thoughts and delayed interpretations)	C – consequences
Receiving an unexpected visitor	*I won't be able to understand what they say or speak properly. I'll have to offer them a cup of tea and they will see me making a mistake.* *I can't bear for people to see me like this!*	Anxiety, apprehension, sweating, couldn't concentrate, felt dizzy
Telephone ringing	*Why is someone calling me? They are checking up on me. They'll ask me questions that I can't answer and I'll look stupid.* *I can't stand it – why can't they leave me alone?*	Frustration, anxiety, despair; didn't answer the phone – but then felt more anxious about what might happen
Mishearing the bus driver (I thought he asked for my fare, but he asked 'How has your day been?')	*He thinks I'm rude – or even worse, that I'm stupid.* *I can't trust myself to function any more!*	Depressed, anxious, embarrassed, felt uptight on the bus and dreaded walking past him to get off

Figure 6.2 Examples of Janelle's ABC diary entries

intervention assessment identified a marked reduction in her level of social anxiety and depression, and her social interaction and activity participation had greatly increased (Ownsworth, 2005).

Adapting CBT for people with brain injury

As reviewed in the previous section, CBT is currently the most researched approach to psychotherapy and has demonstrated efficacy for people with brain injury (e.g., Soo & Tate, 2007; Hsieh et al., 2012a). Although the structured approach of CBT is viewed as beneficial for people with brain injury, there is considerable emphasis on verbal skills, remembering information from previous sessions and transfer of skills into the home environment. Metacognitive and executive impairments may compromise people's self-reflective capacity and ability to regulate their thoughts and behaviour (Hodgson et al., 2005). It therefore is important to adapt psychotherapy according to people's physical, cognitive and behavioural impairments. Although general guidelines for enhancing participation were presented earlier (see Table 6.1), some authors have made more specific suggestions in the context of their treatment approach (e.g., Hodgson et al., 2005; Klonoff, 2010; Medd & Tate, 2000) and description of manualised protocol (e.g., Hsieh et al., 2012a; 2012b). Based on this literature and my own clinical experiences, a summary of recommended adaptations to psychotherapy for people with brain injury is presented in Table 6.6.

Table 6.6 Recommended adaptations to psychotherapy for people with brain injury

Effects of brain injury	Strategy or therapy adaptation	Sources
Low motivation and self-efficacy	• Motivational interviewing: elicit the person's values, explore discrepancies between desired and current states, perform a cost-benefits analysis; recognise previous achievements, develop commitment statements and revisit these regularly • Support people to develop personal mottos to motivate action, provide self-affirmation and assist coping efforts, with visual reminders • Metaphoric identity mapping: develop personal metaphors using the person's own words and analogies, identify obstacles to goals and develop action strategies to support accomplishment	Hsieh et al. (2012a), Klonoff (2010), Ylvisaker & Feeney (2000), Ylvisaker et al. (2008)
Fatigue and reduced attention and processing speed	• Shorten sessions and build in breaks • Provide a clear session plan, and cues to support the person to stay on track • Alternate between cognitive techniques and physical and behavioural exercises • Pacing principles to present information and feedback, with a summary of key points	Ashworth et al. (2011), Hodgson et al. (2005), Hsieh et al. (2012a), Medd & Tate (2000), Wilson et al. (2009)
Memory and learning problems	• Repetition, summary sheets and spaced retrieval of key concepts • Teach new skills using procedural learning and practice in a graduated and systematic fashion • Development of a portfolio of personal background information, major events and achievements to support autobiographical memory • Dictaphones or DVD recordings of therapy content • Multi-modal presentation of important concepts (e.g., mindmaps, written and pictorial aids) • Personal digital assistants (PDAs), cueing devices and other external memory aids to support recall of goals and action strategies	Ashworth et al. (2011), Hsieh et al. (2012a), Klonoff (2010), Wilson et al. (2009)
Planning and organisational difficulties	• Structured therapy folder to organise session handouts and clear and simple homework sheets • Schematic identity maps to link goals and action strategies with everyday routines • Prompts for person to refer to the folder and maps during sessions and develop a routine for completing tasks outside therapy (support with external cues from mobile phone or family member)	Hseih et al (2012a), Klonoff (2010), Ylvisaker & Feeney (2000)

Effects of brain injury	Strategy or therapy adaptation	Sources
Problems with abstract reasoning	• Simplify cognitive techniques, develop user-friendly language and concrete and personally meaningful analogies (e.g., a brick wall to convey obstacles, changing gears to convey mental flexibility) • Use of cartoons as a therapeutic tool (e.g., gypsy and crystal ball to convey mind reading as a cognitive distortion) • Practical assignments to apply new skills in a behavioural or practical sense	Hseih et al (2012a), Klonoff (2010)
Difficulty with idea generation and problem-solving	• Present a small selection of ideas and provide hypothetical problems (initially non-personalised) to practise brain-storming of solutions	Hsieh et al. (2012a), Wilson et al. (2009)
Self-regulation impairments	• Involve significant others to prompt strategy use and reinforce new behaviours in the home and community • Self-instructional training techniques (e.g., stop–think–do, Goal Management Training) • Use of mindfulness techniques and content-free cuing to train people to stop, check, notice and re-direct behaviour in accordance with their goals and values	Hodgson et al. (2005), Levine et al. (2011), Medd & Tate (2000), Ownsworth, Fleming et al. (2006)
Problems with verbal expression	• Use of artwork, photograph montages, DVDs, simplified diagrams (e.g., spider charts, bull's eyes) and symbolic representations of one's life story and brain injury (e.g., see Wilson et al., 2009, p.73)	Klonoff (2010), Lorenz (2010), Wilson et al. (2009)
Emotionality and perseverative thinking	• Teach relaxation and re-direction techniques • Avoid introducing potentially distressing or emotionally laden topics at the end of a session or at the end of a week • To help cognitive shift, use of self-reflection exercises at the end of the session (e.g., 'what have I learnt about myself?')	Klonoff (2010), Ownsworth, Turpin et al. (2008)

Third-wave cognitive and behavioural therapies

As an alternative or adjunct to CBT, the potential of 'third-wave cognitive and behavioural therapies' for enhancing psychological well-being after brain injury has been recognised. Two examples considered here include Acceptance and Commitment Therapy (ACT; Hayes, 2002) and Compassion Focused Therapy (CFT; Gilbert 2010). Kangas and McDonald (2011) proposed that the ACT framework is well suited to addressing psychological difficulties for people with mild to moderate brain injury. The fundamental goal of ACT is to promote people's acceptance of their situation and commitment to living a purposeful life. ACT seeks to improve a person's functionality by focusing on values, valued-guided actions and activity participation that supports well-being (Hayes, 2002). Although there are parallels between ACT and the approaches of CBT and MIM, a main distinction relates to the nature and purpose of cognitive techniques in ACT. Specifically, ACT teaches people to accept and live with their emotions, bodily sensations and thoughts (for a concise introduction to ACT see Harris, 2009). The core processes and skills for enhancing 'psychological flexibility' include:

- Acceptance: accepting that negative and positive thoughts and feelings come and go and are outside one's control;
- Cognitive defusion: observing one's thoughts in a mindful way and viewing these from a different perspective (i.e., allowing thoughts to come and go) without challenging or countering the thought;
- Being in the present moment: focusing attention on one's experiences and interactions within the environment that are present-in-the-moment;
- Self-as-context: taking a step back to observe different aspects of self and how they co-exist (e.g., we are not defined by certain thoughts, feelings or actions);
- Identifying personal values and goals and how these can guide one's actions despite obstacles;
- Committed action: moving in the direction of, and living in accordance with one's values through committed actions (Hayes, 2002; Kangas & McDonald, 2011).

Some neurorehabilitation interventions have incorporated ACT principles; for example, use of mindfulness exercises to promote 'present-mindedness' in Goal Management Training (see Levine et al., 2011). Lundgren, Dahl, Melin and Kies (2006) applied ACT techniques more extensively to improve self-management of seizures and well-being of people with epilepsy. A non-controlled group intervention study by Bédard et al. (2003) evaluated the efficacy of a 12-week mindfulness stress-reduction training programme for people with mild to moderate TBI ($n = 10$). Significant pre–post improvements in quality of life and mood symptoms were reported, although not for depressive symptoms. However, as previously discussed, there is some evidence that group-based mindfulness-based stress reduction improves energy levels and emotional status (Bédard et al., 2012) and quality of life, self-efficacy and cognitive skills after TBI (Azulay et al., 2013). Interventions that trained mindfulness or meditation skills in isolation were not found to improve emotional functioning after brain injury (McMillan et al., 2002; O'Neill & McMillan, 2012). Naturally, it may be argued that the psychological flexibility skills of ACT are just as challenging for people with brain injury to learn as cognitive restructuring skills in CBT. There may be potential to incorporate ACT techniques into neurorehabilitation interventions to enhance their effectiveness (e.g., Levine et al., 2011). More generally, controlled intervention studies are needed to determine the efficacy of therapy approaches based on ACT and factors influencing their effectiveness.

Compassion Focused Therapy (CFT; Gilbert, 2010) has also been described under the rubric of third-wave cognitive and behavioural approaches. The CFT approach represents an integration of theories from neuroscience, attachment theory, and evolutionary psychology and places particular emphasis on emotional experience and affect regulation (see Gilbert, 2010). People's cognitions and emotions are linked to three affect regulation systems, namely: 1) threat and self-protection system (detects threat and activates protective or defensive behaviours); 2) drive and excitement system (provides motivation to gain resources and achieve goals); and 3) soothing and contentment system (promotes feelings of emotional security and calm). Psychological distress is proposed to arise from an imbalance between these systems, for example, excessive activation of the threat system and inadequate stimulation of the soothing and contentment system. This may arise from external (e.g., negative feedback or lack of goal achievement) or internal (e.g., self-criticism) sources of threat, which trigger negative emotions such as anxiety, shame and self-blame. Activity avoidance and social disengagement are safety strategies employed which typically perpetuate the person's distress over time. The CFT framework seems very applicable for people with brain injury given their experience of interpersonal stressors and thwarted goals.

CFT broadly aims to improve the balance between the affect regulation systems. This may entail supporting individuals to find meaning in their lives and achieve personally valued goals, thus stimulating the drive and excitement system. Furthermore, compassionate mind training (CMT) techniques aim to reduce threat processing by activating the soothing–contentment system to promote self-compassion (i.e., kindness and understanding towards one's self) and, ultimately, 'shifting the affective textures to the self' (Ashworth et al., 2011, p. 128). Two case studies have applied CFT within broader psychotherapy interventions for people with TBI (Ashworth et al., 2011) and stroke (Shields & Ownsworth, 2013). For example, Ashworth et al. (2011) found that CBT was of limited effectiveness for managing negative mood for 'Jenny' a woman with severe TBI. CFT was introduced in session 7 and continued for 17 sessions. Techniques included building a CFT-based formulation, psychoeducation on the CFT model, monitoring self-critical thoughts, exploring the source of these thoughts through her life narrative, and learning to self-soothe using CMT (e.g., noticing self-critical thoughts and using imagery of the 'perfect nurturer' to reframe these thoughts). The post-intervention assessment with Jenny indicated a statistically reliable reduction in levels of anxiety and depression and improved self-esteem relative to pre-intervention.

In summary, ACT and CFT frameworks have potential to guide interventions that improve the functionality and emotional well-being of people with brain injury. To date, their utility is supported by Level 3–4 evidence, and therefore controlled intervention studies are required to advance the psychotherapy field.

Project-based interventions

Project-based interventions are based on a well-established theoretical framework and decades of clinical experience of the originators Mark Ylvisaker and Tim Feeney (Ylvisaker & Feeney, 2000; Ylvisaker et al., 2008). Drawing on models of language, metaphor, executive function and cognition, Ylvisaker and Feeney

(2000) advocated for person-centred and context-sensitive interventions. Context-sensitive relates to the need for interventions to be delivered in personally meaningful contexts and based around everyday activities, routines and interactions (e.g., family, peers, teachers and employers) to have a lasting effect. People with brain injury are more likely to achieve deeper learning, skills transfer and autonomy when they engage in meaningful and goal-relevant activities and support is gradually reduced.

The metacognitive contextual interventions developed in our own research similarly focus on training internal self-monitoring and strategy use during daily occupational activities. The efficacy of this approach for improving self-regulation skills is supported by single-case experimental research (Ownsworth, Fleming et al., 2006; Ownsworth, Quinn et al., 2010) and RCTs (Ownsworth, Fleming et al., 2008; Schmidt et al., 2013). However, Ylvisaker and Feeney's project-based learning (PBL) is more identity-oriented because their approach focuses on reconstructing a 'satisfying sense of self' and concurrently targets cognitions, emotions and behaviour. Using the MIM approach outlined earlier, people with brain injury are supported to develop an alternative and compelling schematic mental model of self. PBL provides the opportunity for people to update and consolidate the new identity through positive learning experiences and natural supports. People's association with their updated identity is strengthened by extensive participation in activities that enable them to apply new mental models of self and create a history of successful life experiences.

As described by Feeney and Capo (2010), personally meaningful and sufficiently challenging projects need to be designed that draw upon a person's interests, goals and skills, as opposed to their deficits and limitations. Projects take several weeks or months to complete and produce concrete outcomes or end-products (e.g., community artwork, a multi-media presentation or fundraising target). Projects ideally extend across different life contexts and have a positive impact on others. PBL requires careful planning and organisation, and involves the following steps: 1) specifying desired outcomes; 2) developing an action plan (i.e., logistics, resources, timeline and supports); 3) anticipating and managing obstacles or setbacks; and 4) reviewing progress and project outcomes. Project management relies upon higher order cognitive processes (e.g., planning, initiation, cognitive flexibility and strategic behaviour), and therefore people learn to develop and apply strategies in a range of contexts. PBL can also improve communication and teamwork skills and establish new group memberships (see Chapter 7).

Overall, PBL represents a theory-guided and practical approach to supporting identity reformation following brain injury. PBL has long been used in clinical practice by its developers, who provide numerous case examples in the literature (see Feeney & Capo, 2010; Ylvisaker et al., 2008). However, controlled intervention studies are needed to strengthen the evidence base for PBL in brain injury rehabilitation. There are some parallels between PBL and the portfolio and project work described by Wilson et al. (2009), and self-narrative approaches (e.g., Lorenz, 2010). Furthermore, the emphasis on fostering optimism, meaningful engagement and personal strengths is consistent with positive psychology principles (see Evans, 2011).

Technological frontiers in brain injury rehabilitation

Technological advances in neurorehabilitation provide novel ways to compensate for cognitive impairments that disrupt everyday activities and continuity of self. In particular, the integration of episodic memories, new learning and prospective remembering supports autobiographical self (Conway, 2005; Tulving, 1985). Impairments in working memory and attentional control can interrupt self-monitoring and self-regulation of behaviour and goal attainment. One of the earliest technological innovations designed to support memory and executive functions after brain injury was the NeuroPage service (Wilson, Evans, Emslie & Malinek, 1997), a reminder system that uses a paging company to send timely text messages to the person's pager or mobile phone. Unlike paper-based aids (e.g., diaries), this alerting system compensates for both memory (retrospective and prospective remembering) and executive function impairments (organisation and goal management). The efficacy of NeuroPage for enhancing home independence and community functioning and reducing caregiver strain is supported by Level 1 (e.g., Fish, Manly, & Wilson, 2008; Teasdale, Emslie, Quirk, Evans, Fish & Wilson, 2009) and Level 2 (Wilson, Emslie, Quirk & Evans, 2001) evidence. In a novel application, Yeates, Hamill et al. (2008) used NeuroPage to prompt more adaptive thoughts regarding post-injury identity and enhance mood in the context of cognitive analytic therapy.

Many commercial technological devices have also demonstrated effectiveness for supporting everyday memory function and goal attainment, including PDAs, smartphones, digital voice recorders and other external cueing devices (e.g., Hart, Hawkey, & Whyte, 2002; Svoboda & Richards, 2009; Svoboda, Richards, Leach & Mertens, 2012). The selection of aids and training in their use needs to be tailored to people's neuropsychological status and level of support available beyond the intervention (Svoboda et al. 2012). The advent of the Short Messaging Service (SMS) represents a particularly accessible technology for use in neurorehabilitation. In an RCT, Culley and Evans (2010) evaluated the effectiveness of SMS texts to support recall of therapy goals. They found that sending SMS texts three times a day for 14 days significantly improved recall of therapy goals relative to the control condition. Of course, drawing people's attention to their goals is only beneficial if this prompts the actions required to complete goal-related tasks. Accordingly, Gracey et al. (2012) found that content-free cueing combined with Goal Management Training (Assisted Intention Monitoring) was effective in supporting the achievement of daily intentions for people with executive function impairments.

In addition to prospective memory and alerting devices, technology to support autobiographical memory has been developed. SenseCam, a sensor augmented wearable stills camera, was developed as a retrospective aid to support recollection of earlier experiences (see Berry et al., 2007). SenseCam can capture several hundred images per day, which can be uploaded to a computer and viewed individually or as an entire sequence. Berry et al. (2007) trialled the use of SenseCam with a woman (Mrs B) with severe amnesia after limbic encephalitis. Mrs B wore SenseCam to remember events that were considered interesting or non-routine. They found that viewing the images and discussing the events with her husband was more effective (i.e., 80 per cent retention) than diary recordings of events (49 per cent retention). Mrs B expressed that she felt less anxious about remembering important events when she wore SenseCam (Berry et al., 2007). Remarkably, the events supported by SenseCam were retained several months afterwards. Functional neuroimaging indicated that successful recognition of the SenseCam rehearsed images was associated with frontal and posterior cortical activation (i.e., regions subserving episodic memory) (Berry et al., 2009). Therefore, SenseCam appears to enhance rehearsal and reconsolidation processes that support autobiographical recollection.

SenseCam has also been used in the context of psychotherapy as a memory aid for a man with social phobia and panic symptoms after TBI (Brindley, Bateman & Gracey, 2011). SenseCam was used to record 'emotional trigger events' to support rehearsal and improve retrieval of details regarding the emotional event and his associated thoughts and feelings. The results of a single-case experiment indicated that retention of emotional trigger events was greater with SenseCam (94 per cent) than with conventional recording sheets (22 per cent) or no strategy (39 per cent). Although the participant's level of depression and anxiety did not change between the initial and follow-up assessments, some improvement in self-esteem was evident. The participant's feedback also suggested that self-efficacy about improving his memory had increased, which enhanced his 'sense of hope for the future' (p. 753).

Overall, technological aids that support prospective remembering and autobiographical recall show great promise in supporting people to accomplish their goals and recall salient everyday experiences. In turn, this may support their continuity of self and enhance self-worth. Further evaluation of the application of technological aids to support cognitive and emotional functions and the impact on sense of self would advance the field.

Conclusions

The effectiveness of identity-orientated therapy depends in part on the quality of the therapeutic alliance and people's engagement in therapy. Psychoeducation and feedback on naturalistic tasks can help to people to recognise changes in their abilities and improve their self-regulation skills. The use of client-centred goal setting can increase engagement in therapy and facilitate goal attainment. Although there are many psychotherapy frameworks applied in brain injury rehabilitation, CBT is currently the most evidence-based approach. Overall, there is growing evidence that CBT interventions can improve psychological well-being after brain injury, although few studies have assessed the impact of CBT on broader notions of self (i.e., self-concept and identity). Third-wave cognitive and behavioural approaches also show potential for enhancing psychological well-being, but are yet to be rigorously evaluated. Project-based learning combines metaphoric identity mapping with neurorehabilitation techniques to support people to establish a realistic and adaptive self-identity. Technological aids that support memory and executive functions present new possibilities for supporting continuity of self and goal achievement. The next chapter focuses on the provision of rehabilitation and support in a social context through group and community-based initiatives.

7 Group and community-based interventions

After brain injury, people often experience a loss of roles, relationships and activities and general depletion of their social network. This affects people's sense of belonging, connection to others, and contribution to society. The importance of social factors in adjustment has long been recognised, and group interventions have been the cornerstone of holistic rehabilitation programmes since the 1970s. Social identity perspectives on brain injury rehabilitation emphasise the importance of social connection for supporting people to rediscover a personally meaningful place in the world. This chapter reviews group and community-based approaches that contribute to identity reconstruction of adults with brain injury. Approaches include structured group interventions, holistic neuropsychological programmes, and developing sustainable networks of support through work re-entry, volunteering, advocacy, collaborative group projects and leadership initiatives in the local community. The chapter concludes by discussing the potential for social media to enhance social functioning and well-being after brain injury.

The impact of social identification on well-being

Chapter 6 provided a review of interventions supporting individuals to make sense of and cope with the impact of brain injury. Theoretical perspectives on identity change after brain injury emphasise that the personal self and social self are inherently linked (Klonoff, 2010; Walsh et al., 2012). As covered in Chapter 2, sense of self is largely based on the meaning we derive from our social interactions, roles and group memberships (Jetten et al., 2012; Walsh et al., 2012). Identification with valued groups can help people to feel as though they belong and matter to others, can receive support and contribute to others' well-being. A wealth of studies has highlighted the implications of group membership for health and well-being (see review by Haslam, Jetten, Postmes & Haslam, 2009). Conversely, social threat and exclusion has been found to have negative physiological and psychological consequences (Eisenberger, Lieberman, & Williams, 2003). Social loss (e.g., relationship breakdown, job loss) has been described as one of the most distressing and painful experiences in life due to devaluation of the self. Social disconnection affects people emotionally (e.g., feelings of hurt and grief) and on a neurochemical level. Indeed, research has found that the experience of social loss or rejection is linked to the same neural circuitry (i.e., dorsal anterior cingulate cortex and anterior insula) as the affective component of physical pain. Further, individuals with low self-esteem and high interpersonal sensitivity demonstrate greater psychological and neurochemical reactivity to actual or perceived social exclusion (Eisenberger, 2012).

Social identity theory proposes that people derive their sense of self from group memberships whereby the status and meanings associated with the 'in-group' influence their self-perceptions (Haslam et al. 2009). The more closely that people identify with a social group, the greater impact it has on their sense of self or how they define themselves. The change in status from various pre-injury roles and groups (e.g., worker, student, driver, husband) to that of a person with brain injury (i.e., a new in-group) can have negative psychological consequences due to the stigma attached, and self-stereotyping that ensues from identification. For example, a man with stroke expresses that because of his 'disability' he will always be 'a second class citizen', and reports feeling a sense of inferiority and shame. In contrast, viewing one's group membership differently, for example, as a 'survivor' of brain injury (i.e., beaten the odds, a second chance at life) may produce feelings of pride and stimulate personal growth (Jones et al., 2011; Levack et al., 2010).

Social networks represent people's health-related social capital, whereby social identification influences health and well-being through symptom perception, health-related norms, coping and social support (Haslam et al., 2009). Therefore, social engagement and group memberships can function as a 'social cure' in the context of adversity and illness (Jetten et al., 2012). Many empirical studies have demonstrated the protective biological and psychological effects of social connection. For example, social support and connection has been found to influence the progression of breast cancer (Nausheen, Gidron, Peveler & Moss-Morris, 2009), self-esteem and life satisfaction after heart surgery (Haslam, O'Brien, Jetten, Vormedal & Penna, 2005), life satisfaction after stroke (Haslam et al., 2008) and emotional well-being after TBI (Douglas, 2012; Kendall & Terry, 2009). Therefore, stronger ties with one's family, friends, work and community can promote better physical and psychological health.

As previously reviewed in Chapter 3, social identity perspectives have been applied to understand identity changes after brain injury (Walsh et al., 2012). Social interaction and group memberships are known to diminish after brain injury (Douglas, 2012). For example, in a study investigating email use Todis, Sohlberg, Hood and Fickas (2005) found that only 25 per cent of their brain injury sample engaged in socially interactive activities on a daily basis; instead, solo activities were most commonly reported. Haslam et al. (2008) identified that membership in multiple groups before stroke increased the likelihood of maintaining some memberships after stroke, which in turn was associated with greater life satisfaction. They proposed that groups support people to understand their place in the world, and hence retaining these memberships enhances one's sense of continuity (Haslam et al., 2008). However, cognitive deficits compromised people's ability to maintain their pre-stroke social memberships. Levack et al. (2010) identified that people with TBI commonly experience 'social disconnection', or a marked reduction of their social world due to loss of intimate relationships, friends and employment.

Similar to Haslam et al. they found that TBI reduced people's capacity to form new relationships and access social opportunities. This was attributed to changes in appearance and associated stigma and discrimination, and emotional and behavioural changes. Levack et al. (2010) emphasised the need for interventions to support people to overcome social disconnection and reconstruct their place in the world.

There are two broad rehabilitation approaches relevant to social identity reconstruction. The first more traditional approach focuses on improving physical, cognitive, behavioural and emotional competencies as a basis for pursuing valued social roles (e.g., to return to work and parenting). Group interventions can have the benefits of improving self-knowledge and skill development whilst promoting social interaction and engagement of members. Groups can be conducted at any phase of rehabilitation, although the focus often varies between early and long-term interventions. As shown in Figure 7.1, hospital-based groups mainly focus on improving functional competencies (e.g., communication and cognitive skills) to resume pre-injury activities and life roles during community-reintegration (e.g., Appleton et al., 2011; Thickpenny-Davis & Barker-Collo, 2007). Group interventions in the post-acute phase may also target functional skills, but particularly aim to improve personal and social resources (e.g., self-knowledge and strategies) to engage in new activities and social roles (e.g., Kendall, Catalano, Kuipers, Posner, Buys & Charker, 2007; Muenchberger, Kendall, Kennedy & Charker, 2011; Ownsworth et al., 2000; Ownsworth, Fleming et al., 2008).

The second approach, based on the Social Identity Model of Identity Change (see Haslam et al., 2008; Jetten & Pachana, 2012), focuses specifically on social identity reconstruction through maintaining existing social ties or building

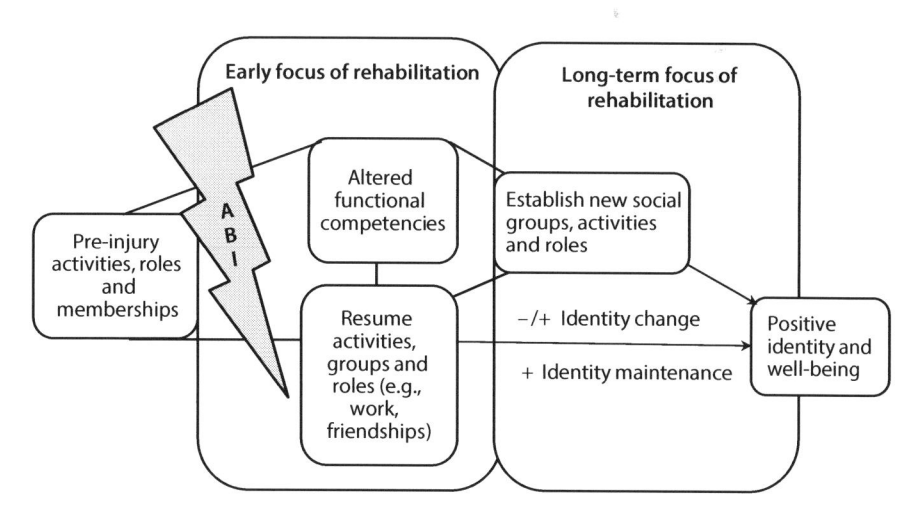

Figure 7.1 Early and long-term focus of interventions contributing to identity maintenance and change after brain injury (adapted from Haslam et al., 2008)
Note: ABI = acquired brain injury

new ones to enhance well-being after brain injury. Continuity of self can be enhanced by supporting people to maintain pre-injury activities and group memberships. Alternatively, where this is not possible or sufficient, people can be supported to develop altered identities by establishing new social groups and activities after their injury (Douglas, 2012). These new memberships can support people to develop a stronger sense of who they are and what they stand for, in light of their experience of brain injury (Jones et al., 2011; Shadden & Koski, 2007). The identity maintenance and identity change pathways are depicted in Figure 7.1. Importantly, these are not mutually exclusive because most people are likely to maintain some existing group memberships, but also develop new ones after brain injury. As noted by Jetten and Pachana (2012), the compatibility of former and new identities, or how well these can be assimilated (i.e., the old and the new me) appears key to people's adjustment and well-being. Group and community-based interventions that contribute to the identity reformation process are now reviewed.

Overview of community rehabilitation

Prior to reviewing group and community-based interventions, it is useful to consider the broader spectrum of post-acute rehabilitation programmes. To some extent, all forms of rehabilitation have a social dimension because the person with brain injury is typically working with and supported by a team of professionals and their informal support network. Based on reviews of post-acute rehabilitation (see Malec & Basford, 1996; Trexler, 2000; Turner-Stokes, 2008), there are six main approaches that vary according to setting, structure and focus, as follows:

- *Traditional outpatient therapy*: hospital-based multi-disciplinary rehabilitation, individual goal setting focusing on activities of daily living (ADLs) and early community re-entry.
- *Community re-entry and outreach services*: community-based rehabilitation with an emphasis on independent living skills, return to work or school and other avocational activities (often coordinated by a case manager).
- *Holistic neuropsychological rehabilitation*: centre-based structured day programmes with an integrated multi-disciplinary team focus on psychosocial adjustment and cognitive skills to enhance independence, productivity and social function.
- *Residential community programmes*: focus on functional skills training (e.g., ADLs) and skills maintenance within a residential environment (transitional or long-term).
- *Neurobehavioural programmes*: behaviour modification and management of neuropsychiatric problems within a structured environment.
- *Community-based support programmes*: promotion of lifelong quality of life with an emphasis on community integration and sustainable social networks.

Group interventions may be conducted within any of these broader rehabilitation contexts, and are integral to holistic programmes. The following sections review the characteristics and evidence base for group interventions following brain injury.

Group interventions

Brain injury support groups

Providing psychological support, education and skills training in groups is often a cost-effective approach to rehabilitation that capitalises on peer support in a more naturalistic setting. Groups vary in their format, level of structure, and type of facilitation. For example, long-term community support groups usually have an open format, which means that people can join or attend at any point and the meetings may continue over time with typically a small group of core or regular attendees. Brain injury support groups are often affiliated with community organisations (e.g., Headway, Brain Injury Association, Cancer Council, Stroke Association, and Encephalitis Society) and may be facilitated by a health professional or a volunteer, such as a person with brain injury or a family member. The topics and focus of informal support group meetings usually vary in response to participants' needs and preferences although guest speakers may be scheduled to share their knowledge and expertise (e.g., a physiotherapist to talk about fatigue and exercise).

The benefits of brain injury support groups have been examined in qualitative research (e.g., Ch'Ng, French & McLean, 2008; Fleming, Kuipers, Foster, Smith & Doig, 2009; Levack et al. 2010). For example, Hoen, Thelander, Worsley and Wells (1997) found that support groups were a valuable avenue for improving psychological well-being and supporting identity reconstruction of people with aphasia (see also Shadden & Koski, 2007). Interacting with other people with brain injury can normalise and validate people's experience of functional impairment and promote acceptance of the need to use strategies. Within this forum, group members are the experts because they have been 'down the rabbit-hole' and can often closely relate to other members' circumstances. The discovery of shared life experiences can reduce feelings of loneliness and isolation for both people with brain injury and their caregivers (Fleming et al., 2009). At a deeper level, participation in support groups encourages 'ongoing storying of self', or forming a coherent narrative of past, present and future selves as the group and relationships evolve over time (Shadden & Koski, 2007).

Leavitt, Lamb and Voss's (1996) naturalistic observations of nurse-facilitated brain tumour support group meetings revealed that groups provide a 'safe haven' and help people to maintain morale through stressful periods. People with brain tumour and their family members felt able to share their stories and express their greatest fears about the illness, treatment and the future. In our research we also found that people with brain tumour perceived psychological benefits from attending support groups and sharing their personal story in a newsletter. However, it is noteworthy that a woman with malignant brain tumour found support group meetings distressing because several people with the same type of tumour as hers passed away, which intensified her anxiety about dying (Ownsworth, Chambers et al., 2011).

Other possible disadvantages of open and less structured support groups is that there is potential for disharmony if some people's views and preferences are expressed and accommodated more than others. Like all social groups, some members may not relate well or like each other. Brain injury support groups are no different to other groups in this sense; however, people with brain injury can experience greater challenges with social interaction, such as reduced communication, perspective-taking and emotion regulation skills (Douglas, 2012; McDonald & Flanagan, 2004). My own experience with a brain injury social group illustrates this point. As a psychology student I volunteered for a brain injury organisation that funded community outings (e.g., bush walking, bowling and barbeques) for people with brain injury. Facilitated by a leisure coordinator, the group was mainly attended by men who were many years post-injury and had experienced family breakdown, loss of employment, and social isolation. During most outings group members would argue and their conversation focused on what they had lost since their injury. New members joining the group for an outing would typically not attend further meetings. Feedback sought from current and past attendees identified the need for a more constructive forum that supported people to improve their self-confidence, skills and life situation.

Structured group interventions

Inspired by the positive psychosocial outcomes of earlier group interventions studies (e.g., Delmonico, Hanley-Peterson & Englander, 1998; Prigatano et al., 1984), we developed the Awareness Support Programme (ASP) to improve self-awareness and psychosocial functioning of people with long-term brain injury (Ownsworth et al., 2000). The group was facilitated by a psychologist and conducted over 16 weeks, with one 90-minute session each week. Four groups were formally evaluated and group sizes ranged from 7 to 13 members (Ownsworth et al. 2000; Ownsworth & McFarland, 2004). Individuals referred to the ASP were screened for suitability using the combination of a clinical interview, neuropsychological testing and reports from relatives and referring professionals. People were considered suitable if they displayed the following characteristics:

- Adequate cognitive and communication skills to participate in 90-minute group meetings;
- Absence of severe emotional and behavioural dysfunction (e.g., suicidal ideation, psychotic symptoms, major substance abuse issues);
- Awareness of impairments at a basic level (i.e., acknowledges the brain injury and its effects on some aspects of functioning);
- Motivation to meet other people, be part of a group and produce change in their lives.

An initial planning meeting was held for group members to introduce themselves and share some level of personal background information, select topics relevant to their goals and daily life and develop guidelines for participation or 'group etiquette'. The latter process involved the group brain-storming potential situations that could arise (e.g., a person feeling upset when discussing a topic or feeling annoyed by another member's comments) and generating shared solutions. The group etiquette was summarised for participants in a brochure and displayed in the group therapy room. The group also discussed confidentiality and options for guest speakers or visitors for some topics. For example, relatives were invited to attend a later session in the programme.

The ASP was designed to be interactive, with the facilitator initially posing open questions for group discussion, and then supplementing participants' collective knowledge and strategy use with research findings and evidence-based strategies. Common topics included: understanding the brain and your injury, attention/concentration, communication and relationships, memory, emotions and coping (spanning several sessions), motivation, work, leisure and social pursuits and self-confidence and assertiveness. Each workshop was structured according to the following components:

- A brief introduction to the area;
- The group's definitions and analogies (e.g., 'what is memory');
- Changes noticed after brain injury and the everyday impact;
- Strategies participants had developed to improve their functioning;
- Further evidence-based strategies from the literature;
- Practice of skills within the group (e.g., memory exercises, use of role plays and hypothetical scenarios) and planned applications at home.

The ASP employed a combination of therapy techniques, including peer feedback, cognitive restructuring, problem-solving, social skills training, motivational interviewing, relaxation techniques and cognitive rehabilitation (i.e., remedial and compensatory techniques). A short coffee break was provided half way through each workshop, which enabled unstructured social interaction between members. Participants received handouts during each workshop for recording their ideas and experiences, and additionally received a comprehensive booklet at the end of the programme which summarised the main content across the 16 weeks, including ideas and strategies generated by the group. This information was typically recorded by a psychology student volunteer. The facilitator received weekly supervision and support from a clinical neuropsychologist.

Challenging situations often occurred when conducting the ASP groups, which sometimes represented a turning point for a participant or the group as a whole. The following case examples depict some situations encountered during the ASP and how these were managed to enhance group cohesion and relationships.

- Wendy, a 19-year-old woman who sustained her injury as a child, was very socially anxious but keen to meet other people with brain injury. During the first two sessions she stated her name, but otherwise did not speak or make eye contact with other group members. The facilitator offered an individual support session for Wendy to prepare and practise a script. She introduced herself and shared her story in session three, which was met by applause from other group members and reinforced her active contribution in future sessions. According to Wendy's mother, through meeting other people with brain injury and connecting with the group Wendy 'found her voice'.

- On the way to the third group meeting Ian left his mobile phone on the train (his fifth mobile phone lost since his accident). He came in late to the meeting, threw his bag on the table and stated 'I don't want to be part of this disabled group!' Ian left the meeting and had individual support with the facilitator after the group session. In the fourth session he apologised to the group and shared the difficulties he has accepting his brain injury and his sense of failure in being unable to return to work. The other members validated his feelings and shared their own experiences of struggling with the label of 'disability' and social exclusion. Ian became a leader of group discussions and after the programme he maintained regular contact with several members of the group.
- In one of the final group meetings Naomi spontaneously asked other group members: 'Would you be comfortable working alongside me as a colleague?' Gerard responded that although he values her friendship, he would find it difficult to work with her every day because of her emotional outbursts. From this feedback and group discussion on emotional changes after brain injury, Naomi recognised the need for individual psychotherapy to improve her emotion regulation.

These case illustrations highlight how identifying with others in a group can provide a positive means to redefine self after brain injury and motivate people to modify their behaviour and support others. Formal evaluation of the ASP (Ownsworth et al. 2000; Ownsworth & McFarland, 2004) identified significant improvements in participants' behavioural functioning (as rated by relatives), self-regulation skills and psychosocial functioning (social interaction, cognitive and emotional functioning and communication) between the pre-intervention and post-intervention assessments. Although there was no control group, a 6-months follow-up indicated that these gains were largely maintained over time. The development of self-regulation skills or ability to anticipate difficulties and apply strategies in daily life was considered a key factor contributing to the maintenance of gains. It is noteworthy that gains in social interaction were less likely to be maintained at follow-up (71 per cent had reliable improvement at post-assessment; 46 per cent had reliable maintenance of gains), potentially because the group itself was no longer a social outlet. Effort was made to encourage ongoing social activities after the 16-week programme; however, contact between group members was not often maintained. As one exception, two participants commenced their own support group, which continues today as an online forum for people with brain injury. Other strategies for sustaining social networks after the completion of group programmes are discussed later in this chapter.

Research investigating the efficacy of group therapy has focused on different aspects of psychological well-being, including self-regulation skills (Lundqvist, Linnros, Orlenius & Samuelsson, 2010), anger (Walker, Nott, Doyle, Onus, McCarthy & Baguley, 2010), depression (Bédard et al., 2003), global health, wellness and life satisfaction (Brenner et al., 2012; Kendall et al. 2007). A systematic review by Cicerone et al. (2011) found robust evidence for the effectiveness of group therapy for enhancing memory, language, social communication skills, and executive functioning.

Group interventions were recommended as a 'practice option' for treating cognitive and communication deficits.

Despite this endorsement, the impact of groups on participants' self-identity or broader notions of self has rarely been examined. As an exception, a pilot study by Vickery and colleagues (2006) evaluated the efficacy of a brief group intervention specifically designed to enhance self-concept after brain injury ($n = 18$). Guided by self-concept theory, their six-session programme (1 hour sessions) focused on enhancing 'self-complexity' and 'importance differentiation'. This entailed increasing participants' knowledge of different aspects of the self (i.e., expanding self-views) and understanding of how the importance of personal attributes to overall happiness is highly subjective (i.e., differentiation). Integration and continuity of self was supported by encouraging participants to identify negative changes (e.g., memory loss) alongside new or ongoing positive self-attributes (e.g., sense of humour). Participants completed the Head Injury Semantic Differential Scale (HISDS) at the start of group sessions 1 and 6. Given the focus on shifting participants' self-descriptions to reflect more positive views, it is perhaps not surprising that self-concept on the HISDS significantly improved between these time points. Positive changes were most evident for the following attributes: attractiveness, boredom, hopefulness, self-confidence and cooperativeness.

The pilot intervention by Vickery et al. (2006) is noteworthy as the first study to specifically evaluate the impact of group therapy on self-identity. However, limitations include the omission of a control group, lack of independence between the delivery of the group and evaluation of outcome, and use of a single outcome measure. It is also unknown whether the improvements in self-concept evident in the final session were maintained over time, and hence reflect deeper changes in self-schema.

A review of controlled group interventions in the literature identified that only a small number of RCTs (i.e., OCEBM Level 2 evidence) included measures of self-esteem or self-concept, and these were typically secondary outcomes. Rath, Simon, Langenbahn, Sherr, and Diller (2003) compared the efficacy of a 24-session CBT problem-solving skills group ($n = 27$) with conventional group rehabilitation ($n = 19$) for people with mild to severe TBI (1–6 years post-injury). The groups were designed to be equivalent in intensity (2 hours of group therapy per week) and format, and included an additional one-hour session each week to either consolidate the group material (problem-solving group) or conduct individual cognitive remediation (conventional group). Within-group analyses indicated that participants in the problem-solving group were more likely to show significant gains on the subjective and objective indices of problem-solving abilities and global self-esteem (assessed by the RSES). However, the changes in self-esteem represented a very small effect size (Cohen's $d = .22$), and the study is limited by a lack of statistical comparison between the two groups.

Self-esteem has often been measured as a secondary outcome of group therapy targeting cognitive appraisals and coping skills. For example, a 10-session coping skills group for people with TBI ($n = 31$) was found to significantly increase use of adaptive coping strategies relative to wait list controls, but no significant changes were evident for self-esteem on the RSES (Anson & Ponsford, 2006b). Similarly, 20 hours of group CBT (treatment $n = 8$; wait list $n = 9$) was found to be effective for reducing hopelessness (primary outcome), but there were no significant gains in self-esteem on the RSES (Simpson, Tate, Whiting & Cotter, 2011).

Some authors have recognised the importance of involving family caregivers to maximise the long-term effects of therapy (see also Chapter 8). For example, Backhaus, Ibarra, Klyce, Trexler and Malec (2010) evaluated the efficacy of a 12-session CBT-based coping skills group (group treatment $n = 10$; controls $n = 10$ dyads) on perceived self-efficacy and mood. The main therapy approaches included psychoeducation, psychotherapy, and stress management and problem-solving training. At post-assessment and 3-months follow-up participants with brain injury in the treatment group reported significantly greater self-efficacy, or increased ability to understand the effects of TBI and manage these effects. Although there were no differences in mood at post-treatment, control participants were more likely to report increased distress at follow-up, suggesting that the gains in self-efficacy may have acted as a stress buffer for the coping skills group. The impact of the programme on family members' well-being was not assessed.

More recently, Kelly, Ponsford and Couchman (2013) evaluated the efficacy of a family-focused group intervention for improving self-concept of people with brain injury. Forty-one individuals and their caregivers participated in a 12-week McFarlane Multifamily Group intervention, with multi-dimensional measures of self-concept (TSCS; see Chapter 5) and self-esteem (RSES) administered at pre- and post-assessment. There were no significant gains found for any self-concept domain or global self-esteem based on a comparison with a matched nonclinical control group who did not receive the intervention.

The positive impact of exercise groups on mood and self-esteem after brain injury has been demonstrated in a number of studies. An RCT by Blake and Batson (2009) found that eight sessions of Tai Chi Qigong (described as a mindful exercise with lower demands on cognitive and physical abilities than Tai Chi) was associated with significant improvements in mood and physical self-concept relative to controls. Other group exercise interventions found to improve broader self-concept after brain injury include aquatic aerobics (Driver, Rees, O'Connor & Lox, 2006) and kayaking (Fines & Nichols, 1994). Thus, a combination of group interaction and active leisure and fitness may increase feelings of personal competency and self-worth.

Overall, a review of current literature provides only limited support concerning the efficacy of group interventions for supporting identity reconstruction after brain injury, as measured by gains in self-concept. In part, this may be due to the lack of sensitivity of tools employed, particularly those assessing global self-esteem. As reviewed in Chapter 5, tools that were developed specifically for the brain injury population and capture different dimensions of self (e.g., current self-concept and self-discrepancy) may have greater utility for assessing intervention effects. However, a further issue is that some group interventions may not be sufficiently intensive to support changes in self-schema, which requires both updating and consolidating the new identity. Future research needs to determine the characteristics of groups (i.e., format, focus of sessions and intensity) that best facilitate enduring changes in self-concept.

Holistic neuropsychological rehabilitation

As discussed in Chapter 6, self-identity reconstruction is a gradual process that involves updating self-knowledge and consolidating a new identity through social interaction and activities that reinforce more adaptive and realistic notions of self (Gracey et al., 2009). A combination of therapy approaches that simultaneously target physical, cognitive and emotional functioning over time and promote social and occupational re-engagement is considered optimal. Consistent with this view, identity reconstruction is at the heart of holistic neuropsychological rehabilitation programmes which integrate cognitive rehabilitation and psychotherapy approaches within a supportive therapeutic community (Prigatano, 1999). The concept of 'therapeutic milieu' refers to the formation of a structured and supportive social and physical environment that fosters a sense of safety, trust and cooperation between clients and staff (Wilson et al., 2009). The first therapeutic milieu for brain injury was founded by Ben-Yishay and colleagues (i.e., the New York University Day Program), and was strongly influenced by Goldstein's (1959) perspectives on neuropsychological rehabilitation (see Ben-Yishay & Diller, 2011). Ben-Yishay (2008) described identity reconstitution as a hierarchical process with successive overlapping stages, namely: engagement, awareness, mastery, control, acceptance, and reconstituted ego-identity. He noted that not all clients will progress through each stage to attain a 'unified sense of selfhood' (p. 517), and that premorbid characteristics influence this process.

The multiple interacting elements within the milieu that support the identity reformation process include: development of a strong working alliance and shared understanding between the therapy team, person with brain injury and their family; individualised goal setting and psychotherapy; peer feedback and group collaboration on projects; psychoeducation and specific therapies for the functional consequences of brain injury; cognitive remediation and training in effective compensatory approaches; and family counselling (Ben-Yishay & Diller, 2011; Fordyce & Roueche, 1986; Klonoff, 2010). In the later stages of the programme, there is increasing focus on activities to support home independence, work/study re-entry and social re-engagement (Wilson et al., 2009). Although holistic rehabilitation may be guided by different theoretical orientations, programmes ultimately share the following characteristics:

- Rigorous admission assessment to determine suitability for the programme;
- Multi-disciplinary team meetings, case meetings and rehabilitation planning;
- Intensive day treatment (i.e., 4–6 hours per day for 4–5 days per week) over 3–7 months;
- Individualised goal setting and a neuropsychologically oriented programme of individual and group therapies coordinated by a lead clinician;
- Focus on developing a shared understanding and collaboration between clients and staff members, with clients involved in the day-to-day running of the centre;
- Involvement of families in assessment, rehabilitation and counselling interventions;

- Provision of, or linkage to, vocational rehabilitation and placement services;
- Monitoring and evaluation of psychological adjustment and vocational and community outcomes beyond the programme (Trexler, 2000).

An in-depth description of the background, philosophy and clinical approaches of holistic rehabilitation is available from leaders in their respective centres around the world (e.g., Ben-Yishay & Diller, 2011; Christensen, 1999; Coetzer, 2008; Prigatano, 1999; Sarajuuri & Koskinen, 2006; Wilson et al., 2009). Evaluation of holistic programmes has predominantly involved case series and quasi-experimental designs. A study by Cicerone et al. (2008) is noteworthy as the first RCT of holistic rehabilitation in the post-acute phase. A sample of 68 individuals with mild to severe TBI were randomly allocated to a holistic rehabilitation programme or standard neurorehabilitation (i.e., individual discipline-specific therapies and individual cognitive rehabilitation). Both programmes were conducted for 15 hours a week over 16 weeks. The holistic programme involved individual and group therapies that focused on development of metacognitive, emotional regulation, interpersonal and functional skills. An outcome evaluation identified that improvement in neuropsychological functioning was comparable between the groups; however, participants in the holistic programme demonstrated significantly greater gains in community functioning, employment (47 per cent vs. 21 per cent), self-efficacy, and life satisfaction than those receiving standard neurorehabilitation.

In a systematic review of rehabilitation approaches for behavioural and psychosocial disorders, Cattelani, Zettin & Zoccolotti (2010) concluded: 'Despite the variety of methodological concerns, results indicate that the greatest overall improvement in psychosocial functioning is achieved by [comprehensive holistic neuropsychological rehabilitation]' (p. 52). Furthermore, systematic reviews by both Cattelani et al. (2010) and Cicerone et al. (2011) recommended holistic brain injury programmes as a practice standard for post-acute rehabilitation. There is a general consensus that holistic rehabilitation is better suited to clients in the post-acute phase than in the acute phase. However, Cicerone et al. (2011) proposed that the rehabilitation model is optimal for people with moderate to severe brain injury, whilst Wilson et al. (2009) advocated their programme for people with mild to moderate brain injury.

Overall, it is clear from outcome evaluations that when clients meeting entry criteria receive holistic rehabilitation marked improvements in independence, psychological, interpersonal and social role functioning can be achieved (Cattelani et al., 2010; Trexler, 2000). Despite the demonstrated clinical utility and cost-effectiveness of holistic programmes (see Prigatano & Pliskin, 2003), this model may not be feasible in many rehabilitation contexts due to the intensity and duration of therapeutic input and low client to staff ratio. More research is needed to investigate the most active components of holistic rehabilitation and client characteristics and programme factors (e.g., staffing, length, intensity) that influence the psychological and social outcomes observed. Guided by theoretical advances (e.g., Y-shaped model; Gracey et al. 2009), an empirical understanding of the impact of holistic rehabilitation on self-identity reformation is needed. Such work is under way at the

Oliver Zangwill Centre (OZC), which employs a personal construct approach to examine changes in self-discrepancy and self-concept throughout rehabilitation (see Gracey et al., 2008; Wilson et al., 2009). As a major service development, holistic brain injury programmes for children have also been developed (Marcantuono & Prigatano, 2008) and are discussed in Chapter 8.

Coetzer (2008) described a model of holistic community-based rehabilitation that entails lower intensity of therapy for a longer duration than traditional programmes. This model evolved in part because of the logistics of community-based rehabilitation (e.g., rural location, travel time for home visits, client heterogeneity), but there are also particular advantages of this approach. Specifically, flexible delivery of services over a longer period may be optimal to facilitate the gradual process of adjustment and identity reformation after brain injury. The capacity to deliver rehabilitation in the home and community in addition to the rehabilitation unit provides greater opportunity to promote generalisation of skills. In this context, there is less emphasis on the therapeutic milieu and more on therapy in real-life settings with natural supports and lifelong access to services.

In summary, holistic rehabilitation focuses on supporting people with brain injury to re-establish a satisfying place in the world through intensive multi-disciplinary therapy within a therapeutic milieu. Although most programmes are centre-based, holistic rehabilitation can also be delivered in the community in a less intensive mode to provide long-term support on a more flexible 'as needs' basis. Other models of post-acute rehabilitation that focus on developing sustainable networks of support are now considered.

Developing sustainable networks of support for people with brain injury

As noted throughout this chapter, a key challenge for clinicians is how to support people with brain injury to maintain functional and psychosocial gains achieved in rehabilitation, particularly in the face of ongoing stressors and life transitions. Different approaches for maximising rehabilitation gains and well-being in the long-term include:

- Targeting the development of personal and social resources (e.g., self-efficacy, coping and social support) to support community reintegration and the expansion of people's social networks (Backhaus et al., 2010; Kendall et al., 2007);
- Programming for maintenance and generalisation of skills through the use of multiple training exemplars, application in real-life contexts and tapering of support (Feeney & Capo, 2010; Ownsworth, Fleming et al., 2006);
- Post-programme monitoring and follow-up with booster sessions as needed, for example, during transitions (Coetzer, 2008; Ownsworth, 2010);
- Case management services facilitating long-term access to support (Radford et al., 2013);
- Providing education and training to members of the person's natural support network, including family members, job coaches, employers, and public services

(Behn, Togher, Power & Heard, 2012; Ownsworth, 2010; Radford et al., 2013; Togher, McDonald, Tate, Power & Rietdijk, 2013);

- Creating long-term support avenues through continued involvement in community projects, forums, advocacy, volunteering and leadership (Kennedy, Turner & Kendall, 2011; Wilson et al., 2009).

The maintenance and generalisation of skills is a particular issue for vocational rehabilitation services, which aim to support people to achieve durable and satisfying job placements.

Work re-entry

The ability to work and engage in a meaningful vocation is closely linked to people's self-identity and broader quality of life (Ownsworth & McKenna, 2004; Prigatano, 1989). A synthesis of qualitative studies by Stergiou-Kita, Dawson and Rappolt (2012) identified four main themes concerning people's perspectives on returning to work after TBI. The first theme, 'meaning of work' related to perceptions of work providing a sense of normality, purpose and contribution, and a way for people to structure their day and achieve economic independence. Work also represented a valued social outlet and way of gaining respect from others. Secondly, the return to work process provided an avenue for 'reconciling a new identity'. People initially experimented with or tested their capabilities on work tasks. In recognising changes to personal competencies, there was often a struggle to maintain former notions of self in light of conflicting information. As people accepted changes to self, they were able to adjust their goals and develop strategies to support their abilities. The third theme, 'opportunities to try versus risk of failure' related to the importance of work trials for developing insight into one's abilities and receiving feedback. However, risks were perceived in participating in work trials too early due to the impact of poor performance evaluations on the person's emotional adjustment and social perceptions (e.g., co-workers). The final theme of 'significance of support' highlighted the importance of receiving guidance, feedback and practical and emotional support throughout the process. Members of people's support network also benefited from education about the effects of brain injury to guide their expectations and understanding of their role.

In a systematic review we identified that access to vocational rehabilitation services was a key predictor of return to work after brain injury (Ownsworth & McKenna, 2004). Established models of vocational rehabilitation for people with brain injury include comprehensive or holistic programmes, case coordination and supported employment (see review by Fadyl & McPherson, 2009). Services are typically structured to provide ongoing monitoring and intervention beyond the initial job placement to maximise retention. The focus on long-term outcomes is important because various personal and environmental factors have been found to influence people's capacity to maintain their employment position. For example, Sale, West, Sherron and Wehman (1991) found that interpersonal and emotional regulation problems were main factors related to job separations after the placement.

Conversely, environmental factors found to enhance job retention six months after a placement include positive contact with co-workers, availability of support, perceived mobility options and a good person–job match (Sale et al., 1991).

Overall, the vocational literature indicates that personal resources (e.g., pre-existing employment skills, self-awareness and strategy use) interact with environmental factors to influence long-term employment outcomes after brain injury (Ownsworth & McKenna, 2004; Stergiou-Kita et al., 2012). Hence, vocational rehabilitation needs to incorporate different levels of intervention to facilitate durable employment and support networks. Interventions include: pre-vocational counselling and skills training, advocacy and case management, education and support for family and employers, work trials, job placement, on-the-job support and work retention strategies.

As an example of this approach, we developed a metacognitive contextual approach to facilitate return to work and other occupational activities after brain injury (Ownsworth, 2010; Ownsworth, Fleming et al., 2008). Three participants (2 with TBI, 1 with stroke) in long-term unemployment participated in a 16-session programme (see Ownsworth, 2010) comprised of the following interventions:

- *Group-based skills training* (8 × 2 hour sessions): psychoeducation, peer support and feedback, development and practice of strategies to enhance cognitive performance, social skills training (e.g., interview skills and assertiveness), management of emotions, motivational problems and fatigue, and work/family balance. Participants were videotaped in a simulated job interview with self-reflection and peer feedback.
- *Individual sessions* (5 × 2 hour sessions): focus on training self-awareness and self-regulation skills on activities in the home, community and work settings.
- *Family involvement and support* (1 × 3 hour session): one group session with parents, partners and children present to discuss work/family balance, family input and need for support regarding changes in routine.
- *Disability employment service training* (2 × 3 hour sessions): 1) a group session with all participants, disability employment case managers and job coaches to provide general brain injury education; 2) participant-specific education and training with the participant, disability employment case manager, job coach, neuropsychologist and occupational therapist. Participants outlined their post-injury strengths, difficulties, strategies, goals and work preferences.
- *Work sampling:* a work skills assessment to gauge work readiness and job suitability, and provide feedback to participants.
- *Employer education and support*: the type and amount of support varied, but typically included: a) brain injury education for employers and supervisors and tailored information on participant's strengths, difficulties and strategies; b) telephone support and onsite visits by occupational therapists to observe work performance; and c) on-the-job support as needed over the first six months.

The 16-session programme supported each participant to achieve a paid job placement (12–25 hours per week), and maintain these positions for over 6 months. The disability employment service provided ongoing support for two years post-placement and supported transitions (e.g., change of supervisor and work duties). Although these outcomes are promising, caution is needed in generalising results from a case series.

A recent UK study by Radford et al. (2013) compared long-term outcomes of specialised TBI vocational rehabilitation ($n = 40$) and usual care ($n = 54$). Groups were based on residential area, and hence were not randomised. The specialised rehabilitation group received case management, which commenced at 4 weeks post-discharge with varied multi-disciplinary input and contact based on individuals' needs. Components included assessment, participant and family education, community reintegration training, pre-work training and liaison with employers to provide education and monitor the return to work plan and job coaching. Outcome assessments at 3, 6 and 12 months identified that people receiving the specialised vocational rehabilitation were more likely to return to work compared with those receiving usual care (e.g., 75 per cent vs. 60 per cent at 12 months), and this difference was greater for those with moderate to severe TBI. Individuals who returned to work reported lower levels of anxiety and depression and better quality of life irrespective of their group. A cost-effectiveness analysis identified that specialised vocational rehabilitation cost substantially less to return people to work than costs associated with usual care.

The ability to return to work has many benefits for the person with brain injury and society as a whole. However, vocational re-entry is not a feasible or desired goal for many. Return to work can have detrimental psychological consequences if the work is perceived to be highly stressful, incompatible with one's interests and capabilities and lacking in personal meaning or sense of fulfilment (Ownsworth & McKenna, 2004; Tsaousides, Ashman & Seter, 2008). Therefore, initiatives that facilitate engagement in other valued occupational roles and social groups are essential.

Community participation initiatives

A brief description of four distinct approaches for enhancing community participation and developing sustainable social networks after brain injury is presented in Table 7.1. Based on a social model of disability, Circles of Support is a well-established approach guided by a strengths-based model of practice after brain injury (see Rowlands, 2001; Willer, Allen, Anthony & Cowlan, 1993). The premise of Circles of Support is that people are best enabled to live the life they want when they have a network of supportive relationships systematically built around them. The circles include family, friends, neighbours, community services, volunteers, paid carers and professionals. As natural support networks become well established, the level of intervention from professionals (e.g., the facilitator) is gradually decreased.

Focusing on leisure activities, Douglas, Dyson and Foreman (2006) investigated whether involvement in community activities and becoming socially connected improves emotional well-being after severe brain injury. The intervention involved regional agencies supporting people with brain injury ($n = 25$) to pursue leisure activities of their own choosing and develop natural supports in their community. The events and transport were coordinated by the agency to overcome practical barriers to participation. The activities people could sample or participate in the long term included various sports (e.g., sailing, kayaking, bowling), creative arts, cooking, dancing, computers and games. Some activities already existed in the community for people with disability whilst others were specifically developed for the intervention. A 6-months follow-up evaluation identified three different participation outcomes: 1) people maintained their increased community participation; 2) people temporarily increased their participation but did not maintain their activities; and 3) people did not participate in activities. The group that sustained their participation demonstrated significant gains in social integration and improved mental health. The effects of sustained engagement were also evident from qualitative analysis, which indicated enhanced self-confidence, mood, friendships and sense of belonging.

Brain injury case management models share similar principles to Circles of Support, whereby case managers aim to link people to resources, build support networks within the community and reduce long-term reliance on professionals. The Skills To Enable People and communitieS (STEPS; Kennedy et al., 2011) was initially developed as a project within a case management service (Acquired Brain Injury Outreach Service [ABIOS]) in Queensland, Australia, and now receives recurrent government funding. STEPS is run by local people who are trained, supported and supervised by STEPS staff (occupational therapists) to become Leaders, and co-facilitate the 6-week group programme. Leaders can be people with a brain injury, family members or friends, local service providers or other members of the community. Leaders and group participants decide collaboratively how they want to run their group in their own local community both during and after the programme. A unique feature of this programme is that there is a combined focus on the personal skill development of STEPS participants and growth experiences of peer leaders (Kennedy et al., 2011).

The Clubhouse model is a longstanding consumer-driven programme that facilitates return to work by providing a range of transitional, supported and independent employment training and placement opportunities for its members (Jacobs & Demello, 1996). Clubhouses typically operate in collaboration with local businesses and receive some government funding or sponsorship through health services. Members share the direction and responsibility for the everyday running of the Clubhouse, which typically aims to become as self-sustaining as possible. Jacobs (1997) proposed that for people with brain injury the supportive social milieu may reduce the interpersonal and behavioural difficulties that can be experienced as product of both their injury and environment. Members of the Clubhouse have a collaborative relationship with staff, and support is provided on an 'as-needed' basis. The approach aims to establish a positive identity for its members, offering flexible and lifelong participation and supporting different levels and pathways of vocational participation (Jacobs, 1997).

Other participant-driven initiatives described in the literature include collaborative PBL activities by Feeney and Capo (2010), as outlined in Chapter 6. When performed in a group, projects promote regular socialisation, development of communication and teamwork skills, social recognition of skills and expertise, and a shared sense of achievement over the final 'product'. Examples of group projects include a

Table 7.1 Summary of community-based initiatives to develop sustainable social networks for people with brain injury

Initiative	Brief description	Objectives and benefits	Empirical support
Circles of Support intervention (e.g., Rowlands, 2001; Willer et al., 1993)	Development of an inclusive community of supportive relationships around the person with brain injury: • 1st circle – intimacy, closest friends and family • 2nd circle – friendships and extended family • 3rd circle – participation, clubs and community groups • 4th circle – exchange, professionals and community contacts. A facilitator supports the person to develop their circles of support and achieve their goals through the interactive roles of circle members	• Intervenes at the social network level rather than seeking to addressing the person's deficits • Aims to empower the person with brain injury by focusing on strengths and abilities, guided by principles of dignity, autonomy, respect, equality and reciprocity • Capitalises on natural supports to make decisions and use their resources to find solutions • Facilitators aim to fade support and promote independence over time as appropriate to the person's needs	Qualitative studies involving case level analysis support the efficacy of Circles of Support interventions (see review by Rowlands, 2001)
Clubhouse model of support (see Jacobs, 1997; Jacobs & DeMello, 1996)	A consumer-driven programme that facilitates return to work and provides education, advocacy, socialisation and support for people with brain injury. The community location enables independent access for members and the daily organisation is structured into work units to involve a small to large number of members (e.g., 15–100)	• Member-directed participation: all aspects are managed by members who share the overall direction and responsibilities • Abilities over disabilities: opportunities for skill development and contribution, positive interactions and peer feedback to reduce the impact of interpersonal and behavioural difficulties • Long-term supports: Clubhouse recognises that learning is gradual, and membership is lifelong	Clubhouse surveys and qualitative studies indicate high levels of satisfaction and improved quality of life of members (Jacobs, 1997)

Initiative	Brief description	Objectives and benefits	Empirical support
The Oliver Zangwill Centre User Group (Wilson et al., 2009)	After the OZC programme, clients are encouraged to maintain contact with the Centre through visits, letters, forums and annual social events	• Fosters a sense of reciprocity, whereby past clients help to improve aspects of service delivery for current and future clients • Maintains sense of connection to others and contribution (e.g., fundraising and promotion) • Opportunity for peer leadership, advocacy and professional education	Positive client feedback (see Wilson et al., 2009); yet to be formally evaluated
Skills To Enable People with brain injury and their communitieS (STEPS; Kennedy et al., 2011)	A 6-week community-based self-management programme for people with brain injury and family members. Groups are led by professionals or trained local peer leaders in multiple communities across Queensland, Australia	• Focus on development of personal and social resources (i.e., how I look after myself; how I live in the community; how I work with services) • Shared group goal to develop break-up activity (social outing or activity) fostering collaboration, cognitive and social skills • People with brain injury and family members can be trained as leaders to facilitate the programme	A large case series ($n = 52$) found that males were more likely to benefit from STEPS (e.g., lower stress and greater self-management) than females, although some gains were not maintained at follow-up (Muenchberger et al., 2011). Peer leaders were found to derive psychological benefits (Kennedy et al., 2011)

fundraising event, fishing tournament, community vegetable garden and building a boat (Feeney & Capo, 2010). Group projects can enhance people's social identity through meaningful engagement in the community and establishing a pattern of pro-social behaviour and reciprocal interactions with others.

A central theme in the Clubhouse and PBL literature is that people with brain injury have unique skills and life experiences that contribute to betterment of the community. Initiatives that promote people's active involvement in community education, staff training and service delivery have many advantages. For example, Pearl, Sage and Young (2011) found that involvement in volunteering not only conferred benefits for people with aphasia (i.e., status, independence, skill development, self-esteem and confidence), but also their family and friends, other people with brain injury, and community organisations. The opportunity to advocate for and inspire others and influence resource development, service delivery and community attitudes can have a powerful effect on self-identity (Pearl et al., 2011).

The OZC User Group (Wilson et al. 2009) is a service initiative for supporting past clients to maintain contact and have continued involvement in the Centre. Influenced by a course run by 'Connect', a UK communication network for people with aphasia, the OZC seeks client feedback to improve aspects of service delivery for current and future clients. Clients have an opportunity to contribute to advocacy, fundraising and promotion, and education of professionals through conferences and forums. For example, at the 10th anniversary conference of the OZC in 2006 previous clients shared their experiences of the programme and long-term outcomes. Similarly, in 2013 a panel of five former clients presented at the annual OZC conference on identity and survivor stories. A number of OZC clients have been supported by staff to publish their personal stories or contribute to journals articles as co-authors.

In the metacognitive contextual programmes run by our group (Ownsworth, Fleming et al., 2008; Ownsworth, 2010), people with brain injury were involved in providing specialised education and training to psychology and occupational therapy students, and staff at a disability employment service. This occurred through guest lectures, writing their personal stories, making DVDs and contributing consumer perspectives to educational resources (e.g., treatment manuals and tip sheets). Collaborative partnerships between people with brain injury, family members, professionals and services are vital to improve the quality of rehabilitation and long-term community support. The involvement of people with brain injury in their community encourages 'transcendence', or an extension of self to enrich others' welfare and environment (see Allport, 1961; Ben-Yishay, 2008).

In summary, community rehabilitation initiatives aim to strengthen people's social identity after brain injury by promoting a sense of belonging, reciprocity and connection to others. Such programmes also emphasise the importance of occupation, or recognising self through doing, and thus help to consolidate new notions of self through everyday interactions and routines (Feeney & Capo, 2010; Turner et al., 2009). Although most approaches to developing sustainable support described here have been evaluated as part of service delivery, the process by which these programmes assist people to re-establish a new identity requires further research, guided by the Social Identity Model of Identity Change (Haslam et al., 2008).

Social media applications in brain injury rehabilitation

The final approach to neurorehabilitation considered in this chapter is social media, or use of the internet to improve social functioning of people with brain injury. Social media denotes a major cultural shift in how people interact and establish and maintain relationships on a global scale. This includes email and social network sites (e.g., Facebook, MySpace and Twitter), which are Web-based services that enable people to set up a public or semi-public profile and establish a list of users (i.e., 'friends') with whom one shares information such as biographical details, photos, videos and life experiences (Boyd & Ellison, 2007). Mobile phone technology and internet accessibility allows people to connect 24 hours a day and in virtually any location. Depending on site restrictions (i.e., open or closed to particular audiences), these sites encourage people to continually build their social network through their list of 'friends' and identification of shared acquaintances or new ones. Due to the instant messaging capability and advanced audio-visual features, social media can be highly immersive.

Research indicates that social networking influences people's identity by enabling them to construct an online profile or self-representation using visual aids and narrative (e.g., photos, interests and likes/dislikes). In particular, effort to enhance 'friendship performance' is a common strategy to validate one's social worth (Boyd & Ellison, 2007). Participating in social network sites has been found to increase sense of social connection, friendship satisfaction and support (Baker & Moore, 2008). Posting entries on internet logs (i.e., 'blogging') has been identified as a form of self-therapy, and may have potential to enhance mental health (Tan, 2008). However, negative effects of online relationships (e.g., cyber bullying, harassment and privacy concerns) have also been identified (Boyd & Ellison, 2007).

In view of this worldwide phenomenon, it is important to consider the potential advantages and disadvantages of internet use and social networking for people with brain injury. Research indicates that access to a computer after brain injury is very common (i.e., approximately 80 per cent; Todis et al., 2005), although less than half of those with access use the internet (Vaccaro, Hart, Whyte, & Buchhofer, 2007). Todis et al. (2005) found that people with brain injury perceived the following advantages of using email:

- Quick and inexpensive means of communicating with people who live far away, ability to reach multiple partners simultaneously and have frequent daily contact;
- Less intrusive than telephone calls and reduced pressure to quickly process and respond in conversation (i.e., people have time to read and compose messages);
- Ability to control level of disclosure regarding disability, or manage their social presentation better than face-to-face or telephone interaction;
- The record of emails sent and received serves a memory aid function, allowing people to check their recollection and track ongoing conversations.

Use of the internet more broadly can provide access to knowledge, information and products, and represents an avenue for building one's social network and occupying time. For example, online forums and virtual communities enable people with brain injury to access resources, share experiences and receive support (Todis et al., 2005; Vaccaro et al., 2007). People with brain injury who use the internet have been found to report higher levels of social integration than non-users (Vaccaro et al., 2007). Fraas and Balz (2008) found that expressive online journaling was associated with greater social integration and quality of life after brain injury. However, empirical research also suggests that there can be various barriers to using social media after brain injury. Lack of computer or internet use has been found to be associated with more severe injuries, sensory impairment (Todis et al., 2005) and literacy difficulties (Vaccaro et al., 2007). Other factors contributing to non-use include lack of comfort with technology, financial restrictions, and visuo-motor problems (Todis et al., 2005; Vaccaro et al., 2007). Despite these barriers, Vaccaro et al. (2007) found that 76 per cent of non-users were interested in using the internet.

Tsaousides, Matsuzawa and Lebowitz (2011) investigated Facebook use after TBI and found that 60 per cent of their sample ($n = 96$) were regular users. Of the non-users, security concerns and cognitive deficits were the most common perceived barriers to using Facebook. Only a small proportion (i.e., 10 per cent) expressed that they would rather connect in person. Approximately half of non-users were keen to learn how to use Facebook, and both users and non-users were interested in receiving training. It is noteworthy that this was an online survey, and hence participants are likely to have possessed a reasonable degree of computer literacy. There is broad consensus in the literature that barriers to using email or social networking after brain injury include:

- Finding the technology too confusing or complicated;
- Lack of internet access, expensive start-up costs and tying up the telephone line;
- Unwanted messages, advertising and privacy concerns;
- Difficulty reading social cues and understanding informal communication (e.g., phonetic spelling, abbreviations and 'emoticons');
- Cognitive-linguistic impairments (e.g., concentration, written comprehension and expression) affecting online interaction and the ability to learn instructions or passwords;
- Lack of drive, frustration and impulsivity;
- Limited access to support or training to deal with technical and instructional issues (Egan, Worrall & Oxenham, 2005; Kilov, Togher, Power & Turkstra, 2010; Todis et al., 2005; Tsaousides et al., 2011; Vaccaro et al., 2007).

Various strategies have been recommended to improve ease of use and functionality of computers after brain injury (Todis et al., 2005; Vaccaro et al., 2007). A main recommendation is the provision of specific training that incorporates demonstration, practice and feedback on skills. A systematic review by Kilov et al. (2010) identified three studies that have examined the effects of internet training (e.g., basic internet skills, use of email) or technological modifications (i.e., customised email interfaces) for people with brain injury. These studies employed a case series and provide preliminary support concerning the benefits of internet-based training and tailored resources. One study by Egan et al. (2005) evaluated the efficacy of specialised internet training for people with cognitive-linguistic impairments after TBI ($n = 7$). They found that concentration, memory, and motivation difficulties presented more barriers to training than language impairments, potentially because they had adapted their training materials to be 'aphasia friendly'. Their tutor training supported 6 of the 7 participants to achieve moderate to total independence on an internet task. Tasks requiring greater abstract reasoning skills and multiple steps were less likely to be achieved with independence.

Overall, the literature suggests that the benefits of social media for people with brain injury may be enhanced by skills training and the provision of resources and support. At a practical level, basic computer skills, familiarity with online technology and internet access are required. Technological aids may facilitate participation for people with sensory and motor impairments (e.g., a one-handed keyboard or customised email interface). The provision of step-by-step training, visual aids and errorless learning principles may support people with cognitive-linguistic impairments to acquire internet literacy and skills. Such training could include learning how to operate privacy settings and social problem-solving skills to manage challenging situations (e.g., inappropriate requests to share personal information) and cope with negative emotions. In particular, there is potential for people to feel socially disconnected or excluded whilst participating in interactive online sites (Kilov et al., 2010). This may occur if people do not accept their friendship requests (or 'unfriend' them), and either fail to respond or respond negatively to their comments. Assistance to understand how communication on the internet differs from face-to-face contact and support to interpret online interaction, common phrases and symbols is likely to be beneficial.

Family members, friends, educators and rehabilitation professionals all have a potential role in supporting people with brain injury to safely and effectively use the internet (Kilov et al., 2010). There is a paucity of research investigating social networking as an avenue for improving social and emotional functioning after brain injury. Future research may examine the benefits of social networking for both maintaining existing social contacts and joining new social groups. The impact of social networking on identity reconstruction after brain injury is a promising avenue of inquiry.

Conclusions

This chapter has highlighted the importance of social groups and community-based initiatives for supporting identity reconstruction after brain injury. Group participation provides a means of socialisation, skill development and social support, and can foster a sense of belonging, contribution and reciprocity. The development of sustainable social networks can be achieved through various avenues, according to people's goals, skills and interests. These include paid work, volunteering, leisure activities, advocacy, collaborative projects, leadership initiatives and social media. Although many approaches reviewed in this chapter were found to improve social integration and subjective well-being, there is currently limited research investigating the efficacy of group and community programmes for enhancing self-concept and self-identity. Continuing along the social theme, Chapter 8 focuses on the experience of family members and reviews family-based and paediatric interventions.

8 Family and paediatric interventions

> I've actually started to admit to myself he's not the person he used to be ... you've lost that person you've married and you've got to deal with that.
>
> (wife, caregiver)

Brain injury is typically viewed as a family affair because of the pervasive effects on the lives and well-being of parents, partners, children, siblings and extended family of the person with the injury. This chapter initially explores the concept of family identity and considers the impact of brain injury on family functioning and relationships. Factors influencing adjustment of the main caregiver are reviewed, which highlight the importance of caregivers' personal and social resources as a focus for intervention. An overview of interventions is presented according to three broad approaches; namely: 1) involving family members in the intervention for the person with brain injury; 2) interventions designed specifically for family caregivers; and 3) family system approaches that jointly support the person with brain injury and family members. A similar framework is applied to review interventions for children with brain injury, with particular emphasis on family-based or contextualised approaches for supporting developing sense of self.

The impact of brain injury on family identity

Families frequently undergo change, including the addition of new members, loss of members, strain or relationship breakdown and other stressful events that may be acute or chronic in nature, such as illness of a family member. The event of brain injury and its enduring consequences represents a chronic stressor that affects all family members to some degree and in different ways. The impact is related in part to the pre-injury quality of relationships and family cohesiveness.

The concept of 'family identity' is important in this context, although this has generally received little attention after brain injury (Kosciulek, 1997). Bennett, Wolin, and McAvity (1988) define family identity as 'the family's subjective sense of its own continuity over time, its present situation, and its character. It is the gestalt of qualities and attributes that make it a particular family and that differentiate it from other families' (p. 212). The identity of a family is co-constructed by its members and the sense of 'who we are as a family' influences how they interact (e.g., communicate and resolve conflict), spend time together, celebrate events and support each other during tough times. Each family is comprised of multiple identities, including the collective identity (i.e., 'in our family we enjoy ... and argue about ...'), relational identities of smaller groups (e.g., 'as parents we believe that ...', 'my son and I like to ...') and individual identity of each member within the family (e.g., 'I am the peacekeeper in my family'). The nature of interaction differs accordingly, and some members may share closer bonds than others.

Family relationships can change drastically after brain injury with one or more members suddenly assuming a caregiver or support role. These circumstances include a husband or wife becoming his or her spouse's carer, parents caring for their adult child, or children contributing to the care of their injured parent. In addition to the direct care demands (e.g., assistance with ADLs, driving the person to appointments), caregivers usually need to make lifestyle adjustments such as altering their work schedule and taking increased responsibility for managing the home, childcare and supporting the family financially. Consequently, there is less opportunity for their own leisure and social pursuits at a time when such activities could provide much-needed respite. The change in roles and responsibilities of the caregiver not only affects his or her relationship with the person with brain injury, but interactions and dynamics of the entire family system (Degeneffe, 2001; Kreutzer, Kolakowsky-Hayner, Demm & Meade, 2002; Kosciulek, 1997). The impact of brain injury on family functioning has been found to be greater than other medical illnesses, and clinically significant levels of emotional distress and social maladjustment were evident for 30 to 50 per cent of caregivers one year after TBI (Ergh Rapport, Coleman, & Hanks, 2002).

Many factors influence the impact of brain injury on family members' well-being. As conceptualised in models of caregiver adjustment (e.g., Sherwood, Given, Given, Schiffman, Murman & Lovely, 2004), these factors include:

- Relationships prior to brain injury: the pre-existing nature and duration of their relationship with the person with brain injury (e.g., partner, son/daughter, mother/father) and their bond;
- Pre-existing social resources and life circumstances (e.g., socio-economic status, work/education, and concurrent stressors) for the caregiver and family;
- The severity and nature of the brain injury and resulting functional impairments;
- The level and type of care demands (e.g., occasional assistance with transportation versus 24-hour care for activities of daily living and supervision of behavioural concerns) and presence of major behavioural and emotional changes;
- Family members' appraisals and coping resources (e.g., preparedness and mastery) to manage the impact of the person's functional impairments and care needs;
- Availability of support and resources (e.g., social support, access to information, rehabilitation and counselling, financial assistance).

It is clear from the literature that quality of relationships and family cohesion prior to brain injury can vary considerably. Relationships more recently established or those that were previously strained are at greater risk of conflict and breakdown after brain injury (Ownsworth, Chambers et al., 2011). In the paediatric literature (see Chapter 3), family dysfunction is a risk factor for a child sustaining a brain injury (McKinlay et al., 2009) and parents' pre-injury mental health and parenting style are key predictors of children's post-injury outcomes (Anderson et al., 2012; Wade et al., 2011). The impact of brain injury on family members is also likely to differ according to the nature of their relationship with the person with brain injury.

In particular, the parents of a child with brain injury typically experience considerable shock and grief. They may feel a sense of loss of the child they have watched grow up and the future they had anticipated for their son or daughter (e.g., graduating from university, getting married and having children). They can also feel anger, guilt and self-blame about the accident or illness that caused the brain injury, and feel concerned about their child experiencing further injury or harm (Degeneffe, 2001). In our qualitative research (Ownsworth, Turpin, Carlson & Brennan, 2004), the mother of an 18-year-old man expressed: 'He is socially isolated, quite disinhibited and impulsive. He says the wrong things and it gets him into trouble and dangerous situations' (p. 63). The experience of extended parenthood and continued dependency of their adult child with brain injury can affect the quality of relationships with other children and family members (Degeneffe, 2001). For example, a 72-year-old father noted: 'We are concerned that we are getting older; could someone else take over the role of noticing when things need to be done and reminding him, because we have another handicapped son?' (Ownsworth et al., 2004, p. 62).

We found that parents wanted their child to live a normal life as much as possible, and have the opportunity to form relationships naturally. A mother in our study expressed: 'He has company when his carers are there or if I'm there, or if he's home here [at his parents' house]. It would be better if he had friends who would pop in and say hello – he really doesn't have any of that' (Ownsworth et al., 2004, p. 61). Many parents recognised the importance of maximising their child's independence and choice, but struggled with this because of the need for supervision and support; for example: 'I am his mother – he is 35 years old. I'm sure he would love to go out with a group of guys, but I restrict what he is able to do. I think the carers do too; because of his behaviour, you have to restrict it' (Ownsworth et al., 2004, p. 63).

The partner or spouse of a person with brain injury faces unique sources of strain, and in some studies have been found to report higher levels of caregiver burden and distress than parental caregivers (e.g., Gervasio & Kreutzer, 1997). This may be because their relationship before the injury was based on mutual support and intimacy, rather than one person caring for and being responsible for the other as characteristic of parent–child relationships. Major changes in mood and behaviour can be particularly hard for spouses to adjust to, as expressed by the wife of a man with brain tumour: 'I've had to grieve for the man I married even though I've still got him ... It's hard because some days "Ian" is really almost like the old Ian and you could sort of, do you say something to him or not?' (Goadby, 2013).

The impact of brain injury on relational skills (e.g., perspective-taking, empathy and emotional sensitivity) can take a particular toll on spousal relationships (Bowen,

Hall, Newby, Walsh, Weatherhead & Yeates, 2009). Changes in sexual functioning can occur with a reduction in sexual interest and activity most typical. Giaquinto et al. (2003) found that partners' attitudes contributed significantly to the decline in sexual activity after stroke, due to their concern about stroke recurrence, emotional distress and lack of arousal. Many spouses face the distressing decision of whether to stay in the relationship or leave. Some stay out of concern for person with brain injury and lack of alternative support options (Degeneffe, 2001). A relationship that was either well established prior to the injury or formed after the brain injury is more likely to be maintained (Bowen et al., 2009). In a large retrospective study ($n = 977$), Arango-Lasprilla et al. (2008) found that 85 per cent of individuals with TBI who were married at the time of injury had stable marital status at two years post-injury. The strongest predictors of separation and divorce were younger age, the male having the TBI, violent injury and an injury of moderate severity.

Siblings of people with brain injury also experience considerable challenges and strain. In the case of childhood brain injury, siblings can feel traumatised by the circumstances of the injury and confused by the changes in their brother or sister, family routine and their lifestyle (Degeneffe, 2001). In Bursnall's (Brain Injury Association of Queensland, BIAQ, 2002) qualitative study on the experience of 24 siblings of children with brain injury, one sibling noted: 'My brother ... is not himself, he's had a total like different personality change' (p. 128). Because siblings are often excluded from the acute care setting, they often have limited understanding of what has happened and how to respond to post-injury changes. In the case of childhood brain injury, uninjured siblings may feel overlooked, jealous, lonely, and a sense of guilt regarding the accident and their own 'normalcy' (BIAQ, 2002; Sambuco, Brookes & Lah, 2008). A 16-year-old in Bursnall's study (BIAQ, 2002) described her feelings as follows: 'Annoyance, she always had to take all the attention. Like I sort of got jealous, everyone's attention was on her, it was like "excuse me, I am also here", with the family' (p. 125).

A review by Sambuco et al. (2008) found that siblings of children with severe TBI and more functional deficits (especially behavioural impairments) were most at risk of poor psychological adjustment, including internalising and externalising behavioural problems and academic difficulties. Siblings' quality of relationship with their injured brother or sister and their parents was typically reduced (e.g., less close and more negative interaction), particularly during the acute recovery stage (Sambuco et al., 2008). Perhaps most noteworthy, a sibling's support role is usually the longest, and may become that of primary caregiver as parents become elderly (Degeneffe, 2001). In growing up with an injured brother or sister, siblings can feel that their own lives are less carefree and perceive a sense of responsibility and concern for the well-being of their sibling. There may be extra demands placed on children that requires maturity beyond their years (e.g., assisting an older sibling with brain injury to perform a self-care task). Two younger siblings expressed this view as follows: 'Sometimes I do feel older than him, more in control and in charge, responsible' (BIAQ, 2002, p. 130); and 'It keeps impacting every day. It's been an experience ... growing up with Ryan the way he is' (p. 128). Therefore, siblings' role within the family and sense of self can be altered by brain injury (Sambuco et al., 2008).

The impact of having a parent with brain injury can also be profound, especially for young children. The brain injury can affect children's bond and attachment to their injured parent, and they can develop heightened anxiety and fear concerning their parent's behavioural changes, such as reduced frustration tolerance and anger outbursts (Bowen et al., 2009). More generally, children's routine and lifestyle is typically disrupted, with greater expectations placed on them to assist around the house, follow rules and minimise stress in the home (e.g., playing quietly and not having friends over). Their emotional and social development can be affected, as illustrated by Cara's story.

Cara, a 9-year-old girl remembers the night of the home invasion five years ago which led to her father sustaining a very severe TBI. She awoke at 1pm to discover her father lying still in a pool of blood near the front door. She recalls her mother screaming and the ambulance arriving. When she saw her father in hospital weeks later he was unrecognisable. His head was bruised and swollen and there were tubes sticking out of his body. The experience was so terrifying for Cara that her mother did not take her into hospital for several weeks afterwards. She later recalls her father being 'awake' in hospital but not paying her much attention. Cara has a vague memory of her father before the accident. He was an active man who made her laugh and played with her. The father she has now is very different. He is overweight and spends most of his time watching television. She doesn't like to be left alone with him because he often laughs, cries and becomes angry for no reason. Cara won't have friends over because she is embarrassed by how her father looks and the way he acts. She has nightmares about the break in and worries about something happening to her mother. She wishes they could spend more time with just the two of them, but feels guilty for feeling this way because she knows the accident was not her father's fault.

The detrimental effects of TBI on parenting style and children's psychological well-being have been demonstrated in a number of studies (e.g., Pessar, Coad, Linn & Willer, 1993; Uysal, Hibbard, Robillard, Pappadopulos & Jaffe, 1998). In a comparison with control families, Uysal et al. (1998) found that parents with TBI were less likely to use goal setting, encourage skill development and promote rule following, orderliness and work values. They were also less nurturing and had less active involvement with their children. The uninjured parents in families with TBI reported lower feelings of warmth, love and acceptance towards their children. Pessar and colleagues (1993) found that psychological outcomes were poorer for older children with a father with TBI and those with an uninjured parent who was depressed. Parent–child relationships were more strained when there were changes in the parenting style of either the injured or uninjured parent. Such changes included not fulfilling their parental role (e.g., not showing interest in, being responsible for or helping their child), negative behaviours (e.g., yelling, arguing) and fewer positive behaviours (e.g., less praise or having fun with the child). A noteworthy finding of both studies is that children's relationship with the uninjured parent can also be adversely affected by brain injury.

Overall, brain injury often affects multiple relationships within the family and the stability of the entire unit. Nevertheless, families can show remarkable resilience in being able to cope with the stressors of brain injury. Some members also describe positive outcomes of how they have derived meaning from their experience. In our brain tumour research a wife caregiver made the following observation about the relationships in her family: 'I think in some way it's made us closer ... we've been lucky in that we've been able to strengthen those bonds' (Ownsworth, Chambers et al., 2011, p. 131). Similarly, a sibling in Bursnall's (2002) study noted 'there have been sacrifices, but I don't look at it all as losing experiences, I see that I have gained an experience' (p. 131).

As reviewed in the next section, most studies to date have focused on identifying vulnerability or risk factors for poor caregiver adjustment or family dysfunction. It is equally important to recognise protective factors or the conditions most conducive to family adaptation and resilience. More specifically, there is a need to understand the personal and social resources that enhance adjustment to brain injury, and how these can be harnessed to strengthen families.

Factors influencing family adjustment and intervention approaches

The psychological adjustment of the primary caregiver has received a lot more attention in research than family functioning as a whole. Research indicates that degree of strain or burden is a consistent predictor of caregiver psychological well-being (Marsh et al., 2002; Sherwood, Given, Given, Schiffman, Murman et al., 2007). Caregiver strain refers to subjective levels of emotional, physical, financial and social stress placed upon the caregiver as a direct result of their caregiving role (Schumacher, Dodd & Paul, 1993). Certain types of functional impairment appear to produce more strain and distress for caregivers than others. For example, Marsh et al. (2002) found that although physical deficits were related to caregiver strain at 6 months post-injury, cognitive, behavioural and social deficits had the strongest associations with strain at 12 months post-injury. In the context of brain tumour and other cancers, we found that interpersonal and emotional difficulties (but not cognitive impairments or dependency with ADLs) were related to caregiver depression, and that caregiver strain mediated this relationship (Ownsworth, Henderson, Chambers & Shum, 2009). Neurobehavioural impairments have also been found to be the most robust predictor of caregiver distress after TBI (Ergh et al., 2002).

Importantly, caregivers' internal resources (e.g., mastery, coping and resilience) and external resources (e.g., adequacy of social support) have been found to mediate or moderate the impact of care demands on emotional well-being. For example, Sherwood et al. (2007) found that caregiver mastery mediated the relationship between behavioural impairments and caregivers' level of depressive symptoms after brain tumour. Focusing on family schemas (i.e., beliefs, values and goals), Kosciulek (1997) reported that perceptions of manageability and meaningfulness surrounding the injury predicted family adaptation. Further, Simpson and Jones (2013) identified that caregivers with higher resilience reported more positive affect and lower caregiver burden after TBI and spinal cord injury. Social support has been found to have a direct effect on family functioning and also function as a stress buffer. In particular, Ergh et al. (2002) found that caregiver distress increased with greater time since injury when social support was perceived to be low (Ergh et al., 2002). Similarly, in our brain tumour research, caregivers supporting individuals with poor functional status had better psychological well-being when they were highly satisfied with their social support (Ownsworth, Henderson & Chambers, 2010).

Many authors have highlighted reciprocal links between the functioning and well-being of the person with brain injury and their family members' adjustment (e.g., Bowen et al., 2009; Kreutzer et al., 2002; Wade et al., 2011). Accordingly, there has been an increased emphasis in the literature on understanding relationship and family dynamics as a means to providing effective support, rather than considering members' support needs in isolation (e.g., Togher et al., 2013). Nevertheless, because family circumstances differ and individual members' willingness to seek support varies, different modes of intervention need to be considered. Three broad approaches include involving family members in the therapy for the person with brain injury, interventions designed specifically for family members, and couple and family system interventions.

Involving family members in therapy for the person with brain injury

One intervention option is to involve family caregivers in therapy that primarily focuses on improving the well-being of the person with brain injury. Such programmes typically focus on psychoeducation for the person with brain injury and caregiver, and strategies for managing the impact of brain injury on their relationship (e.g., communication, problem-solving). Such training can occur in groups, as exemplified by the coping skills group by Backhaus et al. (2010), or within individual therapy programmes (e.g., Ownsworth, Chambers, Stewart, Casey, Walker & Shum, 2013).

As an example from our own research, the Making Sense of Brain Tumour (MSoBT) Project is a 10-session home-based psychotherapy and rehabilitation programme for people with brain tumour and their caregivers (Ownsworth et al., 2013). Approximately 60 per cent of people with brain tumour ($n = 50$) involved family members (mainly a spouse) in their therapy. For some families, we found that the well-being and support needs of the person with brain tumour were closely intertwined with that of the caregiver. In particular, the husband of one participant referred to 'our tumour' and 'when we got treated'. Such caregivers were often actively involved from the outset and attended each session. Other caregivers were initially reluctant to be involved, seemingly because they felt their relative with brain tumour needed the support rather than themselves. When these caregivers decided to join later sessions they usually came to recognise the importance of receiving support for their own well-being. A main aim of the therapy was to create a setting conducive to each member expressing their concerns and goals in the programme. Accordingly, a combination of individual, spouse/caregiver and couple therapy sessions was conducted. Common goals included:

- Learning to manage the effects of brain tumour, for example, cognitive difficulties (e.g., memory, concentration, organisation), loss of motivation and fatigue;
- Managing low mood, anxiety, stress and existential issues regarding the diagnosis, uncertain prognosis, re-growth and end-of-life issues;
- Coping with behavioural changes, including anger, impulsivity and apathy;
- Supporting occupational re-engagement and role functioning (e.g., return to work, parenting skills);
- Addressing fears/concerns of the participant's family (e.g., communicating news to children, developing a family care plan, preparing an advanced health directive and palliative care services);
- Improving relationship functioning (e.g., communication, intimacy and sexual functioning, strategies for managing aphasia).

An evaluation of the MSoBT supports the efficacy of home-based therapy (relative to wait list controls) for reducing depression and improving quality of life for people with brain tumour (Ownsworth et al., 2013). Although the outcomes for caregivers are yet to be formally evaluated, feedback obtained from an interview with a psychologist not involved in the intervention suggested that caregivers valued their involvement, as follows:

> We both found it very beneficial. Because the mental side is neglected – it came at the perfect time. [Husband] is able to manage anxiety now. I can't imagine what we'd be like if we didn't do the programme.
>
> (Jennifer, wife)

> I was quite desperate for some help, I felt very alone and I needed someone to talk to. We were lurching from one drama to another and communication between [my husband] and I wasn't very good ... We both felt supported through the programme – learning a new way to communicate with each other. I've learnt how to bring up new subjects without upsetting him.
>
> (Leah, wife)

Interventions specifically designed for family members

As highlighted by Leah's feedback, receiving information about the effects of brain injury and learning how to manage the impact on relationships can enhance caregivers' own well-being. Many interventions have been primarily developed to enhance caregivers' personal and social resources, including their information and emotional support needs and coping skills. A systematic review of family interventions by Boschen, Gargaro, Gan, Gerber and Brandys (2007) identified four controlled intervention studies (OCEBM Level 2) for TBI and seven for stroke which specifically measured the impact on caregiver well-being (e.g., caregiver burden, stress or depression). Overall, there was modest support for the efficacy of educational interventions (e.g., written material, group discussion, videotapes, and personalised feedback on assessment) and support groups for increasing caregivers' knowledge and preparedness to manage the effects of brain injury and reducing caregiver depression. Telerehabilitation (telephone/internet) approaches were effective for improving caregivers' problem-solving skills, preparedness, emotional and social functioning relative to control conditions (Boschen et al., 2007). Case management and family-based liaison was found to enhance caregivers' knowledge and satisfaction with stroke resources. Interestingly, very few intervention studies were found to directly reduce caregiver strain (see exception by Teng, Mayo, Latimer, Hanley, Wood-Dauphinee, Cote & Scott, 2003), but appeared to enhance caregivers' adjustment by improving their knowledge, self-appraisals and coping skills. In the paediatric literature, advocacy training shows potential for enhancing parents' personal and social resources (Glang, McLaughlin & Schroeder, 2007).

Family system interventions

The third broad intervention approach focuses simultaneously on improving the well-being of the person with brain injury and their family members through family system interventions (Gan, Gargaro, Kreutzer, Boschen & Wright, 2010; Klonoff, 2010; Kreutzer et al., 2002), systemic therapy and relational approaches to brain injury (Bowen et al. 2010; Wilson et al. 2009). Family system approaches recognise the connectedness and interdependence of all family members, whereby reciprocal relationships are evident between the functioning and well-being of the person with brain injury and close family members (Bowen et al., 2010; Gan et al., 2010; Wade et al., 2011). Thus, interventions designed to support relationships within the family, and the family system as a whole are considered optimal.

The Brain Injury Family Intervention (BIFI) developed by Kreutzer and colleagues (2002) is a structured approach to supporting families to understand and manage the main concerns and challenges arising from brain injury. The assumptions underlying BIFI can be grouped according to four main themes. Firstly, brain injury disrupts the lives of all members of the family, and most people want their lives to return to normal. Secondly, each person in the family is important and deserves respect. Thirdly, people who are well informed usually make better decisions, and all family members have the right to make choices. Fourthly, family members have a long-term support role and to provide effective support they need to take care of themselves (Kreutzer et al., 2002). Following an initial assessment, the treatment modalities for the family are selected in accordance with the nature of people's concerns or problems (e.g., impairments and distress), goals, practical issues impacting attendance and the willingness of different members to participate. Intervention modalities include family therapy, marital therapy, individual therapy, group therapy and bibliotherapy (provision of written information). Within these different modalities, interventions focus on the following four key issues:

- Recognising and coping with change (e.g., effects of brain injury) and the implications for the family, normalising the emotional impact, and highlighting the importance of self-care;

- Understanding the recovery and rehabilitation process and ways to maximise functional gains in the long term;
- Managing stress by identifying the signs and learning to cope effectively through personal strategies and social support;
- Communicating and working effectively with rehabilitation professionals to gain information, access services and advocate for improvements in the system of care.

A particularly useful strategy within the BIFI curriculum is supporting members to recognise the impact of brain injury on the family through the Family Change Questionnaire (see Kreutzer et al. 2002), an open-ended measure that poses questions such as: 'How has the brain injury affected your plans for the future?' (p. 365) and 'How have other family members reacted to the patient's injury?' (p. 365). In a pilot study, Kreutzer, Stejskal, Ketchum, Marwitz, Taylor & Menzel (2009) demonstrated the effectiveness of a manualised five-session family systems approach for reducing unmet needs and perceived obstacles to accessing services ($n = 53$ families). However, there were no significant changes in level of distress, life satisfaction or family functioning. Using a mixed methods approach to evaluation in a larger sample ($n = 76$), Kreutzer, Stejskal, Godwin, Powell & Arango-Lasprilla (2010) reported high levels of satisfaction regarding the helpfulness of BIFI and the extent to which goals were attained in the sessions.

The BIFI curriculum has also been applied in an acute care context (Marks & Daggett, 2006), and adapted for adolescents with brain injury (BIFI-A; Gan et al., 2010). Topics integrated for adolescents include 'Being a teen and achieving independence' and 'School, transitions and preparing for adulthood' (p. 656). A preliminary evaluation indicated that BIFI-A was well accepted and considered helpful by adolescents, families and professionals. Gan et al. (2010) emphasised the value of the BIFI-A as a face-to-face intervention for adolescents and family members. However, controlled intervention studies need to determine the efficacy of BIFI in comparison with usual care and alternative approaches (e.g., separate interventions for the individual and family members).

A further example of a systems approach includes training communication partners of people with aphasia (see systematic review by Simmons-Mackie, Raymer, Armstrong, Holland & Cherney, 2010). A recent non-randomised controlled trial by Togher et al. (2013) evaluated the efficacy of training communication partners of people with severe TBI. The JOINT intervention focusing on the communication skills of both the partner and individual with TBI was found to improve everyday conversational performance to a greater extent than individual communication training (SOLO) and the wait list condition. The conversational strategies taught to communication partners included positive communication strategies such as elaborative and collaborative techniques (e.g., sharing information, showing understanding, confirming partner's contribution), cognitive support (e.g., use of cues and memory aids), emotional support (e.g., conveying respect, acknowledging difficulties), supportive questioning and turn taking.

As a recent advance in family and couples therapy, Bowen and colleagues (2010) described their Relational Approach to Rehabilitation. Guided by social neuroscience perspectives and systemic family therapy, they emphasise that post-injury changes are co-created through 'brain-to-brain interactions' between the person with brain injury, his or her close others and professionals. Just as sense of self forms through interacting with others, the 'relational space' can facilitate or impede adaptation and support continuity or discontinuity of self. The emphasis of therapy is on understanding the shared experience or co-constructed reality of the dyad, developing a collaborative approach to communication, and using strategies to circumvent impairments and enhance interpersonal relationships. The application of the relational approach has been illustrated through case studies (see Bowen et al., 2010; Yeates, Hamill et al., 2008), but is yet to be formally evaluated through a controlled study.

Overall, the evidence base supporting the efficacy of family system interventions for brain injury is relatively sparse, although the past two decades have witnessed theoretical advances that capitalise on social neuroscience and systemic theory. By focusing on the needs of all family members and their relationship dynamics, family system and relational approaches have the potential to facilitate positive identity transition for the family as a whole. As described in Klonoff's Family Experiential Model (2010) 'family reconstitution' occurs when members are able to recognise and accept that some things have changed and grieve these losses, and when they re-establish meaningful and fulfilling relationships both within and outside the family. This process requires good communication, timely access to support, and developing appropriate coping strategies so that all members can enjoy meaningful lives.

Interventions for children and adolescents with brain injury

As reviewed in Chapter 3, the impact of brain injury on developing sense of self has been largely overlooked in paediatric research, with most studies focusing on the cognitive, behavioural and social outcomes of paediatric brain injury. Very few studies have assessed psychological consequences such as self-concept for children or adolescents (Beardmore et al., 1999; Hawley, 2012). Chapter 2 highlighted that development of self-awareness and sense of self occurs as a product of both one's biology and socio-cultural context. Specifically, children learn about themselves and form their self-concept through social interaction and by developing age-appropriate competencies, as supported by brain development. Research on paediatric TBI highlights the interactive influence of premorbid functioning, developmental factors (age at injury), the severity and nature of brain injury and social environment on behavioural and psychosocial outcomes (Anderson & Catroppa, 2006; Sambuco et al., 2008; Wade et al., 2011; Yeates et al., 2010). Despite the lack of research focusing specifically on self-concept following paediatric brain injury, based on the literature reviewed in Chapter 3, key themes relevant to interventions supporting children's emerging sense of self are as follows:

- Children with brain injury often lack knowledge about their injury and impairments, which is influenced by developmental factors (e.g., understanding of normal body and brain functioning), their neurocognitive status and access to information (Beardmore et al., 1999; Hanten et al., 2000; Jacobs, 1993).

- Lack of awareness of post-injury changes is related to higher self-esteem (Beardmore et al., 1999); hence, impaired awareness may serve to protect children's self-esteem.
- Children with brain injury report lower self-esteem and poorer social functioning than their peers (Andrews, Rose & Johnson, 1998; Hawley, 2012).
- Lower self-esteem is related to greater behavioural problems and higher levels of parental stress (Hawley, 2012). Parental responsiveness and parenting style influence behavioural outcomes, with warm responsiveness associated with more favourable outcomes (Wade et al., 2011), and permissiveness and authoritarian parenting associated with poorer long-term outcomes (Yeates et al., 2010). The relationship between parenting style and children's self-esteem after brain injury is yet to be examined.
- A high level of support and accommodations (e.g., reduced expectations and assistance on tasks) may help to ensure that children with brain injury mainly experience success at home and school, and hence, is likely to have positive effects on self-esteem (Ylvisaker, Feeney et al., 1998). However, it is unclear what impact this 'shielding' approach has in the long term, as realistic self-appraisal of one's strengths and difficulties influences strategy development and the ability to set achievable goals and pursue a meaningful life path (Mealings & Douglas, 2010).
- For adolescents, the presence of supportive relationships and a sense of belonging may help to maintain or re-establish a positive identity despite changes in functioning and activities (Mealings & Douglas, 2010; Todis & Glang, 2008).
- Impairments in executive control, the ability to 'read people' and solve problems during social interaction may underlie various maladaptive behaviours arising from TBI (Ganesalingam et al., 2007; Levin et al., 2009; Warschausky et al., 1997). The experience of peer rejection and poor social integration can negatively impact on sense of self (Mealings & Douglas, 2010).

The implications for intervention related to these themes are that approaches targeting children's knowledge of brain injury, self-awareness and social cognition need to consider the potential effects on self-esteem. In particular, children and adolescents with greater self-awareness and social perception skills may be more likely to experience self-discrepancies, or unfavourable temporal comparisons (i.e., pre- and post-injury selves) or social comparisons (i.e., self–other comparisons) (Harter, 2012; Wall et al., 2011). Nonetheless, social cognition impairments contribute to behavioural problems, which in turn can negatively affect self-esteem and social functioning.

Developmental literature highlights that the emergence of a realistic and adaptive sense of self is fostered by close and nurturing relationships, positive learning experiences and the opportunity to derive a sense of achievement and form a meaningful life path (Berk & Andersen, 2000; Harter, 2012; Marcia, 1980). Accordingly, it is well-recognised that paediatric brain injury interventions need to be developmentally sensitive and delivered in, or applied to real-life contexts (Cole, Paulos, Cole & Tankard, 2009; Braga, Da Paz & Ylvisaker, 2005; Gardner, Bird, Maguire, Carreiro &

Abenaim, 2003; Ylvisaker, Turkstra & Coelho, 2005). Rehabilitation approaches that focus on maximising children's physical, cognitive, behavioural, social and emotional competencies all ultimately contribute to forming a stable and adaptive identity in adulthood. Anderson and Catroppa (2006) classified models of paediatric brain injury intervention into the following broad approaches:

- *Restorative interventions*: targeting underlying skills or consequences of brain injury (e.g., repetitive training of cognitive skills);
- *Functional adaptation*: training in the use of compensatory strategies such as memory aids and cuing devices;
- *Environmental modification*: minimising the impact of impairments by adapting the naturalistic setting (e.g., classroom), use of technological aids and education and training of parents and teachers;
- *Psychoeducation or informational support*: provision of oral or written information about the effects of paediatric brain injury (e.g., Beardmore et al., 1999) and impact on parents' well-being (e.g., Singer, Glang & Nixon, 1994);
- *Psychological therapy*: applied behavioural analysis and positive behaviour support (see review by Ylvisaker et al., 2005);
- *Family-based interventions* (e.g., Family Problem-Solving; Wade, Carey & Wolfe, 2006) and other *context-sensitive approaches* (e.g., Feeney & Ylvisaker, 2003; Gardner et al., 2003): incorporating positive behaviour supports with cognitive, communication and executive strategies for the child and their natural supports.

The approaches considered most relevant to supporting self-concept after paediatric brain injury are those that are holistic, family-based and context-sensitive. Such interventions typically integrate psychoeducation, environmental modification, psychological and behavioural treatments within children's everyday settings. In a review of family interventions, Cole et al. (2009) presented the following guidelines for people working with families of children and adolescents with brain injury:

a. Choose interventions that are developmentally appropriate, taking into account the impact of the timing of injury on children's developmental stage and related social expectations of their skills and behaviour;
b. Tailor the intervention to the family's needs and functioning (e.g., readiness, distress level and goals);
c. Provide advocacy and case management to link families to resources and community supports;
d. Provide comprehensive education about the child's brain injury;
e. Support family realignment or reorganisation of the family system, including modified roles, communication and support for siblings;
f. Facilitate adjustments and support in the child's environment (e.g., structure of the home and school routine and positive behaviour supports);
g. Provide skills training to the child and their family members (e.g., stress management, coping, problem-solving and communication skills).

In developing these guidelines, Cole et al. classified d) injury education as 'efficacious' with respect to current empirical support, but also noted that 'educational interventions alone are not sufficient in producing substantial changes and that family support and skills training should be added to maximise impact' (p. 163). They classified the guidelines c), f), and g) as 'probably efficacious'; and guidelines a), b) and e) as 'promising, but not yet validated' (Cole et al., 2009, p. 161).

A relatively recent advance in paediatric rehabilitation is centre-based holistic neuropsychological rehabilitation programmes (Fletcher-Janzen & Kade, 1997; Marcantuono & Prigatano, 2008). A paediatric brain injury service based on the adult holistic neuropsychological model was first developed by Fletcher-Janzen and Kade (1997). Established for a post-acute inpatient population, their model is based on neurodevelopmental and neuropsychological rehabilitation principles and incorporates Ben-Yishay's six stages (i.e., engagement, awareness, mastery, control, acceptance and identity formation). Marcantuono and Prigatano (2008) also described a holistic brain injury rehabilitation programme for school-aged children at the Children's Specialised Hospital in New Jersey, USA. Set up in 2003, their service was designed for children with severe brain injury who have the capacity to return to the school environment. The four-day-per-week treatment programme is set up as a classroom environment with 'students' divided into age groups (6–12 years and 13–21 years) or according to their functional status. Children are admitted on an open enrolment basis and programme length varies in accordance with their needs and progress. Their developmental approach recognises that sense of self is emerging for children at the time of their brain injury and they require considerable support to develop a realistic and adaptive sense of self after brain injury. Components of their holistic approach include:

- Staff members of the multi-disciplinary team are referred to as 'coaches' who form 'apprenticeships' with children to support their skill development.
- Use of evidence-based rehabilitation techniques such as: goal setting (poster displays), modelling, scaffolding, verbal mediation, self-prediction and reflection, behavioural experiments, problem-solving and graduated task difficulty.
- Involvement of families in conferences, goal setting, support groups, psychotherapy, transition planning and reinforcing strategies at home.
- Goals to increase children's understanding of their strengths and limitations and develop a sense of mastery and control over their impairments that enables them to effectively manage their deficits in everyday living.
- Diverse therapeutic activities including focus groups (start of the day), orientation group, group counselling or play therapy, and multiple groups on different aspect of cognitive function (e.g., attention, memory), language, sensory/motor function, socialisation/community, ADLs, academic skills and self-advocacy.
- Specific preparation for school re-entry through individual tutoring and tailoring of rehabilitation goals to the academic curriculum.

After participating in the holistic programme, children are typically followed for up to five years. Marcantuono and Prigatano (2008) highlighted that both the clinical utility and cost-effectiveness of these programmes need to be evaluated. They recommended four main clinical outcomes related to friendships, academic performance, parental well-being, and teachers' ability to work effectively with the child. Controlled intervention studies similar to those employed in the adult literature (e.g., Cicerone et al., 2008) would be valuable, although this research is difficult to conduct for many reasons, including the challenge of identifying a meaningful control group. Further validation of measures of self-awareness and self-concept for children with brain injury (see Chapter 5) would support an evaluation of the impact of holistic rehabilitation on developing sense of self.

Many authors have emphasised the importance of contextualised (i.e., home, school and community-based) intervention to enhance the personal and social resources (e.g., knowledge, skills and strategies) of children and adolescents and their natural supports, such as parents and teachers (Feeney & Ylvisaker, 2003; Gardner et al., 2003; Woods, Catroppa, Giallo, Matthews & Anderson, 2012; Ylvisaker et al., 2005). A summary of context-sensitive child and family interventions and their outcomes is presented in Table 8.1.

Interventions for younger children

Developmental perspectives highlight the key influence of stimulating, supportive and empathic parent–child interactions on children's learning, sense of autonomy and emerging self-concept (Fonagy et al., 2004; Harter, 2012). Interventions targeting parents' knowledge and skills are therefore particularly important for young children after brain injury. As summarised in Table 8.1, Braga and colleagues (2005) compared the efficacy of clinician-delivered rehabilitation and family-based rehabilitation for a 12-month period. The family-based intervention that involved educating and training family to implement rehabilitation in the home with professional input yielded significantly greater improvement in children's physical and cognitive outcomes. Such findings indicate that with the support of multidisciplinary professionals family members can be trained to effectively deliver rehabilitation in real-life contexts and stimulate neurodevelopment of children with TBI. Further, given parents' lifelong involvement in their children's lives, their active involvement and empowerment in the rehabilitation process is essential. These principles underlie paediatric rehabilitation services at the SARAH Network of Rehabilitation Hospitals in Brazil (Braga et al., 2005).

These ecological principles also underpin context-sensitive approaches in the literature, such as positive behavioural supports (PBS) in family and school life (Ylvisaker et al., 2005). In contrast to traditional applied behaviour analysis, PBS focuses primarily on bringing about satisfying lifestyle changes for the person with brain injury and their close relationships. The intervention combines behaviour management with cognitive, social-communication and executive strategy training for the child and members of their support network (Feeney & Ylvisaker, 2003; 2006). Behavioural management through antecedent control and environmental modification (e.g., positive communication, increasing sense of control and choice) helps to establish a pattern of positive behaviours in the context of everyday activities and routines which become naturally reinforcing. Personally meaningful pursuits and skills for gaining competency are focused on in a gradual sense to gain 'behavioural momentum' (i.e., start with easy and preferred challenges and build up to more difficult ones). In time, children's social participation can increase and coincide with positive changes to sense of self. The efficacy of PBS has been demonstrated through Level 1 evidence involving single-case experimental designs (e.g., Feeney & Ylvisaker, 2003; 2006). The application of PBS to educational and vocational settings is discussed in the section on adolescent interventions.

In line with the ecological principles of contextualised intervention, the efficacy of family problem-solving (FPS) has received the most attention to date in the paediatric literature, with Level 1–2 evidence. A systematic review of parenting interventions by Brown, Whittingham, Boyd and Sofronoff (2012) identified eight studies (4 pre-post designs, 4 RCTs) that evaluated FPS. Common components of FPS included parent education and training in behavioural management. However, the main intervention target is problem-solving, or supporting families to identity problem areas, learn new skills and implement effective solutions for stressful situations related to the injury (i.e., ABCDE: Aim, Brainstorm, Choose, Do it and Evaluate skills). As summarised in Table 8.1, FPS has been evaluated by Wade and colleagues (2005; 2006; 2008; 2009; 2010) through pilot studies and RCTs of both face-to-face and online delivery. Brown et al. (2012) concluded that there was modest evidence (i.e., mainly small to medium effect sizes) from the RCTs concerning the efficacy of FPS interventions for improving child behavioural and emotional outcomes and parenting skills and adjustment.

As summarised in Table 8.1, child and family interventions typically combine various modes of delivery, including individual face-to-face, group, telephone, video-conferencing and self-guided sessions. For example, in the RCT of online FPS by Wade, Carey et al. (2006), there was an initial face-to-face meeting followed by videoconferencing and 14 self-guided online sessions (i.e., didactic content, video clips modelling the problem-solving skills and family exercises to practise the skill). This intervention focused broadly on children aged 5–16 years. Eight core sessions covered problem-solving, communication and antecedent behaviour management. The remaining six sessions were flexibly tailored to specific issues experienced by a family (e.g., sibling concerns, marital communication). There was a significantly greater improvement in parental distress, depression and anxiety after FPS, but no significant difference in problem-solving skills (or mediating effect of problem-solving skills on outcomes) between the intervention and control conditions. Therefore, the specific mechanisms underlying intervention gains are unclear.

In a further intervention study, Wade, Oberjohn, Burkhardt and Greenberg (2009) examined the feasibility and efficacy of I-InTERACT (Internet-based Interacting Together Everyday: Recovery After Childhood TBI), designed for nine parents of children aged 3–9 years. Their Web-based programme provided 15 sessions (10 core and 5 supplemental) on positive parenting skills training and psychoeducation. Sessions included audio recordings of other parents' experiences and videos of parent modelling of skills. Videoconferences were held with therapists between the Web-based sessions to review material and receive coaching. As summarised in Table 8.1, there is preliminary support for the efficacy of this approach for improving positive parenting behaviours based on blinded observer ratings of parenting behaviours. Further, there

Table 8.1 Overview of contextualised interventions focusing on child and/or parent emotional and behavioural outcomes after brain injury

Intervention	Brief description	Study and design	Findings
Family-based rehabilitation: educating and training family members to implement rehabilitation in the home with support from professionals (Braga et al., 2005)	12-month intervention for 87 children with moderate to severe TBI (5–12 years)	RCT of direct clinician delivered rehabilitation ($n = 43$) and family-based rehabilitation ($n = 44$)	The family-based intervention yielded significantly greater improvement in children's physical and cognitive outcomes.
Family Problem Solving (FPS): primary focus on problem-solving skills, with psychoeducation, behaviour management and tailored sessions supporting specific family issues	Online (12–14 sessions), self-guided Web-based sessions with fortnightly videoconferencing	Wade et al. (2005), pre-post ($n = 6$); age: 5–16 years Wade, Carey et al. (2006); RCT comparing online FPS ($n = 20$) with internet resources ($n = 20$); age: 5–16 years	Significant reduction in antisocial behaviour, but not executive function, social function or depression. Significant effect for child self-management and compliance, but not other behavioural and emotional outcomes. Older children and those with lower SES made greatest gains.
	7 sessions of face-to-face FPS over 6 months	Wade, Michaud et al. (2006); RCT comparing FPS ($n = 16$) with usual care ($n = 16$), age: 5–16 years	Significant effect for child internalising behaviours (depression, anxiety and withdrawal), but not externalising behaviours.
	I-INTERACT: up to 13 videoconferences held fortnightly and self-guided Web-based FBS based on parent–child interaction therapy, incorporating live observation and feedback	Wade et al. (2009); pre-post ($n = 5$); age: 3–8 years	Non-significant trend towards reduction in child problem behaviours and significant increase in positive parenting behaviours (e.g., giving praise) and decrease in negative behaviours (objective measure).
	Teen Online Problem Solving (TOPS); 10 core sessions and up to 4 supplementary sessions	Wade et al. (2008); pre-post ($n = 9$); age: 11–18 years. Wade et al. (2011); RCT of TOPS ($n = 16$) compared with internet resources ($n = 19$), adolescents aged 11–14 years	Significant improvements in adolescents' internalising symptoms and depression. Significantly lower parent–teen conflict (parent rated). Improvements in parent-reported externalising and internalising behaviour were greater for adolescents with severe TBI.

Intervention	Brief description	Study and design	Findings
Positive Behaviour Supports, combining communication, cognitive and executive strategy training	Intensive multi-component intervention with family, peer, school and community focus	Single-case designs (ABAB) of two young children (6 & 7 years, Feeney & Ylvisaker, 2003).	Significant reduction in aggressive behaviours. Eight-year follow-up indicated no major behavioural concerns and sound academic progress.
		Single-case design (ABCA), 3 adolescents with aggressive behaviour (Feeney & Ylvisaker, 1995)	Marked reduction in aggressive behaviour and increased productivity at school. All three participants gained employment.
		Long-term observational case studies of two adolescents with chronic behaviour challenges (Gardner et al., 2003)	Reduction of target behaviours to zero, increased school participation and self-management after support was withdrawn.
Signposts for Building Better Behaviour programme (Woods et al., 2012), 9 information booklets, a DVD and workbook	48 families of children aged 2–12 years elected to receive Signposts in either group ($n = 23$) or telephone ($n = 25$) support format over 5 months	Post-intervention ratings of feasibility and satisfaction	Feasibility and satisfaction ratings were high for both intervention formats.
Stepping Stones (Brown et al., 2013) parenting programme with an initial stress management component	2 group sessions on mindfulness for parents, 6 group sessions and 3 telephone calls	RCT with two arms: intervention ($n = 30$) and wait list controls ($n = 29$); age: 2–12 years	Significantly lower number and intensity of child behavioural, emotional and peer problems. Significant improvement in parents' emotional state (anxiety and stress) and positive parenting style. Most gains were maintained at 6-months follow-up.

were high ratings for the ease of use, therapeutic alliance and satisfaction with the Web-based programme. This online mode of therapy overcomes various barriers to accessing support such as time, distance, and the unavailability of skilled providers.

In a group therapy context, Brown, Sofronoff, Whittingham, Boyd and McKinlay (2013) evaluated a combination of parent stress management and Stepping Stones (an extension of the Triple P programme) for parents of children aged 2–12 years who displayed behavioural and emotional problems after brain injury. Their RCT compared Stepping Stones Triple P ($n = 30$) with a wait list control condition ($n = 29$). Parents (90 per cent mothers) in the intervention group initially attended two sessions of stress management based on ACT principles, and then participated in six group sessions (2 hours) focusing on positive parenting strategies for managing child emotional and behavioural problems. Parents also received three 30-minute telephone calls to support the application of intervention strategies in the home. The outcome evaluation indicated a significantly greater reduction in level of behavioural, emotional and peer problems for children, and greater improvements in positive parenting (i.e., reduced laxness, over-reactivity and hostility) and parental emotional well-being (anxiety and stress, but not depression) after the intervention than the wait list period. Most gains were maintained at 6-months follow-up. The inclusion of parent stress management prior to the parenting programme is a novel feature, although further research is needed to determine the influence of different intervention components to outcome.

It is likely that multiple mechanisms underlie the effectiveness of family-based interventions (Braga et al., 2005). In particular, the context-sensitivity of training and tailoring of content to each family's circumstances are key features (Cole et al., 2009; Wade, Carey et al., 2006). Further, professional support to transfer skills beyond the training session into everyday interactions and routines of family life most likely contributed to durable gains (Brown et al., 2013). The increase in positive parenting behaviours and reduction in child behavioural problems and parental stress are likely to have mutually enhancing or reciprocal benefits on parent–child relationships and well-being (Wade et al., 2011; Ylvisaker et al., 2005). Understanding the specific contribution of these features of intervention and their interaction would be beneficial for advancing treatment theory and intervention planning.

Overall, there is Level 1–2 evidence that PBS and FPS interventions can improve the psychological well-being of children with brain injury and/or their parents. However, the impact of these interventions on children's sense of self is yet to be investigated. Use of behavioural observation (e.g., parent–child interactions; see Wade et al., 2011) in combination with significant-other ratings and child self-report measures of self-concept would strengthen the methodology and evidence base for psychological interventions for young children after brain injury.

Interventions for adolescents

Whilst most intervention studies have focused on younger children, studies focusing on the unique needs of adolescents with brain injury are emerging (e.g., Gan et al., 2010; Wade, Walz et al., 2010). Adolescence is pivotal time for identity formation, during which the views and reactions of one's peers become important sources of self-definition. Adolescents typically have more complex notions of self than young children due to their more extensive autobiographical memories and related capacity to reflect on their past and future selves (Harter, 2012). The impact of brain injury at early versus later developmental stages (i.e., early childhood versus mid-adolescence) was illustrated by the case studies of Dan and Jasmine in Chapter 3. Backhouse and Rodger (1999) found that adolescents with brain injury expressed many hopes and dreams for the future (e.g., career aspirations), which often reflected their pre-injury abilities and did not take into account their injury-related impairments. Their parents expressed concern about their children's vocational prospects and options, and the lack of support to transition into the workforce. Therefore, whilst interventions for adolescents still focus on family relationships and fostering home independence, there is often a shift in focus from the home and family interaction to peers, school and vocational pursuits.

With these developmental issues in mind, modification of the BIFI (i.e., BIFI-A; Gan et al., 2010) involved integrating topics for adolescents such as 'Being a teen and achieving independence' and 'School, transitions and preparing for adulthood' (p. 656). Similarly, in their Teen Online Problem-Solving (TOPS) intervention, Wade et al. (2008; 2011) adapted their FPS approach for adolescents to target self-regulation and social skills that promote successful functioning in adulthood. More emphasis was placed on the adolescent monitoring and managing their own behaviour, with parents providing positive behavioural support. New session content focused on social problem-solving, language pragmatics and nonverbal communication. Supplementary modules included 'working with the school', 'planning for after high school' (Wade et al., 2008) and 'parent–teen communication' (Wade et al., 2010). Both adolescents and parents participated in the initial face-to-face and subsequent video-conferencing and self-guided sessions.

Based upon leading research in the field (Blosser & De Pompei, 2003; Glang et al., 2004; Ylvisaker et al., 2001), some broad recommendations for supporting students with brain injury at school and in vocational placements include:

- Development of an individualised education programme (IEP) or tailored curricula for students, which includes access to specialised resources and therapies to enhance their learning and behaviour management.
- Use of proactive teaching strategies such as: linking students' skill development to their personal goals, setting clear and logically sequenced directions on tasks, using pacing and errorless learning principles, developing organisational strategies (e.g., external cuing aids, mind maps) and providing consistent feedback on strengths and suggestions for improvement.
- Increase students' tolerance to stress by teaching coping behaviours and social skills (e.g., communication, emotion regulation and social problem-solving) that will enhance their opportunity to participate in desired activities, thus providing natural reinforcement.
- Use of a behavioural momentum approach that initially focuses on behaviours that students find easy or are more willing to perform to ensure success before moving onto behaviours that are more difficult to perform.
- Modify the environment to avoid high risk situations or identified triggers for distress, frustration and escalation to aggressive behaviour.
- Teach metacognitive skills by training online awareness and self-instructional strategies (e.g., Stop–Think–Do) to improve behaviour regulation with the aim of gradually removing external supports for these strategies.
- Provide TBI-specific education and training to natural communication partners (e.g., parents, teachers, teacher's aides and guidance counsellors) in positive behaviour support strategies, including collaborative communication techniques and increasing choice and sense of control over their environment.

Glang and colleagues (2004) highlighted the importance of the student, parents, therapists and educators working in a partnership to support successful school re-integration, but also noted that such relationships can become strained due to different expectations and goals. It is beneficial for parents and teachers to understand that late developing problems can emerge as academic and developmental demands increase for the student (Cronin, 2001). Rehabilitation and case management services that are able to monitor students in the long term and provide developmentally sensitive interventions around key transition periods have been found to improve outcomes (see Blosser & De Pompei, 2003; Ylvisaker et al., 2001). Transitions refer to changes in status and roles, such as those involved with the student transitioning from hospital to the community, between year levels, between schools, from school to work, and from home to more independent living situations. Increasing adolescents' choice and influence over decisions during transition is essential to promote their active participation and willingness to trial strategies and accept support (Feeney & Ylvisaker, 1995; Mealings & Douglas, 2010).

A key role of support services in providing education and support for parents, school/university, and vocational networks is to minimise misconceptions (e.g., about behavioural problems), address unrealistic expectations and recommend evidence-based strategies for learning and behavioural problems. Goals for a particular transition need to be developed collaboratively between students and members of their support network (Blosser & De Pompei, 2003). In relation to the latter, it may be beneficial for a student's peers to be involved in the school re-integration process through awareness and sensitivity training (see the case study of Jasmine in Chapter 3). Accessible education about brain injury in school-aged children is important, such as the Centres for Disease Control and Prevention's 'Heads Up to Schools: Know Your Concussion ABCs', which is available as a webinar and interactive website (http://www.cdc.gov/concussion/headsup/schools.html). There is some evidence to support team-based interventions such as 'BrainSTARS' for children with brain injury (Dise-Lewis, Lewis & Reichardt, 2009). Using a pre-post single group design, Dise-Lewis et al. evaluated the efficacy of specialised paediatric brain injury education and meetings between parents, regular and special educators and school personnel. The intervention was found to increase participants' perceived competency in supporting students with brain injury and ratings of the students' performance.

There is currently limited literature on the transition from school to work or higher education for adolescents after brain injury. This transition reflects a major rite of passage for all young adults and is commonly associated with heightened stress and uncertainly as they seek to establish their place in the world (Marcia, 1980). Adolescents with brain injury typically face additional challenges, including a lack of understanding of their abilities, cognitive and behavioural impairments and unrealistic goals. They may cope reasonably well with the structure and support provided in their school and parents' home, but lack the skills needed to live independently, manage the demands of university or employment and establish and maintain relationships (Backhouse & Rodger, 1999; Mealings & Douglas, 2010). Continued or increased dependency on parents is common, with some parents assuming advocacy roles to seek work, study and social opportunities for their child (Backhouse & Rodger, 1999). The importance of collaboration and coordination between school and post-school services has been emphasised as key to successful transition. Similar recommendations have been made in the broader transition literature for youth with disabilities, with a recommendation that transition planning begin no later than age 14 (Cobb & Alwell, 2009). Their review concluded that student-focused transition planning can greatly improve student outcomes. Outcomes are maximised when students are actively involved in the process, have peer advocates or mentors and opportunity to gain work experiences and develop their social skills in applied settings.

Some research provides Level 1 or Level 2 evidence that PBS is effective for managing behavioural issues that impact on adolescents' school and work functioning (Feeney & Ylvisaker, 1995; Gardner et al., 2003). Two studies that employed single-case experiments or long-term observational studies to evaluate PBS are summarised in Table 8.1. For example, Feeney and Ylvisaker (1995) evaluated a PBS intervention for three adolescents with aggressive behaviour in the high school and prevocational setting. The multi-component intervention focused on strategies for managing students' cognitive impairments through routine and organisation and addressed behavioural issues by increasing choices and involvement in decisions and enhancing opportunity for success based on behavioural momentum principles. All three participants displayed a marked reduction in aggressive episodes and increased productivity. Moreover, the participants engaged in employment or further study with minimal or no support.

Despite these promising findings there is a dearth of literature on the transition from school to work or higher education for adolescents with brain injury. The process of transition and factors influencing outcomes and efficacy of vocational interventions for adults injured during childhood represent much-needed areas of research. Other key gaps in the literature for adolescents with brain injury relate to interventions for independent living, friendships, intimacy and sexuality.

One promising avenue of intervention for children and adolescents with brain injury involves internet-based social networking. Computer-mediated communication (e.g., Facebook, blogging) represents a dominant method of communication for adolescents and young adults worldwide. As previously discussed in Chapter 7, there may be potential to improve people's friendship networks and access to brain injury resources (e.g., TBI education and forums) through this means. However, Kilov et al. (2010) stressed the need to weigh up the relative benefits and risks of online interaction for adolescents. Specifically, due to cognitive-linguistic and behavioural impairments associated with brain injury this mode of communication has various challenges (e.g., interpreting jargon and graphic representation of emotion) and there are risks for safety and self-esteem (e.g., bullying and social rejection). They highlighted the importance of training programmes for adolescents and their supports (e.g., teachers, clinicians and parents) to increase awareness of safety and pragmatic issues and how to manage these. Further development and evaluation of brain injury specific training packages for enhancing participation in online social networking would advance the field (Egan et al., 2005). Such developments are not limited to people with brain injury, as the opportunity to connect with others with similar experiences in a flexible manner may reduce the sense of isolation and improve the well-being of family members, including parents, siblings and children.

Conclusions

Brain injury can have a profound impact on family functioning and the wellness of individual members. As reviewed in this chapter, family members can be supported through different approaches, including their involvement in an intervention for a child or adult with brain injury, programmes specifically designed for family caregivers and family system interventions that concurrently support the person with brain injury and family members. For children with brain injury, the efficacy of contextualised interventions (i.e. family problem-solving and positive behaviour supports) has received most empirical support to date. There is a need for further research to evaluate the impact of contextualised interventions on family identity and children's emerging sense of self.

9 Summary and future directions

Understanding of the impact of brain injury on sense of self has greatly improved over the last two decades, stimulated by developments in many fields including social psychology and cognitive neuroscience. Empirical research on children and adults with brain injury underscores the interplay of premorbid characteristics, neuro-cognitive functions and social environmental factors in the adjustment process. However, there are few validated assessment tools and interventions focusing specifically on self-identity. A multi-level approach to intervention is recommended that incorporates individual, group, community and family-based support. This chapter summarises key developments in the self-identity and brain injury literature and provides suggestions for future research.

This book has highlighted how brain injury can have a major impact on how people see themselves. Changes in abilities and lifestyle can alter personal and social identity in both negative and positive ways. For example, some people express that they feel 'useless', 'misunderstood' and 'isolated' after brain injury, while others perceive that the injury helped them to recognise what really matters in life and increased their compassion and desire to help others. Importantly, people can simultaneously experience losses, growth, and sameness or continuity of self (Gelech & Desjardins, 2011; Secrest & Zeller, 2007). Self-perceptions may fluctuate in response to different stressors, learning opportunities and goal achievement (Cantor et al., 2005; Douglas, 2013; Kristensen, 2004). More generally, the process of redefining one's self after brain injury may continue indefinitely (Muenchberger et al., 2008; Nochi, 2000). This idea is consistent with Allport's (1955) concept of 'becoming' and the view that self is an ongoing construction (Conway, 2005; D'Argembeau et al., 2008). Such advances in conceptualising self-identity change have important implications for rehabilitation approaches that seek to support people to re-establish a meaningful and satisfying life after brain injury. The following section summarises key developments in understanding self-identity after brain injury and gaps in the literature that represent priorities for future research.

Leading developments in self-identity and brain injury research

It is difficult to conceive how something as complex as self-identity is represented in the brain. Social neuroscience research has made considerable progress in identifying neural substrates supporting the self and social identification. As described in Chapter 2, an integrated subcortical-cortical midline system has been consistently implicated in self-referential processing, as measured by tasks that require people to make judgements on or respond to self-related stimuli (Northoff et al., 2011). Although reflection on self-related stimuli (e.g., faces, psychological traits) cannot be equated to the more complex notion of self-identity, particularly given the greater focus on objective aspects of self than subjective aspects (see Christoff et al., 2011), the pattern of activation supports a dissociation between areas underlying current self and past and future selves. Reflecting on current self has been found to activate a neural region (i.e., medial prefrontal cortex) distinct from the system involved in remembering one's past and projecting self into the future (D'Argembeau et al., 2010; Rathbone et al., 2011). Cortical midline structures support self-reflection across time and processing of changes to one's self from the past to the present (D'Argembeau et al., 2008). Thus, a coordinated neural system produces an ongoing sense of self that is continually updated through life experiences and influenced by one's goals (Conway, 2005; Damasio, 1999).

The discovery of mirror neurons and their role in self–other representations (e.g., imitation and empathy) provides a possible basis for understanding social identification processes or our experience of 'we' and 'us' (Rizzolatti & Craighero, 2005). More specifically, this research suggests that shared activation of neural circuits supports our sense of connection with others, allowing mutual meanings, intentions and feelings to form (Platek et al., 2004). Lesion studies support that damage to different brain regions produces varied deficits that impact on the experience of self in the world (i.e., 'neuropathologies of self'), including bodily self, relational self and autobiographical self (Feinberg, 2011b). The most profound alterations in personal identity result from lesions to the right hemisphere and damage to the medial-frontal or orbito-frontal areas (Feinberg, 2011b). Guided by research on neurological disorders, neuropsychological accounts depict the interplay between cognition, emotion, language and culture that support higher level self-representations (e.g., Agnew & Morris, 1998; Conway, 2005; Damasio, 1999; Stuss, 2007; Teasdale & Barnard, 1993). These models have been applied to understand disorders of self-awareness and identity changes in the context of brain injury (Gracey & Ownsworth, 2012; Ownsworth, Clare et al., 2006; Ylvisaker & Feeney, 2000).

Chapters 3 and 4 adopted a biopsychosocial perspective to consider how neuropathology interacts with premorbid personality and aspects of the social environment to influence psychological adjustment after brain injury. In particular, research indicates that cognitive impairments interfere with people's ability to understand their brain injury and perceive changes in their functioning (Cooper-Evans et al., 2008; Nochi, 1998). Metacognitive impairments restrict the capacity to accurately self-evaluate performance on tasks and compare pre-injury and post-injury abilities. In turn, awareness deficits may preserve one's pre-existing self-schema and protect self-esteem (Beardmore et al., 1999; Carroll & Coetzer, 2011; Cooper-Evans et al., 2008). However, poor self-awareness impacts on the ability to make sense of changes to one's life circumstances (e.g., understand reasons for not being able to drive or work) and develop strategies to maintain participation in valued activities. Conversely, individuals with heightened awareness of their impairments who make unfavourable comparisons between their pre-injury and post-injury selves are more likely to perceive threat in everyday situations, use avoidant coping and develop depression (Cantor et al., 2005; Medley et al., 2010; Ownsworth, 2005). Therefore, people who present with either poor self-awareness or negative self-discrepancy may struggle to develop a realistic and adaptive self-identity over time. This perspective needs to be specifically examined in prospective longitudinal research on the role of self-awareness, self-discrepancy and coping behaviours in identity transition after brain injury.

Future advances in research on self-identity processes after brain injury are reliant on access to reliable and valid tools. In Chapter 5 it was recommended that self-report measures be used in conjunction with collateral information (e.g., family and therapist ratings) and performance-based measures. This is potentially more achievable for assessing self-awareness (e.g., Schmidt et al., 2013) and coping strategies (e.g., Krpan et al., 2011) than self-concept or identity. The Head Injury Semantic Differential Scale (HISD III) has most frequently been used to assess changes in self-concept (i.e., self-discrepancy) after brain injury, whereas the Rosenberg Self-Esteem Scale (RSES) was employed in most studies to measure global self-esteem (e.g., Anson & Ponsford, 2006a; 2006b; Kelly et al., 2013). Further psychometric analysis of the HISD III is needed, including test–retest reliability, factor analysis and sensitivity to change. The HISD III may have greater potential to reflect change in response to intervention than the RSES because of the scope to assess change across individual attributes as well as current self and the discrepancy between past and current self (Vickery et al., 2005). A direct comparison of the responsiveness to change of these tools is needed within the same study.

Only preliminary research has been conducted on self-awareness and self-esteem of children with brain injury and most researchers have employed measures developed for the general paediatric population (e.g., Coopersmith Self-Esteem Inventory and Piers–Harris Children's Self-Concept Scale). The suitability of these generic measures for assessing children's developing sense of self after brain injury needs to be examined longitudinally. Additionally, the psychometric properties of tools specifically developed or modified for paediatric brain injury such as the Knowledge Interview for Children (Beardmore et al., 1999) and Social-Emotional Questionnaire for Children (Wall et al., 2011) require further investigation. Interview schedules (e.g., Self-Understanding Interview) and observation of children and adolescents in their naturalistic social environment may also provide valuable insight into their self-awareness and self–other perceptions (Mealings & Douglas, 2010; Wade et al., 2011).

When using self-report measures with children, inferences made about 'insight' or self-awareness need to take into account the process of normal development or age-related differences in self-understanding (see Chapter 2). The process by which children and adolescents evaluate themselves over time (i.e., temporal comparison) and in comparison to their peers (self–other comparisons) represents a key area for future research. More generally, it would be valuable to understand the extent to which brain injury influences children's self-definition, sense of continuity versus change, perception of strengths and difficulties, and their goals and hopes for the future.

The lack of validated tools for assessing children's self-perceptions after brain injury may partly account for the paucity of research in this area. As reviewed in Chapter 3, the small body of paediatric brain injury literature on self-awareness and self-esteem suggests that developmental, neuro-cognitive and social factors have an interactive influence on developing sense of self. In particular, Jacobs (1993) found that children aged 7–15 years lacked understanding of their brain injury, which was attributed in part to their low knowledge of normal body and brain functioning. Similar to the self-descriptions of children without brain injury (Harter, 2012), their self-understanding was greater for observable physical changes (e.g., mobility and appearance). Lack of understanding of brain injury is also related to memory impairment (Beardmore et al., 1999). Children with poorer memory function are likely to be more reliant upon their parents' recollections of events to build their autobiographical self (Harter, 2012), thus highlighting the key influence of parenting style and responsiveness (Wade et al., 2011; Ylvisaker, Feeney et al., 1998). Also consistent with developmental literature (Harter, 2012), children with less realistic perceptions of their abilities were found to report higher self-esteem (Beardmore et al., 1999).

Children with brain injury are generally found to experience poorer self-esteem and social functioning than their peers (Andrews et al., 1998; Hawley, 2012). In one study, low self-esteem was related to greater behavioural problems and parental stress (Hawley, 2012). Although not specifically investigated, it is possible that social cognition deficits influence the relationship between behavioural problems and poor self-esteem. In particular, impairments in the ability to read people and solve social problems are likely to affect children's ability to interact appropriately with their peers and family, which in turn produces negative social experiences (e.g., peer rejection and family conflict) that affects their self-worth. Wade et al. (2011) found that parenting styles characterised by greater warmth and responsiveness and lower negativity were associated with fewer internalising and externalising behavioural problems. Therefore, a supportive home environment is more likely to foster positive self-concept in children after brain injury, although this is yet to be specifically examined.

The limited research on adolescents' sense of self after brain injury has mainly focused on the school re-integration process. Similar to young children, adolescents may lack awareness of their post-injury changes and have difficulty relating to their peers (Wall et al., 2011; Wilson et al., 2011). When returning to school, adolescents can struggle to fit in, make sense of changes to their abilities and establish meaningful and realistic goals (Mealings & Douglas, 2010; Sharp et al., 2006). The presence of transition support services is considered vital to facilitate school re-integration and students' entry into work and higher education placements (Backhouse & Rodger, 1999; Todis & Glang, 2008). As discussed in Chapter 8, factors influencing the success of the school-to-work transition and related interventions represent a major gap in the literature.

In Chapter 6 it was emphasised that interventions combining psychotherapy and neurorehabilitation techniques are optimal for supporting identity reconstruction, or the process of updating and consolidating a new identity (Gracey et al., 2009; Feeney & Capo, 2010). As part of this process, the importance of building the therapeutic alliance and the value of client-centred feedback and goal-directed interventions was highlighted. A review of controlled studies of psychotherapy for people with brain injury identified that CBT approaches can be effective for reducing and preventing emotional distress (e.g., Hseih et al., 2012; Watkins et al., 2007; 2011). Few studies have specifically examined the impact of psychotherapy on sense of self after brain injury. The findings of the CALM stroke intervention by Thomas et al. (2013) are noteworthy in this respect because they found that behavioural therapy was effective for improving self-esteem and reducing depression in people with aphasia and low mood. The efficacy of project-based learning (PBL) for facilitating identity reconstruction has been exemplified through case studies, but requires more rigorous evaluation through controlled studies (i.e., Level 1–2 evidence). The application of technological aides in psychotherapy represents a cutting-edge development in the field. Electronic devices can support people to remember and act on their intentions, achieve personal goals and recollect their success. In doing so, these devices have the potential to improve people's self-agency and self-worth (Brindley et al., 2011).

Further promising therapy developments include the application of positive psychology techniques and third-wave cognitive and behavioural therapies in brain injury rehabilitation (e.g., Azulay et al., 2013; Bédard et al., 2012; Evans, 2011). ACT and positive psychotherapy approaches have a shared focus on human flourishing, valued living, personal strengths and finding meaning (Kashdan & Ciarrochi, 2013). A major premise of positive psychology is that well-being is related to satisfaction with one's past, flow and happiness in the present, and optimism and growth in the future (Csikszentmihalyi, 2000). Accordingly, people with brain injury can be supported to reach their unique potential through positive learning experiences, close and supportive relationships and fulfilling occupation (Evans, 2011; Kangas & McDonald, 2011). Adopting a growth perspective after brain injury can help shift focus from treating (and researching) impairments and dysfunction to identifying and promoting personal strengths and meaning after brain injury. This view was particularly reflected in the discussion of PBL in Chapter 6 and community-based initiatives in Chapter 7.

It is well recognised that social loss and disconnection (e.g., friends, family, clubs and work) after brain injury has detrimental consequences for subjective well-being (Douglas, 2012; Haslam et al., 2008; Walsh et al., 2012). As discussed in Chapter 7, greater recognition of the link between social networks and psychological adjustment following adversity has stimulated group and community-based interventions to support people to maintain or rebuild their social identity after brain injury (e.g., Douglas et al., 2006; Kennedy et al., 2011). In terms of people's informal support network, the impact of brain injury on family identity has received little empirical attention (see Kosciulek, 1997) when compared with the large body of research on primary caregivers' adjustment (Boschen et al., 2007). As described in Chapter 8, family-system interventions that focus on relationship dynamics (e.g., communication and problem-solving skills) and enhancing dimensions of a person's social environment (e.g., positive behaviour supports) can improve the well-being of the person with brain injury and their family members (Feeney & Ylvisaker, 1995; Togher et al., 2013; Wade, Michaud et al., 2006; 2010). Further research guided by the Social Identity Model of Change (SIMIC; Haslam et al., 2008; Jetten & Pachana, 2012) is needed to investigate the two proposed social pathways to enhancing well-being after brain injury: namely, identity maintenance (retaining group memberships) and identity change (building new group memberships), and implications for interventions. Social media applications discussed in Chapters 7 and 8 represent a potential avenue for maintaining social connections and forming new ones for individuals and family members.

A key challenge for researchers in the neurorehabilitation field is to understand not only whether an intervention is effective but *how* or *why* it works (Whyte & Hart, 2003). For interventions reviewed in Chapters 6–8 the mechanisms or active ingredients of effective intervention were often unclear because of multiple components of treatment that differed from control interventions (e.g., Brown et al., 2013; Thomas et al., 2013; Wade et al., 2006). Some studies have been able to 'partial out' the contribution of these components through carefully designed RCTs (e.g., Schmidt et al., 2013). Greater use of dismantling designs and single-case experimental methodology (e.g., alternating treatments design) may advance treatment theory and guide selection of treatment strategies in clinical practice.

Future research directions

To build upon these developments in the self-identity and brain injury field, key priorities for future research include:

- Validating tools for assessing the impact of brain injury on sense of self, particularly for children and adolescents;
- Modelling the identity transition process and biopsychosocial factors influencing reconstruction of identity over time (e.g., application of SIMIC);
- Determining factors related to successful transition from school to work or higher education for adolescents with brain injury;
- Investigating the impact of brain injury on family identity and evaluation of different levels of family-system intervention (e.g., support programmes for siblings);
- Conducting controlled studies of the efficacy of identity-oriented interventions (e.g., PBL, ACT, social media and community initiatives) and identifying the active components and characteristics of effective treatment.

Conclusions

Brain injury can alter people in the most fundamental way – their sense of self. This book set out to provide a comprehensive account of the impact of brain injury on self-identity. To help achieve this, the theoretical underpinnings of self and social neuroscience perspectives were initially reviewed. After reviewing literature on self-identity after brain injury, the book provided assessment and intervention guidelines and strategies for clinicians. This final chapter summarised major developments in the field and recommendations for future research. It is hoped that the ideas conveyed in this book contribute to improving the quality of rehabilitation and support for individuals and families affected by brain injury.

Appendix A
Head Injury Semantic Differential III

Name:...............	Dob:............	Date:...............	Past / Present / Future	
Bored	:	:	:	:	:	:	:	Interested
Unhappy	:	:	:	:	:	:	:	Happy
In Control	:	:	:	:	:	:	:	Helpless
Worried	:	:	:	:	:	:	:	Relaxed
Satisfied	:	:	:	:	:	:	:	Dissatisfied
Despondent	:	:	:	:	:	:	:	Hopeful
Self Confident	:	:	:	:	:	:	:	Lacks Confidence
Unstable (1)	:	:	:	:	:	:	:	Stable
Attractive (2)	:	:	:	:	:	:	:	Unattractive*
Of Value	:	:	:	:	:	:	:	Worthless*
Aggressive	:	:	:	:	:	:	:	Unaggressive
Calm	:	:	:	:	:	:	:	Irritable
Capable	:	:	:	:	:	:	:	Incapable
Dependent	:	:	:	:	:	:	:	Independent
Inactive	:	:	:	:	:	:	:	Active
Withdrawn	:	:	:	:	:	:	:	Talkative
Friendly	:	:	:	:	:	:	:	Unfriendly
Patient	:	:	:	:	:	:	:	Impatient

(1) Emotionally (2) As a Person
* Items Attractive–Unattractive & Of Value–Worthless are replaced in relatives' version
Reproduced with the author's permission (Andy Tyerman)

Appendix B
The Brain Injury Grief Inventory

This questionnaire is designed to help your clinician to know how you feel. Read each item below and underline the response which comes closest to how you have been feeling in the past week.

If you find it difficult reading and filling in the items, you can ask someone else to read each question out to you.

Don't take too long over your replies; your immediate reaction to each item will probably be more accurate than a long, thought-out response.

Name: _____ Date: _____

Please rate each statement below as 'never', 'sometimes' or 'mostly'.

Please underline one only.

	F1	F2
1. I try to avoid thinking and reminding myself about having had a brain injury Never Sometimes Mostly	☐	
2. I am able now to think through what the brain injury means to my life Never Sometimes Mostly		☐
3. I feel angry that I had a brain injury Never Sometimes Mostly	☐	
4. Although life has changed for me, I feel able to get on with my life now Never Sometimes Mostly		☐
5. I am upset by things that remind me about my injury, e.g. the anniversary Never Sometimes Mostly	☐	
6. I have stopped comparing how things were before my brain injury Never Sometimes Mostly		☐

7. I have found myself longing for the time before my injury occurred
   Never   Sometimes   Mostly   ☐

8. I am less preoccupied with the effects of my brain injury now than I was before
   Never   Sometimes   Mostly   ☐

9. I have a strong desire to talk about my injury and the effects it had on me
   Never   Sometimes   Mostly   ☐

10. I feel I can reach out to people   ☐
    Never   Sometimes   Mostly

11. I miss the things I cannot do since I had my injury   ☐
    Never   Sometimes   Mostly

12. I think I have overcome the losses resulting from my brain injury   ☐
    Never   Sometimes   Mostly

13. I have been feeling low since my injury   ☐
    Never   Sometimes   Mostly

14. I feel it is unfair that I had a brain injury   ☐
    Never   Sometimes   Mostly

15. I think I understand what has happened to me   ☐
    Never   Sometimes   Mostly

16. I think about my brain injury so much that I find it difficult to do other things   ☐
    Never   Sometimes   Mostly

17. I do not feel sad or depressed   ☐
    Never   Sometimes   Mostly

18. I feel less able to care for other people since my injury   ☐
    Never   Sometimes   Mostly

19. I have accepted the fact that I have a brain injury   ☐
    Never   Sometimes   Mostly

20. Life is empty since my injury   ☐
    Never   Sometimes   Mostly

F1   *F2*

Thank you for completing this questionnaire.

© B. R. Coetzer, North Wales Brain Injury Service, Conwy & Denbighshire NHS Trust, Colwyn Bay Hospital, Hesketh Road, Colwyn Bay, LL29 8AY, United Kingdom.

Reproduced with author's permission.

References

Abreu, B.C., Seale, G., Scheibel, R.S., Huddleston, N., Zhang, L., & Ottenbacher, K.J. (2001). Levels of self-awareness after acute brain injury: how patients' and rehabilitation specialists' perceptions compare. *Archives of Physical Medicine, 82*, 49–56.
Adler, A. (1954). *Understanding human nature*. New York: Fawcett Publications.
Adler, A. (1964). *The individual psychology of Alfred Adler*. H. L. Ansbacher and R. R. Ansbacher (Eds). New York: Harper Torchbooks.
Agnew, S.K., & Morris, R.G. (1998). The heterogeneity of anosognosia for memory impairment in Alzheimer's disease: A review of the literature and a proposed model. *Aging & Mental Health, 2*, 7–19.
Allen, C.C. & Ruff, R.M. (1990). Self-rating versus neurophysiological performance of moderate versus severe head-injured patients. *Brain Injury, 4*, 7–17.
Allport, G.W. (1955). *Becoming; Basic considerations for a psychology of personality*. London: Yale University Press.
Allport, G.W. (1961). *Pattern and growth in personality*. New York: Holt, Rinehart and Winston.
Anderson, S., & Tranel, D. (1989). Awareness of disease states following cerebral infarction, dementia, and head trauma: standardised assessment. *Clinical Neuropsychologist, 3*, 327–339.
Anderson, S., Damasio, H., & Tranel, D. (1990). Neuropsychological impairments associated with lesions caused by tumor or stroke. *Archives of neurology, 47*, 397–405.
Anderson, V., & Catroppa, C. (2006). Advances in postacute rehabilitation after childhood-acquired brain injury: A focus on cognitive, behavioral, and social domains. *American Journal of Physical Medicine & Rehabilitation, 85*, 767–778.
Anderson, V., Brown, S., Newitt, H., & Hoile, H. (2009). Educational, vocational, psychosocial, and quality-of-life outcomes for adult survivors of childhood traumatic brain injury. *Journal of Head Trauma Rehabilitation, 24*, 303–312.
Anderson, V., Catroppa, C., Morse, S., Haritou, F., & Rosenfeld, J. (2005). Functional plasticity or vulnerability after early brain injury? *Pediatrics, 116*, 1374–1382.
Anderson, V., Godfrey, C., Rosenfeld, J.V., & Catroppa, C. (2012). Predictors of cognitive function and recovery 10 years after traumatic brain injury in young children. *Pediatrics, 129*, 254–261.
Andrews, T.K., Rose, F.D., & Johnson, D.A. (1998). Social and behavioural effects of traumatic brain injury in children. *Brain Injury, 12*, 133–138.
Anson, K., & Ponsford, J. (2006a). Coping and emotional adjustment following traumatic brain injury. *Journal of Head Trauma Rehabilitation, 21*, 248–259.
Anson, K., & Ponsford, J. (2006b). Evaluation of a coping skills group following traumatic brain injury. *Brain Injury, 20*, 167–178.

Appleton, S., Browne, A., Ciccone, N.A., Fong, K., Hankey, G., Lund, M., ... Yee, Y. (2011). A multidisciplinary social communication and coping skills group intervention for adults with acquired brain injury (ABI): A pilot feasibility study in an inpatient setting. *Brain Impairment, 12*, 210–222.

Arango-Lasprilla, J.C., Ketchum, J.M., Dezfulian, T., Kreutzer, J.S., O'Neil-Pirozzi, T.M., Hammond, F., & Jha, A. (2008). Predictors of marital stability 2 years following traumatic brain injury. *Brain Injury, 22*, 565–574.

Ashman, T., & Tsaousides, T. (2012). Cognitive Behavioral Therapy for Depression Following Traumatic Brain Injury: Findings of a Randomized Controlled Trial. Paper presented at the 9th Annual Conference of the Neuropsychological Rehabilitation Special Interest Group of the World Federation of Neurorehabilitation, July 2–3, Bergen, Norway.

Ashworth, F., Gracey, F., & Gilbert, P. (2011). Compassion focused therapy after traumatic brain injury: Theoretical foundations and case illustration. *Brain Impairment, 12*, 128–139.

Australian Institute of Health and Welfare (2008). *Austrralia's health 2008*. (Cat. no. AUS 99). Canberra: AIHW.

Azulay, J., Smart, C., Mott, T., & Cicerone, K. (2013). A pilot study examining the effect of Mindfulness-Based Stress Reduction on symptoms of chronic mild traumatic brain injury/postconcussive syndrome. *Journal of Head Trauma Rehabilitation, 28*, 323–331.

Babikian, T., & Asarnow, R. (2009). Neurocognitive outcomes and recovery after pediatric TBI: meta-analytic review of the literature. *Neuropsychology, 23*, 283–296.

Bachman, J.G., O'Malley, P.M., Freedman-Doan, P., Trzesniewski, K.H., & Donnellan, M.B. (2011). Adolescent self-esteem: Differences by race/ethnicity, gender, and age. *Self and Identity, 10*, 445–473.

Backhaus, S.L., Ibarra, S.L., Klyce, D., Trexler, L.E., & Malec, J.F. (2010). Brain injury coping skills group: A preventative intervention for patient with brain injury and their caregivers. *Archives of Physical Medicine and Rehabilitation, 91*, 840–848.

Backhouse, M., & Rodger, S. (1999). The transition from school to employment for young people with acquired brain injury: Parent and student perceptions. *Australian Occupational Therapy Journal, 46*, 99–109.

Bäckman, L., & Dixon, R.A. (1992). Psychological compensation: A theoretical framework. *Psychological Bulletin, 112*, 259–283.

Baker, J.R., & Moore, S.M. (2008). Blogging as a social tool: a psychosocial examination of the effects of blogging. *Cyberpsychological Behaviour, 11*, 747–749.

Baltes, P. (1987). Theoretical propositions of life-span developmental psychology: On the dynamics between growth and decline. *Developmental Psychology, 23*, 611–626.

Bandura, A. (1989). Human agency in social cognitive theory. *American Psychologist, 44*, 1175–1184.

Bandura, A. (2001). Social cognitive theory: An agentic perspective. *Annual Review of Psychology, 52*, 1.

Barker, D., Reid, D., & Cott, C. (2004). Acceptance and meanings of wheelchair use in senior stroke survivors. *American Journal of Occupational Therapy, 58*, 221–230.

Barker-Collo, S.L. (2007). Depression and anxiety 3 months post stroke: Prevalence and correlates. *Archives of Clinical Neuropsychology, 22*, 519–531.

Bartlett, R.C., & Collins, S.D. (2011). *Aristotle's nicomachean ethics*. Chicago: University of Chicago Press.

Beardmore, S., Tate, R., & Liddle, B. (1999). Does information and feedback improve children's knowledge and awareness of deficits after traumatic brain injury? *Neuropsychological Rehabilitation, 9*, 45–62.

Beck, A.T. (1967). *Depression: Clinical, experimental, and theoretical aspects*. New York: Hoeber.

Beck, A.T. (2005). The current state of cognitive therapy: A 40-year retrospective. *Archives of General Psychiatry, 62*, 953–959.

Bédard, M., Felteau, M., Marshall, S., Dubois, S., Gibbons, C., Klein, R., & Weaver, B. (2012). Mindfulness-based cognitive therapy: benefits in reducing depression following traumatic brain injury. *Advances in Mind-Body Medicine, 26*, 14–20.

Bédard, M., Felteau, M., Mazmanian, D., Fedyk, K., Klein, R., Richardson, J., … Minthorn-Biggs, M.-B. (2003). Pilot intervention of a mindfulness-based intervention to improve quality of life among individuals who sustained traumatic brain injuries. *Disability and Rehabilitation, 25*, 722–731.

Bedian, A.G., Teague, R.J., & Zmud, R.W. (1977). Test-retest reliability and internal Consistency of a short-form of Coopersmith's Self Esteem Inventory. *Psychological Reports, 41*, 1041–1042.

Behn, N., Togher, L., Power, E., & Heard, R. (2012). Evaluating communication training for paid carers of people with traumatic brain injury. *Brain Injury, 26*, 1702–1715.

Bell, K., Temkin, N., Esselman, P., Doctor, J., Bombardier, C., Fraser, R., Hoffman, J., Powell, J., & Dikmen, S. (2011). The effect of a scheduled telephone intervention on outcome after moderate to severe traumatic brain injury: a randomized trial. *Archives of Physical Medicine Rehabilitation, 86*, 851–856.

Bennett, L.A., Wolin, S.J., & McAvity, K.J. (1988). Family identity, ritual, and myth: A cultural perspective on life cycle transitions. In C.J. Falicov (Ed.), *Family transitions* (pp. 211–234). New York: Guilford Press.

Bennett-Levy, J., Westbrook, D., Fennell, M., Cooper, M., Rouf, K., & Hackmann, A. (2004), Behavioural experiments: historical and conceptual underpinnings. In *Oxford Guide to Behavioural Experiments in Cognitive Therapy* (pp.1–20). Oxford: Oxford University Press.

Ben-Yishay, Y. (2008). Foreword. In F. Gracey and T. Ownsworth (Eds). *The self and identity in rehabilitation: A special issue of the journal Neuropsychological Rehabilitation, 18*, 513–521.

Ben-Yishay, Y., & Diller, L. (2011). *Handbook of holistic neuropsychological rehabilitation*. New York: Oxford University Press.

Ben-Yishay, Y., Rattok, J., Lakin, P., Piasetsky, E., Ross, B., Silver S.L., Zide, E., & Ezrachi, O. (1985). Neuropsychological rehabilitation: The quest for a holistic approach. *Seminars in Neurology, 5*, 252–259.

Berk, M.S., & Andersen, S.M. (2000). The impact of past relationships on interpersonal behavior: behavioral confirmation in the social-cognitive process of transference. *Journal of Personality and Social Psychology, 79*, 546–562.

Bernabeu, M., Laxe, S., Lopez, R., Stucki, G., Ward, A., Barnes, M., … Cieza, A. (2009). Developing core sets for persons with traumatic brain injury based on the international classification of functioning, disability, and health. *Neurorehabilitation and Neural Repair, 23*, 464–467.

Berry, E., Hampshire, A., Rowe, J., Hodges, S., Kapur, N., Watson, P., … Owen, A. (2009). The neural basis of effective memory therapy in a patient with limbic encephalitis. *Journal of Neurology, Neurosurgery, and Psychiatry, 80*, 1202–1205.

Berry, E., Kapur, N., Williams, L., Hodges, S., Watson, P., Smyth, G., & Wood, K. (2007). The use of a wearable camera, SenseCam as a pictorial diary to improve autobiographical memory in a patient with limbic encephalitis: A preliminary report. *Neuropsychological Rehabilitation, 17*, 582–601.

BIAQ (Brain Injury Association of Queensland). (2002). *Surviving acquired brain injury* (pp. 118-139). Milton, Australia: Brain Injury Association of Queensland.

Blake, H., & Batson, M. (2009). Exercise intervention in brain injury: a pilot randomized study of Tai Chi Qigong. *Clinical Rehabilitation, 23*, 589–598.

Blosser, J.L., De Pompei, R. (2003). *Pediatric Traumatic Brain Injury: Proactive intervention*, 2nd edition. Delmar: Clifton Park NY.

Bodiam, C. (1999). The use of the COPM for the assessment of outcome on a neurorehabilitation unit. *British Journal of Occupational Therapy, 62*, 123–126.

Bolognini, M., Plancherel, B., Bettschart, W., & Halfon, O. (1996). Self-esteem and mental health in early adolescence: development and gender differences. *Journal of Adolescence, 19*, 233–245.

Bombardier, C.H., Bell, K.R., Temkin, N.R., Fann, J.R., Hoffman, J., & Dikmen, S. (2009). The efficacy of a scheduled telephone intervention for ameliorating depressive symptoms during the first year after traumatic brain injury. *Journal of Head Trauma Rehabilitation, 24*, 230–238.

Bombardier, C., Fann, J.R., Temkin, N.R., Esselman, P.C., Barber, J., & Dikmen, S.S. (2010). Rates of major depressive disorder and clinical outcomes following traumatic brain injury. *Journal of the American Medical Association, 303*, 1938–1945.

Borgaro, S.R., & Prigatano, G.P. (2003) Modification of the PCRS for use in an acute neurorehabilitation unit: the PCRS-NR. *Brain Injury, 17*, 847–853.

Bornstein, R.F. (2005). Reconecting psychoanalysis to mainstream psychology. Challenges and opportunities. *Psychoanalytic Psychology, 22*, 323–340.

Boschen, K., Gargaro, J., Gan, C., Gerber, G., & Brandys, C. (2007). Family interventions after acquire brain injury and other chronic conditions: A critical appraisal of the quality of evidence. *NeuroRehabilitation, 22*, 19–41.

Bouwens, S.F.M., van Heugten, C.M., & Verhey, F.R.J. (2009). The practical use of goal attainment scaling for people with acquired brain injury who receive cognitive rehabilitation. *Clinical Rehabilitation, 23*, 310–320.

Bovend'Eert, T.J.H., Botell, R.E., & Wade, D.T. (2009). Writing SMART rehabilitation goals and achieving goal attainment scaling: a practical guide. *Clinical Rehabilitation, 23*, 352–361.

Bowen, C., Hall, T., Newby, G., Walsh, B., Weatherhead, S., & Yeates, G. (2009). The impact of brain injury on relationships across the lifespan and after school, family and work contexts. *Human Systems: The Journal of Therapy, Consultation & Training, 20*, 62–77.

Bowen, C., Yeates, G., & Palmer, S. (2010). *A Relational Approach to Rehabilitation: Thinking about Relationships after Brain Injury*. London: Karnac Books.

Bowlby, J. (1977). The making and breaking of affectional bonds. I. Aetiology and psychopathology in the light of attachment theory. An expanded version of the Fiftieth Maudsley Lecture, delivered before the Royal College of Psychiatrists, 19 November 1976. *British Journal of Psychiatry, 130*, 201–210.

Boyd, D.M., & Ellison, N.B. (2007). Social network sites: Definition, history, and scholarship. *Journal of Computer-Mediated Communication, 13*, 210–230.

Braga, L.W., Da Paz, A.C., & Ylvisaker, M. (2005). Direct clinician-delivered versus indirect family-supported rehabilitation of children with traumatic brain injury: a randomized controlled trial. *Brain Injury, 19*, 819–831.

Bramham, J., Morris, R.G., Hornak, J., Bullock, P., & Polkey, C.E. (2009). Social and emotional functioning following neurosurgical prefrontal cortex lesions. *Journal of Neuropsychology, 3*, 125–143.

Brenner, L.A., Braden, C.A., Bates, M., Chase, T., Hancock, C., Harrison-Felix, C., … Staniszewski, K. (2012). A health and wellness intervention for those with moderate to severe traumatic brain injury: a randomized controlled trial. *Journal of Head Trauma Rehabilitation, 27*, 57–68.

Brindley, R., Bateman, A., & Gracey, F. (2011) Exploration of use of SenseCam to support autobiographical memory retrieval within a cognitive behavioural therapeutic intervention following acquired brain injury. *Memory*, *19*, 745–757.

Brinthaupt, T.M., & Erwin, L.J. (1992). Reporting about the self: issues and complications. In T.M. Brinthaupt and R.P. Lipka (Eds) *The self: Definitional and methodological issues* (pp. 137–71). Albany, NY: State University of New York Press.

Brinthaupt, T.M., & Lipka, R.P. (1992). *The self: Definitional and methodological issues*. Albany: State University of New York.

Broomfield, N.M., Laidlaw, K., Hickabottom, E., Murray, M.F., Pendrey, R., Whittick, J.E. & Gillespie, D.C. (2010). Post-stroke depression: The case for augmented, individually tailored cognitive behavioural therapy. *Clinical Psychology and Psychotherapy*, *18*, 202–217.

Brown, F.L., Sofronoff, K., Whittingham, K., Boyd, R., & McKinlay, L. (2013). Stepping Stones Triple P for parents of children with acquired brain injury: A randomised controlled trial. Paper presented at the 36th Annual Brain Impairment Conference, Hobart, Tasmania (2–4 May, 2013).

Brown, F., Whittingham, K., Boyd, R., & Sofronoff, K. (2012) A Systematic Review of Parenting Interventions for Traumatic Brain Injury: Child and Parent Outcomes. *Journal of Head Trauma Rehabilitation*. May 28, Epub ahead of print.

Brunner, J. (2002). Freud's (de)construction of the conflictual mind. *Thesis Eleven*, *71*, 24–39.

Bryant, R.A., Moulds, M.M., Guthrie, R., & Nixon, R.D.V. (2003). Treating acute stress disorder following mild traumatic brain injury. *American Journal of Psychiatry*, *160*, 585–587.

Bucholtz, M., & Hall, K. (2003). Language and identity. In A. Duranti (Ed.), *A companion to linguistic anthropology*. Oxford: Blackwell.

Bugental, J., & Zelen, S. (1950). Investigations into the self-concept: The W-A-Y technique. *Journal of Personality*, *18*, 483–498.

Bullock, L.M., Gable, R.A., & Mohr, J.D. (2005). Traumatic brain injury: A challenge for educators. *Preventing School Failure*, *49*, 6–10.

Butler, R.J. & Gasson, S.L. (2005). Self-esteem/self-concept scales for children and adolescents: A review. *Child & Adolescent Mental Health Journal*, *10*, 1–12.

Cantor, J.B., Ashman, T.A., Schwartz, M.E., Gordon, W.A., Hibbard, M.R., Brown, M., ... Cheng Z. (2005). The role of self-discrepancy theory in understanding post-traumatic brain injury affective disorders: A pilot study. *Journal of Head Trauma Rehabilitation*, *20*, 527–543.

Carroll, E., & Coetzer, R. (2011). Identity, grief and self-awareness after traumatic brain injury. *Neuropsychological Rehabilitation*, *21*, 289–305.

Carver, S.C., Scheier, M.F., & Weintraub, J.K. (1989). Assessing coping strategies: A theoretically based approach. *Journal of Personality and Social Psychology*, *56*, 267–283.

Cattelani, R., Zettin, M. & Zoccolotti, P. (2010) Rehabilitation treatments for adults with behavioral and psychosocial disorders following acquired brain injury: A systematic review. *Neuropsychological Review*, *20*, 52–85.

Cheng, S.K.W. & Man, D.W.K. (2006). Management of impaired self-awareness in persons with traumatic brain injury. *Brain Injury*, *20*, 621–628.

Ch'Ng, A.M., French, D.J., & McLean, N.J. (2008). Coping with the challenges of recovery from stroke: Long term perspectives of stroke support group members. *Journal of Health Psychology*, *13*, 1136–1146.

Christensen, A.-L. (1999). Neuropsychological Rehabilitation. In A-L Christensen & B. Uzzell (Eds), *International Handbook of Neuropsychological Rehabilitation* (pp. 151–163). New York: Kluwer Academic Press/Plenum Publishers.

Christoff, K., Cosmelli, D., Legrand, D., & Thompson, E. (2011). Specifying the self for cognitive neuroscience. *Trends in Cognitive Sciences*, *15*, 104–112.

Cicerone, K.D. (1989). Psychotherapeutic interventions with traumatically brain-injured patients. *Rehabilitation Psychology, 34*, 105–114.

Cicerone, K.D. & Azulay, J. (2007). Perceived self-efficacy and life satisfaction after traumatic brain injury. *Journal of Head Trauma Rehabilitation, 22*, 257–266.

Cicerone, K.D., Langenbahn, D.M., Braden, C., Malec, J.F., Kalmar, K., Fraas, M., ... Ashman T. (2011). Evidence-based cognitive rehabilitation: updated review of the literature from 2003 through 2008. *Archives of Physical Medicine and Rehabilitation, 92*, 519–530.

Cicerone, K.D., Mott, T., Azulay, J., Sharlow-Galella, M.A., Ellmo, W.J., Paradise, S., Friel, J.C. (2008). A randomized controlled trial of holistic neuropsychologic rehabilitation after traumatic brain injury. *Archives of Physical Medicine Rehabilitation; 89*, 2239–2249.

Ciurli, P., Bivona, U., Barba, C., Onder, G., Sivestro, D., Azicnuda, E., ... Formisano, R. (2010). Metacognitive unawareness correlates with executive function impairment after severe traumatic brain injury. *Journal of the International Neuropsychological Society, 16*, 360–368.

Clark, D.A., & Beck, A.T. (1999). *Scientific Foundations of Cognitive Theory and Therapy of Depression.* New York: Wiley.

Clarke, D.M. (2006). *Descartes: A biography.* Cambridge: Cambridge University Press.

Clarke, P., & Black, S.E. (2005). Quality of life following stroke: Negotiating disability, identity and resources. *Journal of Applied Gerontology, 24*, 319–336.

Clare, L. (2008). *Neuropsychological rehabilitation and people with dementia.* Hove, UK: Psychology Press.

Cloute, K., Mitchell, A., & Yates, P. (2008). Traumatic brain injury and the construction of identity: A discursive approach. *Neuropsychological Rehabilitation, 18*, 651–670.

Cobb, R.B., & Alwell, M. (2009). Transition planning/coordinating interventions for youth with disabilities: A systematic review. *Career Development for Exceptional Individuals, 32*, 70–81.

Coetzer, R. (2007). Psychotherapy following traumatic brain injury: Integrating theory and practice. *Journal of Head Trauma Rehabilitation, 22*, 39–47.

Coetzer, R. (2008). Holistic neuro-rehabilitation in the community: Is identity a key issue? *Neuropsychological Rehabilitation, 18*, 1–18.

Coetzer, R. (2010). *Anxiety and mood disorders following traumatic brain injury: Clinical assessment and psychotherapy.* London: Karnac Books.

Coetzer, B.R. & Corney, M.J.R. (2001). Grief and self-awareness following brain injury and effect of feedback as an intervention. *Journal of Cognitive Rehabilitation, 19*, 8–14.

Coetzer, R., Ruddle, J.A., & Mulla, F. (2006). The Brain Injury Grief Inventory: A follow-up study of emotional and functional outcome following traumatic brain injury. *Journal of Cognitive Rehabilitation, 24*, 7–11.

Coetzer, B.R., Vaughan, F.L., & Ruddle, J.A. (2003). The Brain Injury Grief Inventory. Unpublished Manuscript. North Wales Brain Injury Service, Conwy and Denbighshire NHS Trust, UK.

Cole, W.R., Paulos, S.K., Cole, C.A.S., & Tankard, C. (2009). A review of family intervention guidelines for pediatric acquired brain injuries. *Developmental Disabilities Research Reviews, 15*, 159–166.

Collicutt McGrath, J. (2011). Posttraumatic growth and spirituality after brain injury. *Brain Impairment, 12*, 82–92.

Collicutt McGrath, J., & Linley, P.A., (2006). Post-traumatic growth in acquired brain injury: A preliminary small scale study. *Brain Injury, 20*, 767–773.

Conway, M.A. (2005). Memory and the self. *Journal of Memory and Language, 53*, 594–628.

Conway, M.A., & Pleydell-Pearce, C.W. (2000). The construction of autobiographical memories in the self-memory system. *Psychological Review, 107*, 261–288.

Cooley, C.H. (1902). *Human nature and the social order.* New York: Scribner.

Cooper, J.M. (1999). *Reason and emotion: Essays on ancient moral psychology and ethical theory*. Princeton: Princeton University Press.
Cooper-Evans, S., Alderman, N., Knight, C., & Oddy, M. (2008). Self-esteem as a predictor of psychological distress after severe acquired brain injury: An exploratory study. *Neuropsychological Rehabilitation, 18*, 607–626.
Coopersmith, S. (1989). *Self-esteem inventories*. Palo Alto, CA: Consulting Psychologists Press.
Corrigan, J.D., Selassie, A.W., & Orman, J.A. (2010). The epidemiology of traumatic brain injury. *Journal of Head Trauma Rehabilitation, 25*, 72–80.
Crain, R.M. (1996). The influence of age, race, and gender on child and adolescent multidimensional self-concept. In B.A. Bracken (Ed.), *Handbook of self-concept: Developmental, social, and clinical considerations* (pp. 395–420). Oxford: John Wiley & Sons.
Cramer, P. (2000). Defense mechanisms in psychology today: Further processes for adaption. *American Psychologist, 55*, 158–172.
Cramer, P. (2003). Defense mechanisms and physiological reactivity to stress. *Journal of Personality, 71*, 221–244.
Cronin, A.F. (2001). Traumatic brain injury in children: Issues in community function. *American Journal of Occupational Therapy, 55*, 377–384.
Csikszentmihalyi, M. (2000). The contribution of flow to positive psychology. In M.E.P. Seligman & J. Gillham (Eds), *The science of optimism and hope: Research essays in honor of Martin E.P. Seligman* (pp. 387–397). Pennsylvania: Templeton Foundation Press.
Culley, C., & Evans, J.J. (2010). SMS text messaging as a means of increasing recall of therapy goals in brain injury rehabilitation: A single-blind within-subjects trial. *Neuropsychological Rehabilitation, 20*, 103–119.
Curran, C.A., Ponsford, J.L., & Crowe, S. (2000). Coping strategies and emotional outcome following traumatic brain injury: A comparison with orthopedic patients. *Journal of Head Trauma Rehabilitation, 15*, 1256–1274.
Damasio, A.R. (1999). *The feeling of what happens: Body and emotion in the making of consciousness*. New York: Harcourt Brace.
Damasio, A.R. (2003). *Looking for spinoza: Joy, sorrow and the feeling brain*. New York: Harcourt.
Damon, W., & Hart, D. (1982). The development of self-understanding from infancy through adolescence. *Child Development, 53*, 841–864.
Damon, W., & Hart, D.S. (1988). *Self-understanding in childhood and adolescence*. New York: Cambridge University.
D'Argembeau, A., Feyers, D., Majerus, S., Collette, F., Van der Linden, M., Maquet, P., & Salmon, E. (2008). Self-reflection across time: cortical midline structures differentiate between present and past selves. *Social Cognitive and Affective Neuroscience, 3*, 244–252.
D'Argembeau, A., Stawarczyk, D., Majerus, S., Collette, F., Van der Linden, M., & Salmon, E. (2010). Modulation of medial prefrontal and inferior parietal cortices when thinking about past, present, and future selves. *Social Neuroscience, 5*, 187–200.
De Sepulveda, L.I.B., & Chang, B. (1994). Effective coping with stroke disability in a community setting: the development of a causal model. *Journal of Neuroscience & Nursing, 26*, 193–203.
De Wit, L., Putman, K., Baert, I., Lincoln, N.B., Angst, F., Beyens, H., … Feys, H. (2008). Anxiety and depression in the first six months after stroke. A longitudinal multicentre study. *Disability & Rehabilitation, 30*, 1858–1866.
Degeneffe, C.E. (2001). Family caregiving and traumatic brain injury. *Health and Social Work, 26*, 257–268.
Delmonico, R.I., Hanley-Peterson, P., & Englander, J. (1998). Group psychotherapy for persons with traumatic brain injury: management of frustration and substance abuse. *Journal of Head Trauma Rehabilitation, 13*, 10–22.

Dennis, M., Agostino, A., Taylor, H.G., Bigler, E.D., Rubin, K., Vannatta, K., ... Yeates, K.O. (2013). Emotional expression and socially modulated emotive communication in children with traumatic brain injury. *Journal of the International Neuropsychological Society, 19*, 34–43.

Dewar, B.K. & Gracey, F. (2007). 'Am not was': Cognitive behavioural therapy for adjustment and identity change following herpes simplex encephalitis. *Neuropsychological Rehabilitation. 17*, 602–620.

Dirette, D., Plaisier, B.R., & Jones, S.J. (2008). Patterns and antecedents of the development of self-awareness following traumatic brain injury: the importance of occupation. *British Journal of Occupational Therapy, 71*, 44–51.

Dise-Lewis, J.E., Lewis, H.C., & Reichardt, C.S. (2009). BrainSTARS: pilot data on a team-based intervention program for students who have acquired brain injury. *Journal of Head Trauma Rehabilitation, 24*, 166–177.

Doering, B.K., Conrad, N., Rief, W., & Exner, C. (2011). Living with acquired brain injury: Self-concept as mediating variable in the adjustment process. *Neuropsychological Rehabilitation, 21*, 42–63.

Doig, E.J., Fleming, J., Cornwell, P., & Kuipers, P. (2010). Clinical utility of the combined use of the Canadian Occupational Performance Measure and the Goal Attainment Scale. *American Journal of Occupational Therapy, 64*, 904–914.

Doig, E.J., Fleming, J., Kuipers, P., Cornwell, P., & Khan, A. (2011). Goal-directed outpatient rehabilitation following TBI: A pilot study of programme effectiveness and comparison of outcomes in home and day hospital settings, *Brain Injury, 25*, 1114–1125.

Donnellan, C., Hevey, D., Hickey, A., & O'Neill, D. (2006). Defining and quantifying coping strategies after stroke: a review. *Journal of Neurology, Neurosurgery & Psychiatry, 77*, 1208–1218.

Douglas, J. (2012). Social linkage, self-concept, and well-being after severe traumatic brain injury. In J. Jetten, C. Haslam, & A. Haslam (Eds). *The Social Cure* (pp. 237–254). Hove, East Sussex: Psychology Press.

Douglas J., Dyson M., & Foreman, P. (2006). Increasing leisure activity following severe traumatic brain injury: Does it make a difference? *Brain Impairment, 7*, 107–118.

Douglas, J.M. (2013) Conceptualizing self and maintaining social connection following severe traumatic brain injury. *Brain Injury, 27*, 60–74.

Douglas, J.M., & Spellacy, F.J. (2000). Correlates of depression in adults with severe traumatic brain injury and their carers. *Brain Injury, 14*, 71–88.

Driver, S., Rees, K., O'Connor, J., & Lox, C. (2006). Aquatics, health-promoting self-care behaviors and adults with brain injuries. *Brain Injury, 20*, 133–141.

Dumont, C. (2013). Identity. In J.H. Stone & M. Blouin (Eds), *International Encyclopedia of Rehabilitation*. Available online: ttp://cirrie.buffalo.edu/encyclopedia/en/article/156/

Durkheim, E. (1960). *The Division of Labor in Society* (1893). Translated by George Simpson. New York: The Free Press.

Eccles, S., House, A.O., & Knapp, P.R. (1999) Psychological adjustment and self-reported coping in stroke survivors with and without emotionalism. *Journal of Neurology, Neurosurgery and Psychiatry, 67*, 137–138.

Egan, J., Worrall, L., & Oxenham, D. (2005). An Internet training intervention for people with traumatic brain injury: Barriers and outcomes. *Brain Injury, 19*, 555–568.

Eisenberger, N. (2012). Broken hearts and broken bones: A neural perspective on the similarities between social and physical pain. *Current Directions in Psychological Science, 21*, 42–47.

Eisenberger, N.I., Lieberman, M.D., & Williams, K.D. (2003). Does rejection hurt? An fMRI study of social exclusion. *Science, 302*, 290–292.

Eisenstadt, D., & Leippe, M.R. (1994). The self-comparison process and self-descrepant feedback: Consequences of learning you are what you thought you were not. *Journal of Personality & Social Psychology, 67,* 611–626.

Eisenstadt, D., Leippe, M.R., & Rivers, J.A. (2002). Asymmetry and defense in self-comparison: Differential reactions to feedback about the rejected and ideal selves. *Self and Identity, 1,* 289–311.

Elkis-Abuhoff, D.L. (2003). The impact of coping strategies, negative life events and health locus of control for persons living with the pain of osteoarthritis. *Dissertation Abstracts, 63,* 3910.

Ellis, A. (1962). *Reason and emotion in psychotherapy.* New York: Lyle & Stuart.

Ellis-Hill, C.S., & Horn, S. (2000). Change in identity and self-concept: A new theoretical approach to recovery following a stroke. *Clinical Rehabilitation, 14,* 279–287.

Ellis-Hill, C., Payne, S. & Ward, C. (2000). Self-body split: issues of identity in physical recovery following a stroke. *Disability & Rehabilitation, 22,* 725–733.

Epstein, R.S., & Ursano, R.J. (1994). Anxiety disorders. In J.M. Silver, S.C. Yudofsky & R.E. Hales (Eds), *Neuropsychiatry of traumatic brain injury* (pp. 3–41). Washington, DC: American Psychiatric Press.

Ergh, T.C., Rapport, L.J., Coleman, R.D., & Hanks, R.A. (2002). Predictors of caregiver and family functioning following traumatic brain injury: social support moderates caregiver distress. *Journal of Head Trauma Rehabilitation, 17,* 155–174.

Erikson, E.H. (1963). *Childhood and society* (2nd edn.). New York: Norton.

Etkin, A., Egner, T., & Kalisch, R. (2011). Emotional processing in the anterior cingulate and medial prefrontal cortex. *Trends in Cognitive Sciences, 15,* 85–93.

Evans, J. (2011). Positive psychology and brain injury rehabilitation. *Brain Impairment, 12,* 117–127.

Evans, J.J. (2012) Goal setting during rehabilitation early and late after acquired brain injury. *Current Opinion in Neurology, 25,* 651–655.

Ewing, J. (2006). Changing world of neuroscience and clinical practice: A personal perspective (Part 1 – paediatric brain injury). *Brain Impairment, 7,* 33–38.

Ewing-Cobbs, L., Prasad, M.R., Kramer, L., Cox Jr, C.S., Baumgartner, J., Fletcher, S., ... Swank, P. (2006). Late intellectual and academic outcomes following traumatic brain injury sustained during early childhood. *Journal of Neurosurgery, 105,* 287–296.

Fadyl, J.K., & McPherson, K.M. (2009). Approaches to vocational rehabilitation after traumatic brain injury: a review of the evidence. *Journal of Head Trauma Rehabilitation, 24,* 195–212.

Falcone, G., & Chong, J. (2007). Gender differences in stroke among older adults. *Geriatric & Aging, 10,* 497–500.

Fann, J.R., Hart, T., & Schomer, K.G. (2009). Treatment for depression after traumatic brain injury: A systematic review. *Journal of Neurotrauma, 26,* 2383–2402.

Feeney, T.J., & Capo, M. (2010). Making meaning: The use of project-based supports for individuals with brain injury. *Journal of Behavioral and Neuroscience Research, 8,* 70–80.

Feeney, T.J., & Ylvisaker, M. (1995). Choice and routine: Antecedent behavioral interventions for adolescents with severe traumatic brain injury. *Journal of Head Trauma Rehabilitation, 10,* 67–86.

Feeney, T.J., & Ylvisaker, M. (2003). Context-sensitive behavioral supports for young children with TBI: Short-term effects and long-term outcome. *Journal of Head Trauma Rehabilitation, 18,* 33–51.

Feeney, T.J., & Ylvisaker, M. (2006). Context-sensitive cognitive-behavioural supports for young children with TBI: A replication study. *Brain Injury, 20,* 629–645.

Feigin, V.L., Lawes, C.M., Bennett, D.A., Barker-Collo, S.L., & Parag, V. (2009). Worldwide stroke incidence and early case fatality reported in 56 population-based studies: a systematic review. *Lancet neurology, 8*, 355–369.

Feinberg, T.E. (2011a). The nested neural hierarchy and the self. *Consciousness and Cognition, 20*, 4–15.

Feinberg, T.E. (2011b). Neuropathologies of the self: Clinical and anatomical features. *Consciousness and Cognition, 20*, 75–81.

Feinberg, T.E., & Keenan, J.P. (2005). Where in the brain is the self? *Consciousness and Cognition, 14*, 661–678.

Fennell, M.J.V. (2000). Depression. In K. Hawton, P.M. Salkovskis, J. Kirk & D.M. Clark (Eds), *Cognitive behaviour therapy for psychiatric problems* (pp. 169–234). Oxford: Oxford University Press.

Fines, L., & Nichols, D. (1994). An evaluation of a twelve week recreational kayak program: effects on self-concept, leisure satisfaction and leisure attitude of adults with traumatic brain injuries. *Journal of Cognitive Rehabilitation, 12*, 10–15.

Fish, J., Manly, T., & Wilson, B.A. (2008). Long-term compensatory treatment of organizational deficits in a patient with bilateral frontal lobe damage. *Journal of the International Neuropsychological Society, 14*, 154–163.

Fitts, W.H., & Warren, W.L. (1996). *Tennessee self-concept scale, TSCS:2* (2nd edition) [manual]. Los Angeles: Western Psychological Services.

Fleming, J., & Ownsworth, T. (2006). A review of awareness interventions in brain injury rehabilitation. *Neuropsychological Rehabilitation, 16*, 474–500.

Fleming, J.M., Kuipers, P., Foster, M., Smith, S., & Doig, E. (2009). Evaluation of an outpatient, peer group intervention for people with acquired brain injury based on the ICF 'environment' dimension. *Disability & Rehabilitation, 31*, 1666–1675.

Fleming, J.M., Strong, J., & Ashton, R. (1996). Self-awareness of deficits in adults with traumatic brain injury: How best to measure? *Brain Injury, 10*, 1–15.

Fleming, J.M., Strong, J., & Ashton, R. (1998). Cluster analysis of self-awareness levels in adults with traumatic brain injury and relationship to outcome. *Journal of Head Trauma Rehabilitation, 13*, 39–51.

Fleminger, S. (2009). Cerebrovascular Disorders. In A.S. David, S. Fleminger, M.D. Kopelman, S. Lovestone., & J.D.C. Mellers (Eds), *Lishman's Organic Psychiatry* (pp. 473–542). West Sussex, UK: Wiley-Blackwell.

Fleminger, S., & Ponsford, J. (2005). Long term outcome after traumatic brain injury: More attention needs to be paid to neuropsychiatric functioning. *BMJ: British Medical Journal, 331*, 1419.

Fleminger, S., Oliver, D.L., Williams, W.H., & Evans, J. (2003). The neuropsychiatry of depression after brain injury. *Neuropsychological Rehabilitation, 13*, 65–87.

Fletcher-Janzen, E., & Kade, H.D. (1997). Pediatric brain injury rehabilitation in a neurodevelopmental milieu. In C.R. Reynolds & E. Fletcher-Janzen (Eds), *Handbook of child clinical neuropsychology* (2nd edn., pp. 452–481). New York: Plenum Press.

Folkman, S. (1997). Positive psychological states and coping with severe stress. *Social Science Medicine, 45*, 1207–1221.

Folkman, S. & Lazarus, R.S. (1985). If it changes it must be a process: Study of emotion and coping during three stages of a college examination. *Journal of Personality and Social Psychology, 48*, 150–170.

Fonagy, P., Gergely, G., Jurist, E., & Target, M. (2004). *Affect regulation, mentalisation and the development of the self.* New York: Other Press.

Fordyce, D.J., & Roueche, J.R. (1986). Changes in perspectives of disability among patients, staff, and relatives during rehabilitation of brain injury. *Rehabilitation Psychology, 31*, 217–229.

Forster, A., & Young, J. (1996). Specialist nurse support of patients with stroke in the community: a randomised controlled trial. *British Medical Journal, 312*, 1642–1646.

Foucault, M. (1980). *Power/Knowledge: Selected Interviews and Other Writings 1972–1977.* London: Harvester Press.

Fraas, M., & Balz, M.A. (2008). Expressive electronic journal writing: freedom of communication for survivors of acquired brain injury. *Psycholinguistic Research, 37*, 115–124.

Freeman, M. (1992). Self as narrative: The place of life history in studying the life span. In T.M. Brinthaupt & R.P. Lipka (Eds), *The self: Definitional and methodological issues* (pp. 15–43). Albany: State University of New York Press.

Freud, S. (1917). Introductory lectures on psychoanalysis. In J. Strachey (Ed.), *The standard edition of the complete psychological works of Sigmund Freud* (Vol. 15 & 16). London: Hogarth Press and the Institute of Psychoanalysis.

Freud, S. (1923). The ego and the id. In J. Strachey (Ed.), *The standard edition of the complete psychological works of Sigmund Freud* (Vol. 19). London: Hogarth Press.

Friedman, G., Froom, P., Sazbon, L., Grinblatt, I., Shochina, M., Tsenter, J., ... Groswasser, Z. (1999). Apolipoprotein E- 4 genotype predicts a poor outcome in survivors of traumatic brain injury. *Neurology, 52*, 244.

Frydenberg, E., & Lewis, R. (2012). *Coping Scale for Adults.* Camberwell, Melbourne: Australian Council for Educational Research.

Fuentes, B., Ortiz, X., SanJose, B., Frank, A., & Díez-Tejedor, E. (2009). Post-stroke depression: Can we predict its development from the acute stroke phase? *Acta Neurologica Scandinavica, 120*, 150–156.

Gainotti, G. (2012). Brain structures playing a crucial role in the representation of tools in humans and non-human primates. *Behavioral and Brain Sciences, 35*, 224–225.

Gallagher, S. (2000). Philosophical conceptions of the self: implications for cognitive science. *Trends in Cognitive Sciences, 4*, 14–21.

Gan, C., Gargaro, J., Kreutzer, J., Boschen, K., & Wright, V. (2010). Development and preliminary evaluation of a structured family system intervention for adolescents with brain injury and their families. *Brain Injury, 24*, 651–663.

Ganesalingam, K., Yeates, K.O., Sanson, A., & Anderson, V. (2007). Social problem-solving skills following childhood traumatic brain injury and its association with self-regulation and social and behavioural functioning. *Journal of Neuropsychology, 1*, 149–170.

Gangstad, B., Norman, P., & Barton, J. (2009). Cognitive processing and posttraumatic growth after stroke. *Rehabilitation Psychology, 54*, 69–75.

Gardner, R.M., Bird, F.L., Maguire, H., Carreiro, R., & Abenaim, N. (2003). Intensive positive behavior supports for adolescents with acquired brain injury. *Journal of Head Trauma Rehabilitation, 18*, 52–74.

Gelech, J.M., & Desjardins, M. (2011). I am many: The reconstruction of self following acquired brain injury. *Qualitative Health Research, 21*, 62–74.

Gergen, K. (1991). *The saturated self: Dilemmas of identity In contemporary life.* New York: Basic Books.

Gervasio, A., & Kreutzer, J. (1997). Kinship and family member's psychological distress after traumatic brain injury: A large sample study. *Journal of Head Trauma Rehabilitation, 12*, 14–26.

Geyh, S., Cieza, A., Schouten, J., Dickson, H., Frommelt, P., Omar, Z., ... Stucki, G. (2004). ICF core sets for stroke. *Journal of Rehabilitation Medicine, 36*, 135–141.

Giaquinto, S., Buzzelli, S., Di Francesco, L., & Nolfe, G. (2003). Evaluation of sexual changes after stroke. *Journal of Clinical Psychiatry, 64*, 302–307.

Gilbert, P. (2010). *Compassion Focused Therapy: Distinctive Features.* East Sussex, UK: Routledge.
Glang, A., McLaughlin, K., & Schroeder, S. (2007). Interactive multimedia to teach parent advocacy skills: An exploratory study. *Journal of Head Trauma Rehabilitation, 22*, 196–203.
Glang, A., Tyler, J., Pearson, S., Todis, B., & Morvant, M. (2004). Improving educational services for students with TBI through statewide consulting teams. *NeuroRehabilitation, 19*, 219–231.
Glanz, K., Rimer, B.K., & Lewis, F.M. (2002). *Health Behavior and Health Education. Theory, Research and Practice.* San Francisco: Wiley & Sons.
Gluhoski, V.L., & Wortman, C.B. (1996). The impact of trauma on world views. *Journal of Social and Clinical Psychology, 15*, 417–429.
Goadby, E. (2013). A brain tumour means different things: Family caregiver experiences and factors influencing their psychological adjustment. Unpublished Doctorate Thesis. Griffith University, Mt Gravatt, Australia.
Godfrey, H.P.D., Knight, R.G., & Partridge, F.M. (1996). Emotional adjustment following traumatic brain injury: A stress-appraisal-coping formulation. *Journal of Head Trauma Rehabilitation, 11*(6), 29–40.
Godfrey, H.P.D., Partridge, F.M., Knight, R.M., & Bishara, S. (1993). Course of insight disorder and emotional dysfunction following closed head injury: A controlled cross-sectional follow-up study. *Journal of Clinical and Experimental Neuropsychology, 15*, 503–515.
Goffman, E. (1956). *The presenting of self in everyday life.* New York: Anchor Books.
Gogtay, N., Giedd, J.N., Lusk, L., Hayashi, K.M., Greenstein, D., Vaituzis, A.C., ... Thompson, P.M. (2004). Dynamic mapping of human cortical development during childhood through early adulthood. *Proceedings of the National Academy of Sciences of the USA, 25*, 8174–8179.
Goldberg, G., Segal, M.E., Berk, S.N., Schall, R.R., & Gershkoff, A.M. (1997). Stroke transition after inpatient rehabilitation. *Topics in Stroke Rehabilitation, 4*, 64–79.
Goldstein, K. (1943). On so-called war neuroses. *Psychosomatic Medicine, 5*(4), 376–383.
Goldstein, K. (1952). The effect of brain damage on the personality. *Psychiatry, 15*, 245–260.
Goldstein, K. (1959). Notes on the development of my concepts. *Journal of Individual Psychology, 15*, 5–14.
Goverover, Y., Johnston, M.V., Toglia, J., & DeLuca, J. (2007). Treatment to improve self-awareness in persons with acquired brain injury. *Brain Injury, 21*, 913–923.
Gracey, F., & Ownsworth, T. (2008). Editorial. *The self and identity in rehabilitation: A special issue of the journal Neuropsychological Rehabilitation, 18*, 522–526.
Gracey, F., & Ownsworth, T. (2012). The experience of self in the world: the personal and social contexts of identity change after brain injury. In A. Haslam, C. Haslam & J. Jetten (Eds). *The Social Cure* (pp. 273–295). Hove, East Sussex: Psychology Press.
Gracey, F., Evans, J.J., & Malley, D. (2009). Capturing process and outcome in complex rehabilitation interventions: A 'Y-shaped' model. *Neuropsychological Rehabilitation, 19*, 867–890.
Gracey, F., Oldham, P., & Kritzinger, R. (2007). Finding out if 'The "me" will shut down': successful cognitive-behavioural therapy of seizure-related panic symptoms following subarachnoid haemorrhage: a single case report. *Neuropsychological Rehabilitation, 17*, 106–119.
Gracey, F., Palmer, S., Rous, B., Psaila, K., Shaw, K., O'Dell, J., Cope, J., & Mohamed, S. (2008). 'Feeling part of things': Personal construction of self after brain injury. *Neuropsychological Rehabilitation, 18*, 627–650.
Gracey, F., Wilson, B.A., Manly, T., Bateman, A., Fish, J., Malley, D., ... Evans, J. (2012). The effectiveness of brief goal management training (GMT) and SMS text alerts on psychosocial functioning following brain injury: the Assisted Intention Monitoring (AIM) Trial. Paper

presented at the 9th Annual Conference of the Neuropsychological Rehabilitation Special Interest Group of the World Federation of Neurorehabilitation, July 2–3, Bergen, Norway.

Grimm, S., Ernst, J., Boesiger, P., Schuepbach, D., Hell, D., Boeker, H., & Northoff, G. (2009). Increased self-focus in major depressive disorder is related to neural abnormalities in subcortical-cortical midline structures. *Human Brain Mapping, 30*, 2617–2627.

Hackett, M.L., Anderson, C.S., House, A.O., & Halteh, C. (2008). Interventions for preventing depression after stroke. *Stroke, 40*, e485–e486.

Hackett, M.L., Anderson, C.S., House, A.O., & Xia, J. (2008). Interventions for treating depression after stroke. *Cochrane Database of Systematic Reviews, 4*, 1–95.

Hackett, M., Yapa, C., Parag, V., Anderson, C. (2005). Frequency of depression after stroke: a systematic review of observational studies. *Stroke; a Journal of Cerebral Circulation, 36*(6), 1330–40.

Hammell, K.W. (2004). Dimensions of meaning in the occupations of daily life. *Canadian Journal of Occupational Therapy, 71*, 296–305.

Hanten, G., Bartha, M., & Levin, H.S. (2000). Metacognition following pediatric traumatic brain injury: A preliminary study. *Developmental Neuropsychology, 18*, 383–398.

Harris, R. (2006). Embracing your demons: An overview of acceptance and commitment therapy. *Psychotherapy in Australia, 12*, 70–76.

Harris, R. (2009). *ACT made simple: An easy-to-read primer on acceptance and commitment therapy*. Oakland, CA: New Harbinger Publications.

Hart, T., Giovannetti, T., Montgomery, M.W., & Schwartz, M.F. (1998). Awareness of errors in naturalistic action after traumatic brain injury. *Journal of Head Trauma Rehabilitation 13*, 16–28.

Hart, T., Hawkey, K., & Whyte, J. (2002). Use of a portable voice organizer to remember therapy goals in traumatic brain injury rehabilitation: A within-subjects trial. *Journal of Head Trauma Rehabilitation, 17*, 556–570.

Hart, T., Seignourel, P.J., & Sherer, M. (2009). A longitudinal study of awareness of deficit after moderate to severe traumatic brain injury. *Neuropsychological Rehabilitation, 19*, 161–176.

Harter, S. (2012). *The construction of the self* (2nd edition). New York: Guilford Press.

Haslam, C., Holme, A., Haslam, S.A., Iyer, A., Jeyyen, J., & Williams, W.H. (2008). Maintaining group memberships: Social identity continuity predicts well-being after stroke. *Neuropsychological Rehabilitation, 18*, 671–691.

Haslam, S.A., Jetten, J., Postmes, T., & Haslam, C. (2009). Social identity, health and well-being: An emerging agenda for applied psychology. *Applied Psychology, 58*, 1–23.

Haslam, S.A., O'Brien, A., Jetten, J., Vormedal, K., & Penna, S. (2005). Taking the strain: social identity, social support, and the experience of stress. *British Journal of Social Psychology, 44*, 355–370.

Haun, J., & Rittman, M.R. (2008). The continuum of connectedness and social isolation during post stroke recovery. *Journal of Aging Studies, 22*, 54–64.

Hawley, C.A. (2005). Saint or sinner? Teacher perceptions of a child with traumatic brain injury. *Developmental Neurorehabilitation, 8*, 117–129.

Hawley, C.A. (2012). Self-esteem in children after traumatic brain injury: An exploratory study. *NeuroRehabilitation, 30*, 173–181.

Hawley, C.A., & Joseph, S. (2008). Predictors of positive growth after traumatic brain injury: A longitudinal study. *Brain Injury, 22*, 427–435.

Hayes, S.C. (2002). Acceptance, mindfulness, and science. *Clinical Psychology: Science and Practice, 9*, 101–106.

Helffenstein, D.A., & Wechsler, F.S. (1982). The use of interpersonal process recall (IPR) in the remediation of interpersonal and communication skill deficit in the newly brain-injured. *Clinical Neuropsychology, 4*, 139–143.

Hett, W.S. (1936). *Collections English & Greek 1936*. Oxford: Heinemann.
Hibbard, M.R., Uysal, S., Kepler, K., Bogdany, J., & Silver, J. (1998). Axis I psychopathology in individuals with traumatic brain injury. *Journal of Head Trauma Rehabilitation, 13*, 24–39.
Higgins, E.T. (1987). Self-discrepancy: A theory relating self and affect. *Psychological Review, 94*, 319–340.
Hodgson, J., McDonald, S., Tate, R., & Gertler, P. (2005). A randomised controlled trial of a cognitive-behavioural therapy program for managing social anxiety after acquired brain injury. *Brain Impairment, 6*, 169–180.
Hoen, B., Thelander, M., Worsley, J., & Wells, A. (1997). Improvement in psychological well-being of people with aphasia and their families: Evaluation of a community-based programme. *Aphasiology, 11*, 681–691.
Hogg, M.A., & Abrams, D. (1988). *Social identifications: a social psychology of intergroup relations and group processes*. London: Routledge.
Horney, K. (1950). *Neurosis and human growth*. New York: Norton.
House, A. (2000). The treatment of depression after stroke. *Journal of Psychosomatic Research, 48*, 235.
Howes, H., Edwards, S., & Benton, D. (2005). Male body image following acquired brain injury. *Brain Injury 19*, 135–147.
Hsieh, M., Ponsford, J.L., Wong, D.K., Schönberger, M., McKay, A.J.D., & Haines, K.E., (2012a). Development of a motivational interviewing programme as a prelude to CBT for anxiety following traumatic brain injury, *Neuropsychological Rehabilitation, 22*, 563–584.
Hsieh, M., Ponsford, J.L., Wong, D.K., Schönberger, M., Taffe, J.R., & McKay, A.J.D., (2012b) Motivational interviewing and cognitive behaviour therapy for anxiety following traumatic brain injury: a pilot randomised controlled trial. *Neuropsychological Rehabilitation, 22*, 585–608.
Hume, D. (2003). *A Treatise of Human Nature* (2003 edition). New York: Dover Publications.
Hux, K., & Hacksley, C. (1996). Mild Traumatic brain injury: Facilitating school success. *Intervention in School and Clinic, 31*, 158–165.
Jacobs, H.E. (1997). The Clubhouse: Addressing work-related behavioral challenges through a supportive social community. *Journal of Head Trauma Rehabilitation, 12*, 14–27.
Jacobs, H.E., & DeMello, C. (1996). The Clubhouse model and employment following brain injury. *Journal of Vocational Rehabilitation, 7*, 169–179.
Jacobs, M.P. (1993). Limited understanding of deficit in children with brain dysfunction. *Neuropsychological Rehabilitation, 3*, 341–365.
James, W. (1890). *The principles of psychology*. Michigan: H. Holt.
Jenkinson, N., Ownsworth, T., & Shum, D. (2007). Utility of the Canadian Occupational Performance Measure in community-based brain injury rehabilitation. *Brain Injury, 21*, 1283–1294.
Jennings, G.H. (1999). *Passages beyond the gate: A Jungian approach to understanding the nature of American psychology at the dawn of the new millennium*. New York: Ginn Press.
Jeste, D.V., & Harris, J.C. (2010). Wisdom – a neuroscience perspective. *Journal of the American Medical Association, 304*, 1602–1603.
Jetten, J., & Pachana, N. (2012). Not wanting to grow old: A Social Identity Model of Identity Change (SIMIC) analysis of driving cessation among older adults. In J. Jetten, C. Haslam & S.A. Haslam (Eds), *The social cure: identity, health and well-being* (pp. 97–114). New York: Psychology Press.
Jetten, J., Haslam, C., & Haslam, S.A. (2012). *The social cure: identity, health and well-being*. New York: Psychology Press.

Johnson, J., & Pearson, V. (2000). The effects of a structured education course on stroke survivors living in the community including commentary by Phipps M. *Rehabilitation Nursing, 25*, 59–65.

Johnson, M.H. (2001). Functional brain development in humans. *Nature Reviews Neuroscience, 2*, 475–483.

Jones, J.M., Haslam, S.A., Jetten, J., Williams, W.H., Morris, R., & Saroyan, S. (2011). That which doesn't kill us can make us stronger (and more satisfied with life): The contribution of personal and social changes to well-being after brain injury. *Psychology and Health, 26*, 353–369.

Judd, D., & Wilson, S.L. (2005). Psychotherapy with brain injury survivors: an investigation of the challenges encountered by clinicians and their modifications to therapeutic practice. *Brain Injury, 19*, 437–449.

Jumisko, E., Lexell, J., & Soderberg, S. (2005). The meaning of living with traumatic brain injury in people with moderate or severe traumatic brain injury. *Journal of Neuroscience Nursing, 37*, 42–50.

Jung, C. (1954). The development of personality. In *The development of personality*, Collected works (Vol. 16, pp. 53–75). Princeton, NJ: Princeton University Press.

Jung, C.G., & De Laszlo, V.S. (1959). *The basic writings of C.G. Jung.* Princeton: Princeton University Press.

Kabat-Zinn, J. (1990). *Full catastrophe living: Using the wisdom of your body and mind to face stress, pain, and illness.* New York: Delacorte.

Kangas, M., & McDonald, S. (2011). Is it time to act? The potential of acceptance and commitment therapy for psychological problems following acquired brain injury. *Neuropsychological Rehabilitation, 21*, 250–276.

Kangas, M., Williams, J.R., & Smee, R.I. (2011) Benefit finding in adults treated for benign Meningioma brain tumour: Relations with psychosocial well-being. *Brain Impairment, 12*, 105–116.

Karlovits, T., & McColl, M.A. (1999). Coping with community reintegration after severe brain injury: a description of stresses and coping strategies. *Brain Injury, 13*, 845–861.

Kashdan, T., & Ciarrochi, J. (2013). *Mindfulness, Acceptance, and Positive Psychology: The Seven Foundations of Well-Being.* Oakland, CA: New Harbinger.

Keijsers, G.P.J., Schaap, C.P.D.R., & Hoogduin, C.A.L. (2000). The impact of interpersonal patient and therapist behavior on outcome in cognitive-behavior therapy: A review of empirical studies. *Behavior Modification, 24*, 264–297.

Kelly, A., Ponsford, J., & Couchman, G. (2013). Impact of a family-focused intervention on self-concept after acquired brain injury. *Neuropsychological Rehabilitation, 23*, 563–579.

Kelly, G.A. (1955). *Personal construct psychology.* New York: Norton.

Kendall, E. & Terry, D. (2008). Understanding the adjustment following traumatic brain injury: is the goodness of fit coping hypothesis useful? *Social Science and Medicine, 67*, 1217–1224.

Kendall, E., & Terry, D. (2009). Predicting emotional well-being following traumatic brain injury: a test of mediated and moderated models. *Social Science and Medicine, 69*, 947–954.

Kendall, E., Catalano, T., Kuipers, P., Posner, N., Buys, N., & Charker, J. (2007). Recovery following stroke: The role of self-management education. *Social Science and Medicine, 64*, 735–746.

Kendall, E., Shum, D., Lack, B., Bull, S., & Fee, C. (2001). Coping following traumatic brain injury: the need for contextually sensitive assessment. *Brain Impairment, 2*, 81–96.

Kennedy, A., Turner, B., & Kendall, M. (2011). Growth in a 'new world': case studies of peer-leader experiences in the STEPS Program for people with acquired brain injury. *Brain Impairment, 12*, 152–164.

Kennedy, M.R.T., Krause, M.O., & Turkstra, L.S. (2008). An electronic survey about college experiences after traumatic brain injury. *NeuroRehabilitation, 23*, 511–520.
Keppel, C.C., & Crowe, S.F. (2000). Changes to body image and self-esteem following stroke in young adults. *Neuropsychological Rehabilitation 10*, 15–31.
Kesler, S.R., Adams, H.F., Blasey, C.M., & Bigler, E.D. (2003). Premorbid intellectual functioning, education, and brain size in traumatic brain injury: An investigation of the cognitive reserve hypothesis. *Applied Neuropsychology, 10*, 153–162.
Kilov, A.M., Togher, L., Power, E., & Turkstra, L. (2010). Can teenagers with traumatic brain injury use Internet chatrooms? A systematic review of the literature and the Internet. *Brain Injury, 24*, 1135–1172.
Kim, E., Lauterbach, E.C., Reeeve, A., Arciniegas, D.B., Coburn, K.L., Mendez, M.F., Rummans, T.A. & Coffey, E.C. (2007) Neuropsychiatric complications of traumatic brain injury: a critical review of the literature (A report by the ANPA committee on research). *Journal of Neuropsychiatry and Clinical Neuroscience, 19*, 106–127.
King, R.B., Shade-Zeldow, Y., Carlson, C.E., Feldman, J.L., & Phillips, M. (2002). Adaptation to stroke: a longitudinal study of depressive symptoms, physical health, and coping process. *Topics in Stroke Rehabilitation, 9*, 46–66.
Kiresuk, T.J., Smith, A., & Cardillo, J.E. (1994). *Goal Attainment Scaling: Applications, Theory and Measurement.* New Jersey: Lawrence Erlbaum Associates.
Kirschbaum, C., Pirke, K.M. & Hellhammer, D.H. (1993). The 'Trier Social Stress Test' – a tool for investigating psychobiology stress responses in a laboratory setting. *Neuropsychobiology, 28*, 76–81.
Klonoff, P.S. (2010). *Psychotherapy after brain injury: Principles and techniques.* New York: The Guilford Press.
Kohut, H. (1971). *The analysis of the self.* New York: International Universities Press.
Korpelainen, J.T., Nieminen, P., & Myllylä, V.V. (1999). Sexual functioning among stroke patients and their spouses. *Stroke, 30*, 715–719.
Kosciulek, J.F. (1997). Relationship of family schema to family adaptation to brain injury. *Brain Injury, 11*, 821–830.
Koskinen, S., Hokkinen, E.-M., Sarajuuri, J., & Alaranta, H. (2007). Applicability of the ICF checklist to traumatically brain-injured patients in post-acute rehabilitation settings. *Journal of Rehabilitation Medicine, 39*, 467–472.
Krefting, L. (1989). Reintegration into the community after head injury: The results of an ethnographic study. *Occupational Therapy Journal of Research, 9*, 67–83.
Kreutzer, J., Kolakowsky-Hayner, S., Demm, S., & Meade, M. (2002). A structured approach to family intervention after brain injury. *Journal of Head Trauma Rehabilitation, 17*, 349–367.
Kreutzer, J.S., Marwitz, J.H., Walker, W., Sander, A., Sherer, M., Bogner, J., … Bushnik, T. (2003). Moderating factors in return to work and job stability after traumatic brain injury. *Journal of Head Trauma Rehabilitation, 18*, 128–138.
Kreutzer, J., Stejskal, T., Godwin, E., Powell, V., & Arango-Lasprilla, J. (2010). A mixed methods evaluation of the brain injury family intervention. *NeuroRehabilitation, 27*, 19–29.
Kreutzer, J., Stejskal, T., Ketchum, J., Marwitz, J., Taylor, L., & Menzel, J. (2009). A preliminary investigation of the Brain Injury Family Intervention: Impact on family members. *Brain Injury, 23*, 535–547.
Kristensen, O.S. (2004). Changing goals and intentions among participants in a neuropsychological rehabilitation programme: An exploratory case study evaluation. *Brain Injury, 18*, 1049–1062.
Krpan, K., Levine, B., Stuss, D., & Dawson, D.R. (2007). Executive function and coping at one-year post traumatic brain injury. *Journal of Clinical and Experimental Neuropsychology, 29*, 36–46.

Krpan, K.M., Stuss, D.T., & Anderson, N.D. (2011). Planful versus avoidant coping: Behaviour of individuals with moderate-to severe traumatic brain injury during a psychosocial stress test. *Journal of the International Neuropsychological Society, 17,* 248–255.

Kuhn, M.H., & McPartland, T. (1954). An empirical investigation of self-attitudes. *American Sociological Review, 19,* 68–76.

Lambert, M.J. (1992). Psychotherapy outcome research: Implications for integrative and eclectic therapists. In J. Norcross (Ed.), *Handbook of psychotherapy integration* (pp. 94–129). New York: Basic Books.

Langer, K.G. & Padrone, F.J. (1992). Psychotherapeutic treatment of awareness in acute rehabilitation of traumatic brain injury. *Neuropsychological Rehabilitation, 2,* 59–70.

Langlois, J., Rutland-Brown, W., & Thomas, K. (2006). *Traumatic brain injury in the United States: Emergency Department visits, Hospitalizations, and Deaths.* Atlanta, GA: Centers for Disease Control and Prevention, National Center for Injury Prevention and Control.

Lau, S. (1990). Crisis and vulnerability in adolescent development. *Journal of Youth and Adolescence, 19,* 111–131.

Law, M., Cooper, B., Strong, S., Stewart, D., Rigby, P., & Letts, L. (1996). The person-environment-occupation model: a transactive approach to occupational performance. *Canadian Journal of Occupational Therapy, 63,* 9–23.

Lazarus, A.A. (1966). Broad spectrum behaviour therapy and the treatment of agoraphobia. *Behavior Research and Therapy, 4,* 95–97.

Lazarus, R., & Folkman, S. (1984). *Stress, appraisal and coping.* New York: Springer.

Leary, M.R., & Price Tangney, J. (2003). *Handbook of self and identity.* New York: Guilford Press.

Leavitt, M.B., Lamb, S.A., & Voss, B.S. (1996). Brain tumor support group: content themes and mechanisms of support. *Oncology Nursing Forum, 23,* 1247–1256.

LeDoux, J. (1996). *The emotional brain: the mysterious underpinnings of emotional life.* New York: Touchstone.

LeDoux, J. (2000). Emotion circuits in the brain. *Annual Review of Neuroscience, 23,* 155–184.

Lee, A., & Hobson, R.P. (1998). On developing self-concepts: a controlled study of children and adolescents with autism. *Journal of Child Psychology & Psychiatry, 39,* 1131–1144.

Lehman, D.R., Chiu, C.-Y., & Schaller, M. (2004). Psychology and culture. *Annual Review of Psychology, 55,* 689–714.

Lenz, B. (2001). The transition from adolescence to young adulthood: A theoretical perspective. *Journal of School Nursing, 17,* 300–306.

Lev, E.L., & Owen, S.V. (1996). A measure of self-care self-efficacy. *Research in Nursing & Health, 19,* 421–429.

Levack, W.M.M., Kayes, N.M., & Fadyl, J.K. (2010). Experience of recovery and outcome following traumatic brain injury: a metasynthesis of qualitative research. *Disability & Rehabilitation, 32,* 986–999.

Leventhal, H., Benyamini, Y., Brownlee, S., Diefenbach, M., Leventhal, E.A., Patrick-Miller, L., & Robitaille, C. (1997). Illness representations: Theoretical foundations. In K.J. Petrie & J. Weinman (Eds), *Perceptions of health and illness* (pp. 19–46). Amsterdam: Harwood Academic Press.

Levin, H.S. (2012). Long-term intellectual outcome of traumatic brain injury in children: Limits to neuroplasticity of the young brain? *Pediatrics, 129,* 494–495.

Levin, H.S., Hanten, G., & Li, X. (2009). The relation of cognitive control to social outcome after paediatric TBI: Implications for intervention. *Developmental Neurorehabilitation, 12,* 320–329.

Levine, B., Robertson, I.H., Clare, L., Carter, G., Hong, J., Wilson, B.A., Duncan, J., & Stuss, D.T. (2000). Rehabilitation of executive functioning: An experimental-clinical validation of Goal Management Training. *Journal of the International Neuropsychological Society, 6,* 299–312.

Levine, B., Schweizer, T.A., O'Connor, C., Turner, G., Gillingham, S., Stuss, D.T., ... Robertson, I.H. (2011). Rehabilitation of executive functioning in patients with frontal lobe damage with goal management training. *Frontiers in Human Neuroscience, 5*, 1–9.

Li, L., & Liu, J. (2012). The effect of pediatric traumatic brain injury on behavioral outcomes: A systematic review. *Developmental Medicine & Child Neurology, 55*, 37–45.

Lincoln, N.B., & Flannaghan, T. (2003). Cognitive behavioural psychotherapy for depression following stroke: a randomized controlled trial. *Stroke, 34*, 111–115.

Lincoln, N.B., Flannaghan, T., Sutcliffe, L., & Rother, L. (1997). Evaluation of cognitive behavioural treatment for depression after stroke: A pilot study. *Clinical Rehabilitation, 11*, 114–122.

Lincoln, N.B., Kneebone, I.I., Macniven, J.A.B., & Morris, R.C. (2012). *Psychological management of stroke*. West Sussex: John Wiley & Sons.

Locke, J., & Winkler, K. (1996). *An essay concerning human understanding*. Indianapolis, IN: Hackett Publishing.

Loehlin, J.C. (1992). *Genes and environment in personality development*. Newbury Park, CA: Sage.

Longworth, C., Deakins, J., Rose, D., & Gracey, F. (2012). Exploring the nature of self-esteem after acquired brain injury. Paper presented at the 9th Annual Conference of the Neuropsychological Rehabilitation Special Interest Group of the World Federation of Neurorehabilitation, July 2–3, Bergen, Norway.

Lorenz, L.S. (2010). Discovering a new identity after brain injury. *Sociology of Health & Illness, 32*, 862–879.

Lorig, K., Stewart, A., Ritter, P., González, V., Laurent, D., & Lynch, J. (1996). *Outcome Measures for Health Education and other Health Care Interventions* (pp. 24–45). Thousand Oaks, CA: Sage Publications.

Luis, C.A., & Mittenberg, W. (2002). Mood and anxiety disorders following pediatric traumatic brain injury: a prospective study. *Journal of Clinical and Experimental Neuropsychology, 24*, 270–279.

Lundgren, T., Dahl, J., Melin, L., & Kies, B. (2006). Evaluation of acceptance and commitment therapy for drug refractory epilepsy: A randomized controlled trial in South Africa – A pilot study. *Epilepsia, 47*, 2173–2179.

Lundqvist, A., Linnros, H., Orlenius, H., & Samuelsson, K. (2010). Improved self-awareness and coping strategies for patients with acquired brain injury – a group therapy programme. *Brain Injury, 24*, 823–832.

Mahler, M. (1975). *The psychological birth of the human infant*. New York: Basic Books.

Malec, J.F. (2012). *The Perceived Control Scale for Brain Injury*. The Center for Outcome Measurement in Brain Injury. http://www.tbims.org/combi/pcsbi (accessed September 13, 2012).

Malec, J.F., & Basford, J.S. (1996). Post-acute brain injury rehabilitation. *Archives of Physical Medicine and Rehabilitation, 77*, 198–207.

Malec, J.F., Brown, A.W., Moessner, A.M., Stump, T.E., & Monahan, P. (2010). A preliminary model for posttraumatic brain injury depression. *Archives of Physical Medicine and Rehabilitation, 91*, 1087–1097.

Malec, J., Buffington, A., Moessner, A., & Degiorgio, L. (2000). A medical/vocational case coordination system for persons with brain injury: An evaluation of employment outcomes. *Archives of Physical and Medical Rehabilitation, 81*, 1007–1015.

Marcantuono, J.T., & Prigatano, G.P. (2008). A holistic brain injury rehabilitation program for school-aged children. *NeuroRehabilitation, 23*, 457–466.

Marcia, J.E. (1980). Identity in adolescence. In J. Adelson (Ed.), *Handbook of adolescent psychology* (pp. 159–187). New York: Wiley.

Marks, J.P., & Daggett, L.M. (2006). A critical pathway for meeting the needs of families of patients with severe traumatic brain injury. *Journal of Neuroscience Nursing, 38*, 84–89.
Markus, H. (1977). Self-schemata and processing information about the self. *Journal of Personality and Social Psychology, 35*, 63–78.
Markus, H., & Kitayama, S. (1991). Culture and the self: Implications for cognition, emotion, and motivation. *Psychological Review, 98*, 224–253.
Markus, H., & Nurius, P. (1986). Possible selves. *American Psychologist, 41*, 954–969.
Marsh, H.W. (1989). Age and sex effects in multiple dimensions of self-concept: Preadolescence to early adulthhood. *Journal of Educational Psychology, 81*, 417–430.
Marsh, N.V., Kersel, D.A., Havill, J.H., & Sleigh, J.W. (2002). Caregiver burden during the year following severe traumatic brain injury. *Journal of Clinical and Experimental Neuropsychology, 24*, 434–447.
Maslow, A.H. (1943). A theory of human motivation. *Psychological Review, 50*, 370–396.
Maslow, A.H. (1970). *Motivation and personality*. New York: Harper & Row.
Mathews, D.J.H., Bok, H., & Rabins, P.V. (2009). *Personal identity and fractured selves: Perspectives from philosophy, ethics, and neuroscience*. Baltimore, MA: Johns Hopkins University Press.
May, R. (1953). *Man's search for himself*. New York: Norton.
McDonald, S., & Flanagan, S. (2004). Social perception deficits after traumatic brain injury: Interaction between emotion recognition, mentalizing ability, and social communication. *Neuropsychology, 18*, 572–579.
McKinlay, A., Dalrymple-Alford, J.C., Horwood, L.J., & Fergusson, D.M. (2002). Long term psychosocial outcomes after mild head injury in early childhood. *Journal of Neurology, Neurosurgery & Psychiatry, 73*, 281–288.
McKinlay, A., Grace, R., Horwood, J., Fergusson, D., & MacFarlane, M. (2009). Adolescent psychiatric symptoms following preschool childhood mild traumatic brain injury: Evidence from a birth cohort. *Journal of Head Trauma Rehabilitation, 24*, 221–227.
McMillan, T., Robertson, I.H., Brock, D., & Chorlton, L. (2002). Brief mindfulness training for attentional problems after traumatic brain injury: A randomised control treatment trial. *Neuropsychological Rehabilitation, 12*, 117–125.
McPherson, K.M., Kayes, N., & Weatherall, M. (2009). A pilot study of self-regulation informed goal setting in people with traumatic brain injury. *Clinical Rehabilitation, 23*, 296–309.
Mead, G.H. (1934). *Mind, self, and society: From the standpoint of a social behaviorist*. C.W. Morris (Ed.). Chicago: University of Chicago Press.
Mealings, M., & Douglas, J. (2010). 'School's a big part of your life ...': Adolescent perspectives of their school participation following traumatic brain injury. *Brain Impairment, 11*, 1–16.
Medd, J., & Tate, R. (2000). Evaluation of an anger management therapy programme following acquired brain injury: A preliminary study. *Neuropsychological Rehabilitation, 10*, 185–201.
Medley, A.R., Powell, T., Worthington, A., Chohan, G., & Jones, C. (2010). Brain injury beliefs, self-awareness, and coping: A preliminary cluster analytic study based within the self-regulatory model. *Neuropsychological Rehabilitation, 20*, 899–921.
Mellado-Calvo, N., & Fleminger, S. (2009). Cerebral tumours. In A. David, S. Fleminger, M. Kopelman, S. Lovestone & J. Mellers (Eds), *Lishman's organic psychiatry: A textbook of neuropsychiatry* (pp. 281–308). Oxford, UK: Wiley.
Miller, J.G. (2006). Cultural psychology of moral development. In S. Kitayama & D. Cohen (Eds), *Handbook of Cultural Psychology* (pp. 477–499). New York: Guilford Press.
Miller, W.R., & Rollnick, S. (2002). *Motivational interviewing: Preparing people for change* (2nd edn). New York: Guilford Press.

Milner, B. (1970). Memory and the temporal regions of the brain. In K.H. Pribram and D.E. Broadbent (Eds), *Biology of Memory*. New York: Academic Press.

Mograbi, D.C., Brown, R.G., & Morris, R.G. (2009). Anosognosia in Alzheimer's disease – The petrified self. *Consciousness and Cognition, 18*, 989–1003.

Moore, A.D., & Stambrook, M. (1994). Coping following traumatic brain injury (TBI): Derivation and validation of a TBI sample ways of coping revised subscales. *Brain Injury, 7*, 193–200.

Moore, A.D., & Stambrook, M. (1995). Cognitive moderators of outcome following traumatic brain injury: a conceptual model and implications for rehabilitation. *Brain Injury, 9*, 109–130.

Moore, E.L., Terryberry-Spohr, L., & Hope, D.A. (2006). Mild traumatic brain injury and anxiety sequelae: A review of the literature. *Brain Injury, 20*, 117–132.

Morris, P.G., Prior, L., Shoumitro, D., Lewis, G., Mayle, W., Burrow, C.E., & Bryant, E. (2005). Patients' views on outcome following head injury: a qualitative study. *BMC Family Practice, 6*, 30.

Mosig, Y.D. (2006). Conceptions of the self in Western and Eastern psychology. *Journal of Theoretical and Philisophical Psychology, 26*, 39–50.

Moss-Morris, R., Weinman, J., Petrie, K.J., Horne, R., Cameron, L.D., & Buick, D. (2002). The Revised Illness Perception Questionnaire (IPQ-R). *Psychology and Health, 17*, 1–16.

Muenchberger, H., Kendall, E., Kennedy, A., & Charker, J. (2011). Living with brain injury in the community: outcomes from a community-based self-management support (CB-SMS) programme in Australia. *Brain Injury, 25*, 23–34.

Muenchberger, H., Kendall, E., & Neal, R. (2008). Identity transition following traumatic brain injury: A dynamic process of contraction, expansion and tentative balance. *Brain Injury, 22*, 979–992.

Nalder, E., Fleming, J., Cornwell, P., Foster, M., Ownsworth, T., Shields, C., & Haines, T. (2012). Recording sentinel events in the life course of individuals with acquired brain injury: a preliminary study. *Brain Injury, 26*, 1381–1396.

Nausheen, B., Gidron, Y., Peveler, R., & Moss-Morris, R. (2009). Social support and cancer progression: a systematic review. *Journal of Psychosomatic Research, 67*, 403–415.

Neiss, M.B., Sedikides, C., & Stevenson, J. (2006). Genetic influences on level and stability of self-esteem. *Self and Identity, 5*, 247–266.

Neisser, U. (1988). Five kinds of self knowledge. *Philosophical Psychology, 1*, 35–59.

Nochi, M. (1997). Dealing with the 'Void': Traumatic brain injury as a story. *Disability & Society, 12*, 533–555.

Nochi, M. (1998). 'Loss of self' in the narratives of people with traumatic brain injuries: A qualitative analysis. *Social Science and Medicine, 7*, 869–878.

Nochi, M. (2000). Reconstructing self-narratives in coping with traumatic brain injury. *Social Science and Medicine, 51*, 1795–1804.

Northoff, G., Qin, P., & Feinberg, T.E. (2011). Brain imaging of the self – Conceptual, anatomical and methodological issues. *Consciousness and Cognition, 20*, 52–63.

O'Callaghan C., Powell T., & Oyebode J. (2006). An exploration of the experience of gaining awareness of deficit in people who have suffered a traumatic brain injury. *Neuropsychological Rehabilitation, 16*, 579–593.

O'Koon, J. (1997). Attachment to parents and peers in late adolescence and their relationship with self-image. *Adolescence, 32*, 471–482.

O'Neill, M., & McMillan, T.M. (2012). Can deficits in empathy after head injury be improved by compassionate imagery? *Neuropsychological Rehabilitation, 22*, 836–851.

Orlinsky, D.E., & Howard, K.I. (1987). A generic model of psychotherapy. *Journal of Integrative and Eclectic Psychotherapy*, 6, 6–27.

Orth, U., Trzesniewski, K.H., & Robins, R.W. (2010). Self-esteem development from young adulthood to old age: A cohort-sequential longitudinal study. *Journal of Personality and Social Psychology*, 98, 645–658.

Osgood, C.E., Suci, G., & Tannenbaum, P. (1957). *The measurement of meaning*. Urbana, IL: University of Illinois Press.

Ownsworth, T. (2005). The impact of defensive denial upon adjustment following traumatic brain injury. *Neuropsychoanalysis*, 7, 83–94.

Ownsworth, T.L. (2010). A metacognitive contextual approach for facilitating return to work following acquired brain injury: Three descriptive case studies. *Work: A Journal of Prevention, Assessment & Rehabilitation*, 36, 381–388.

Ownsworth, T., & Clare, L. (2006). The association between awareness deficits and rehabilitation outcome following acquired brain injury. *Clinical Psychology Review*, 26, 783–795.

Ownsworth, T., & Fleming, J. (2011). Editorial: Growth through loss after brain injury. Special Issue of *Brain Impairment*, 12, 79–81.

Ownsworth, T., & McFarland, K. (2004). Investigation of psychological and neuropsychological factors associated with clinical outcome following a group rehabilitation programme. *Neuropsychological Rehabilitation*, 14, 535–562.

Ownsworth, T. & McKenna, K. (2004). Investigation of factors related to employment outcome following traumatic brain injury: a critical review and conceptual model. *Disability and Rehabilitation*, 26, 765–784.

Ownsworth, T., & Oei, T.P.S. (1998). Depression after traumatic brain injury: conceptualization and treatment considerations. *Brain Injury*, 12, 735–751.

Ownsworth, T., Chambers, S., Hawkes, A., Walker, D.G. & Shum, D. (2011). Making sense of brain tumour: A qualitative investigation of personal and social processes of adjustment. *Neuropsychological Rehabilitation*, 21, 117–137.

Ownsworth, T., Chambers, S., Stewart, E., Casey, L., Walker, D., & Shum, D. (2013). Effectiveness of the Making Sense of Brain Tumour Program for improving psychological well-being after brain tumour: A randomised controlled trial. Paper presented at the 10th meeting of the Neuropsychological Rehabilitation Special Interest Group of the World Federation of Neurorehabilitation, Maastricht, The Netherlands (July 2013).

Ownsworth, T., Clare, L., & Morris, R. (2006). An integrated biopsychosocial approach to understanding awareness deficits in Alzheimer's disease and brain injury. *Neuropsychological Rehabilitation*, 16, 415–438.

Ownsworth, T., Fleming, J., Desbois, J., Strong, J., & Kuipers, P. (2006). A metacognitive contextual intervention to enhance error awareness and functional performance following traumatic brain injury: A single case experimental design. *Journal of the International Neuropsychological Society*, 12, 54–63.

Ownsworth, T., Fleming, J., Haines, T., Cornwell, P., Kendall, M., Nalder, E., & Gordon, C. (2011). Development of depressive symptoms during early community reintegration after traumatic brain injury. *Journal of the International Neuropsychological Society*, 17, 112–119.

Ownsworth, T.L., Fleming, J., Shum, D., Kuipers, P., & Strong, J. (2008). Comparison of individual, group and combined intervention formats in a RCT for facilitating goal attainment and improving psychosocial function following acquired brain injury. *Journal of Rehabilitation Medicine*, 40, 81–88.

Ownsworth, T., Fleming, J., Strong, J., Radel, M., Chan, W., & Clare, L. (2007). Awareness typologies, long-term emotional adjustment and psychosocial outcomes following acquired brain injury. *Neuropsychological Rehabilitation*, 17, 129–150.

Ownsworth, T., Hawkes, A.L., Chambers, S., Walker, D.G., & Shum, D. (2010). Applying a biopsychosocial perspective to investigate factors related to emotional adjustment and quality of life for individuals with brain tumour. *Brain Impairment, 11*, 270–280.

Ownsworth, T., Hawkes, A., Steginga, S., Walker, D., & Shum, D. (2009). A biopsychosocial perspective on adjustment and quality of life following brain tumor: A systematic evaluation of the literature. *Disability & Rehabilitation, 31*, 1038–1055.

Ownsworth, T.L., Henderson, L., & Chambers, S. (2010). Social support buffers the impact of functional impairments on caregiver psychological well-being in the context of brain tumour and other cancers. *Psycho-Oncology, 19*, 1116–1122.

Ownsworth, T.L., Henderson, L., Chambers, S., & Shum, D. (2009). Functional impairments and caregiver depression in the context of brain tumour and other cancers: a mediating effect of strain. *Brain Impairment, 10*, 149–161.

Ownsworth, T., Hoffmann, T., Evans, E., Stemm, B., Howlett, J., Read, S., & Shum, D. (2011). Early cognitive appraisals and psychotherapy after stroke. Paper presented at the 8th Conference of the Neuropsychological Rehabilitation Special Interest Group of the World Federation of Neurorehabilitation, Rotorua, New Zealand (July 2011).

Ownsworth, T.L., McFarland, K., & Young, McD. (2000). Self-awareness and psychosocial functioning following acquired brain injury: An evaluation of a group support programme. *Neuropsychological Rehabilitation, 10*, 465–484.

Ownsworth, T.L., McFarland, K., & Young, R.McD. (2002). Investigation of factors underlying deficits in self-awareness and self-regulation. *Brain Injury, 16*, 291–309.

Ownsworth, T.L., Quinn, H., Fleming, J., Kendall, M., & Shum, D. (2010). Error self-regulation following traumatic brain injury: A single case study evaluation of metacognitive skills training and behavioural practice interventions. *Neuropsychological Rehabilitation, 20*, 59–80.

Ownsworth, T.L., Turpin, M., Andrew, B., & Fleming, J. (2008). Participant perspectives on an individualised self-awareness intervention following stroke: A qualitative case study. *Neuropsychological Rehabilitation, 18*, 692–712.

Ownsworth, T., Turpin, M., Carlson, G., & Brennan, J. (2004). Perceptions of long-term community-based support following severe acquired brain injury. *Brain Impairment, 5*, 53–66.

Oxford Centre for Evidence-Based Medicine (OCEBM). Levels of Evidence Working Group (2011). The Oxford 2011 Levels of Evidence. Oxford Centre for Evidence-Based Medicine. http://www.cebm.net/index.aspx?o=5653

Pagulayan, K.F., Temkin, N.R., Machamer, J.E., & Dikmen, S.S. (2007). The measurement and magnitude of awareness difficulties after traumatic brain injury: A longitudinal study. *Journal of the International Neuropsychological Society, 13*, 561–570.

Pargament, K. (1997). *The psychology of religion and coping: Theory, research, practice.* New York: Guilford Press.

Paterson, B., & Scott-Findlay, S. (2002). Critical issues in interviewing people with Traumatic brain injury. *Qualitative Health Research, 12*, 399–409.

Patton, M. (2002). *Qualitative Research and Evaluation Methods.* (3rd edn.). California: Sage Publications.

Peacock, E.J., & Wong, P.T. (1990). The Stress Appraisal Measure (SAM): A multidimensional approach to cognitive appraisal. *Stress Medicine, 6*, 227–236.

Pearl, G., Sage, K., & Young, A.M. (2011). Involvement in volunteering: an exploration of the personal experience of people with aphasia. *Disability & Rehabilitation, 33*, 1805–1821.

Pepping, M., & Roueche, J.R. (1991). Psychosocial consequences of significant brain injury. In D.E. Tupper & K.C. Cicerone (Eds), *The neuropsychology of everyday life: Issues in development and rehabilitation* (pp. 215–255). Norwell, MA: Kluwer Academic.

Pessar, L.F., Coad, M.L., Linn, R.T., & Willer, B.S. (1993). The effects of parental traumatic brain injury on the behaviour of parents and children. *Brain Injury, 7*, 231–240.

Pia, L., Neppi-Modona, M., Ricci, R., & Berti, A. (2004). The anatomy of anosognosia for hemiplegia: A meta-analysis. *Cortex, 40*, 367–377.

Piers, E. (1984). *Piers Harris Children's Self-Concept Scale: Revised Manual*, Western Psychological Services: Los Angeles.

Piers, E.V., & Herzberg, D.S. (2002). *Piers–Harris Children's Self-Concept Scale-Second Edition Manual*. Western Psychological Services, Los Angeles.

Platek, S.M., Keenan, J.P., Gallup Jr, G.G., & Mohamed, F.B. (2004). Where am I? The neurological correlates of self and other. *Cognitive Brain Research, 19*, 114–122.

Ponsford, J. (2003). Sexual changes associated with traumatic brain injury. *Neuropsychological Rehabilitation, 13*, 275–289.

Ponsford, J., Cameron, P., Fitzgerald, M., Grant, M., & Mikocka-Walus, A. (2011). Long-term outcomes after uncomplicated mild traumatic brain injury: a comparison with trauma controls. *Journal of Neurotrauma, 28*, 937–946.

Ponsford, J., McLaren, A., Schonberger, M., Burke, R., Rudzki, D., Olver, J., & Ponsford, M. (2011). The association between apolipoprotein E and traumatic brain injury severity and functional outcome in a rehabilitation sample. *Journal of Neurotrauma, 28*, 1683–1692.

Powell, J., Heslin, J., & Greenwood, R. (2002). Community based rehabilitation after severe traumatic brain injury: a randomised controlled trial. *Journal of Neurology, Neurosurgery and Psychiatry, 72*, 193–202.

Powell, T., Ekin-Wood, A., & Collin, C. (2007). Posttraumatic growth after head injury: A long term follow up. *Brain Injury, 21*, 31–38.

Prigatano, G.P. (1989). Work, love, and play after brain injury. *Bulletin of the Menninger Clinic, 53*, 414–431.

Prigatano, G.P. (1999). *Principles of neuropsychological rehabilitation*. New York: Oxford University Press.

Prigatano, G.P. (2010). *The Study of Anosognosia*. New York: Oxford University Press.

Prigatano, G.P. & Altman, I.M. (1990). Impaired awareness of behavioral limitations after traumatic brain injury. *Archives of Physical Medicine and Rehabilitation, 71*, 1058–1064.

Prigatano, G.P. & Leathem, J.M. (1993). Awareness of behavioral limitations after traumatic brain injury: A cross-cultural study of New Zealand Maoris and non-Maoris. *Clinical Neuropsychologist, 7*, 123–135.

Prigatano, G.P., & Pliskin, N. (2003). *Clinical Neuropsychology and Cost Outcome Research: A Beginning*. New York: Psychology Press.

Prigatano, G.P., Fordyce, D., Zeiner, H., Roueche, J., Pepping, M., & Wood, B. (1984). Neuropsychological rehabilitation after closed head injury in young adults. *Journal of Neurology, Neurosurgery, & Psychiatry, 47*, 505–513.

Prigatano, G.P., Fordyce, D.J., Zeiner, H.K., Roueche, J., Pepping, M., & Wood, B. (1986). *Neuropsychological rehabilitation after brain injury*. Baltimore: John Hopkins University Press.

Qin, P., Di, H., Liu, Y., Yu, S., Gong, Q., Duncan, N., ... Northoff, G. (2010). Anterior cingulate activity and the self in disorders of consciousness. *Human Brain Mapping, 31*, 1993–2002.

Radford, K., Phillips, J., Drummond, A., Sach, T., Walker, M., Tyerman, A., ... Jones, T. (2013). Return to work after traumatic brain injury: Cohort comparison and economic evaluation. *Brain Injury, 27*, 507–520.

Rahula, W. (1974). *The heritage of the bhikkhu: A short history of the bhikkhu in educational, cultural, social and political life*. New York: Random House.

Ramanathan, D.M., Wardecker, B.M., Slocomb, J.E., & Hillary, F.G. (2011). Dispositional optimism and outcome following traumatic brain injury. *Brain Injury, 25*, 328–337.

Rath, J.F., Simon, D., Langenbahn, D.M., Sherr, R.L., & Diller, L. (2003). Group treatment of problem-solving deficits in outpatients with traumatic brain injury: A randomised outcome study. *Neuropsychological Rehabilitation, 13*, 461–488.

Rathbone, C.J., Conway, M.A., & Moulin, C.J.A. (2011). Remembering and imagining: The role of the self. *Consciousness and Cognition, 20*, 1175–1182.

Richards, A.D. (1990). The future of psychoanalysis: The past, present, and future of psychoanalytic theory. *Psychoanalytic Quarterly, 59*, 347–369.

Riley, G.A., Brennan, A.J., & Powell, T. (2004). Threat appraisal and avoidance after traumatic brain injury: why and how often are activities avoided? *Brain Injury, 18*, 871–888.

Riley, G.A., Dennis, R.K., & Powell, T. (2010). Evaluation of coping resources and self-esteem as moderators of the relationship between threat appraisals and avoidance of activities after traumatic brain injury. *Neuropsychological Rehabilitation, 20*, 869–882.

Rizzolatti, G., & Craighero, L. (2005). Mirror neuron: a neurological approach to empathy. In J.-P. Changeux, A.R. Damasio, W. Singer & Y. Christen (Eds), *Neurobiology of human values: Research and perspectives in neurosciences* (pp. 107–123). Berlin Heidelberg: Springer.

Rizzolatti, G., Fadiga, L., Gallese, V., & Fogassi, L. (1996). Premotor cortex and the recognition of motor actions. *Cognitive Brain Research, 3*, 131–141.

Robinson, B. (2009). When therapist variables and the client's theory of change meet. *Psychotherapy in Australia, 15*, 60–65.

Robinson-Smith, G., Johnston, M.V., & Allen, J. (2000). Self-care self-efficacy, quality of life, and depression after stroke. *Stroke, 19*, 1101–1107.

Robson, P. (1989). Development of a new self-report questionnaire to measure self-esteem. *Psychological Medicine, 19*, 513–518.

Rochat, P. (2011). The self as phenotype. *Consciousness and Cognition, 20*, 109–119.

Rochette, A., & Desrosiers, J. (2002). Coping with the consequences of a stroke. *International Journal of Rehabilitation Research, 25*, 17–24.

Rochette, A., Bravo, G., Desrosiers, J., St-Cyr-Tribble, D., & Bourget, A. (2007). Adaptation process, participation and depression over six months in first-stroke individuals and spouses. *Clinical Rehabilitation, 21*, 554–562.

Rogers, C.R. (1951). *Client-centered therapy: Its current practice, implications, and theory*. Oxford, UK: Houghton Mifflin.

Roof, R.L., & Hall, E.D. (2000). Estrogen-related gender difference in survival rate and cortical blood flow after impact-acceleration head injury in rats. *Journal of Neurotrauma, 17*, 1155–1169.

Rosamond, W., Flegal, K., Friday, G., Furie, K., Go, A., Greenlund, K., ... Hong, Y. (2007). Heart disease and stroke statistics – 2007 update: a report from the American Heart Association Statistics Committee and Stroke Statistics Subcommittee. *Circulation, 115*, 69–171.

Rosenberg, M. (1965). *Society and the adolescent self-image*. Princeton, NJ: Princeton University Press.

Rotter, J.B. (1954). *Social learning and clinical psychology*. New York: Prentice-Hall.

Rowlands, A. (2001). Ability of disability? Strengths-based practice in the area of traumatic brain injury. *Families in Society, 82*, 273–286.

Ruddle, J.A., Coetzer, R., & Vaughan, F.L. (2005). Grief after brain injury: A validation of the Brain Injury Grief Inventory (BIGI). *Illness, Crisis & Loss, 13*, 235–247.

Rutland-Brown, W., Langlois, J.A., & Thomas, K.E., & Xi, Y.L. (2006). The incidence of traumatic brain injury in the United States, 2003. *Journal of Head Trauma Rehabilitation, 21*, 544–548.

Rutterford, N.A., & Wood, R.L. (2006). Evaluating a theory of stress and adjustment when predicting long-term psychosocial outcome after brain injury. *Journal of the International Neuropsychological Society, 12*, 359–367.

Ryan, R.M., & Deci, E.L. (2001). On happiness and human potentials: a review of research on hedonic and eudaimonic well-being. *Annual Review of Psychology, 52*, 141–166.

Salander, P., Bergenheim, A.T., Hamberg, K., & Henriksson, R. (1999). Pathways from symptoms to medical care: A descriptive study of symptom development and obstacles to early diagnosis in brain tumour patients. *Family Practice, 16*, 143–148.

Sale, P., West, M., Sherron, P. & Wehman, P. (1991). Exploratory analysis of job separations from supported employment for persons with traumatic brain injury. *Journal of Head Trauma Rehabilitation, 6*, 1–11.

Salmond, C.H., Menon, D.K., Chatfield, D.A., Pickard, J.D., & Sahakian, B.J. (2006). Cognitive reserve as a resilience factor against depression after moderate/severe head injury. *Journal of Neurotrauma, 23*, 1049–1058.

Sambuco, M., Brookes, N., & Lah, S. (2008). Paediatric brain injury: A review of siblings' outcome. *Brain Injury, 22*, 7–17.

Sarajuuri, J.M., & Koskinen, S.K. (2006). Holistic neuropsychological rehabilitation in Finland: The INSURE program – a transcultural outgrowth of perspectives from Israel to Europe via the USA. *International Journal of Psychology, 41*, 362–370.

Schmidt, J., Fleming, J., Ownsworth, T., & Lannin, N. (2013). Video-feedback on functional task performance improves self-awareness after traumatic brain injury: a randomised controlled trial. *Neurorehabilitation and Neural Repair, 27*, 316–324.

Schmidt, J., Lannin, N., Fleming, J., & Ownsworth, T. (2011). A systematic review of feedback interventions for impaired self-awareness following brain injury. *Journal of Rehabilitation Medicine, 43*, 673–680.

Schmidt, A.T., Hanten, G.R., Li, X., Orsten, K.D., & Levin, H.S. (2010). Emotion recognition following pediatric traumatic brain injury: Longitudinal analysis of emotional prosody and facial emotion recognition. *Neuropsychologia, 48*, 2869.

Schönberger, M., Humle, F., & Teasdale, T.W. (2006). The development of the therapeutic working alliance, patients' awareness and their compliance during the process of brain injury rehabilitation. *Brain Injury, 20*, 445–454.

Schumacher, K., Dodd, M., & Paul, S. (1993). The stress process in family caregivers of persons receiving chemotherapy. *Research in Nursing and Health, 16*, 395–404.

Schweitzer, R.D., Seth-Smith, M., & Callan, V. (1992). The relationship between self-esteem and psychological adjustment in young adolescents. *Journal of Adolescence, 15*, 83–97.

Secrest, J., & Thomas, S.P. (1999). Continuity and discontinuity: the quality of life following stroke. *Rehabilitation Nursing, 24*, 240–246.

Secrest, J., & Zeller, R. (2003). Measuring continuity and discontinuity following stroke. *Journal of Nursing Scholarship, 35*, 243–247.

Secrest, J., & Zeller, R. (2006). Replication and extension of the Continuity and Discontinuity of Self Scale (CDSS). *Journal of Nursing Scholarship, 38*, 154–158.

Secrest, J., & Zeller, R. (2007). The relationship of continuity and discontinuity, functional ability, depression, and quality of life over time in stroke survivors. *Rehabilitation Nursing, 32*, 158–164.

Seligman, M.E., & Csikszentmihalyi, M. (2000). Positive psychology. An introduction. *American Psychologist, 55*, 5–14.

Senathi-Raja, D., Ponsford, J., & Schönberger, M. (2010). The association of age and time postinjury with long-term emotional outcome following traumatic brain injury. *Journal of Head Trauma Rehabilitation, 25*, 330–338.

Setterlund, M.B., & Niedenthal, P.M. (1993). Who am I? Why am I here?: Self esteem, self-clarity, and prototype matching. *Journal of Personality and Social Psychology, 65*, 769–780.

Shadden, B.B. (2005). Aphasia as identity theft. Theory and practice. *Aphasiology, 19*, 211–223.

Shadden, B.B., & Koski, P.R. (2007). Social construction of self for persons with aphasia: When language as a cultural tool is impaired. *Journal of Medical Speech-Language Pathology, 15,* 99–105.

Shallice, T., & Burgess, P.W. (1996). The domain of supervisory processes and the temporal organisation of behaviour. *Philosophical Transactions of the Royal Society of London B., 351,* 1405–1412.

Sharp, N.L., Bye, R.A., Llewellyn, G.M., & Cusick, A. (2006). Fitting back in: Adolescents returning to school after severe acquired brain injury. *Disability & Rehabilitation, 28,* 767–778.

Sherer, M., Bergloff, P., Boake, C., High, W.M., & Levin, E. (1998a). The Awareness Questionnaire: factor analysis structure and internal consistency. *Brain Injury, 12,* 63–68.

Sherer, M., Bergloff, P., Levin, E., High, W.M., Oden, K.E., & Nick, T.G. (1998b). Impaired awareness and employment outcome after traumatic brain injury. *Journal of Head Trauma Rehabilitation, 13,* 52–61.

Sherer, M., Hart, T., Whyte, J., Nick, T.G., & Yablon, S.A. (2005). Neuroanatomical basis of impaired self-awareness after traumatic brain injury: Findings from early computed tomography. *Journal of Head Trauma Rehabilitation, 20,* 287–300.

Sherer, M., Nick, T.G., Sander, A.M., Hart, T., Hanks, R., Rosenthal, M., … Yablon, S.A. (2003). Race and productivity outcome after traumatic brain injury: Influence of confounding factors. *Journal of Head Trauma Rehabilitation, 18,* 408–424.

Sherwood, P.R., Given, B.A., Charles, C.W., Schiffman, R.F., Murman, D.L., vonEye, A., Lovely, M., Rogers, L.R., & Remar, S. (2007). The influence of caregiver mastery on depressive symptoms. *Journal of Nursing Scholarship, 39,* 249–255

Sherwood, P., Given, B., Given, C., Schiffman, R., Murman, D., & Lovely, M. (2004). Caregivers of persons with a brain tumour: A conceptual model. *Nursing Inquiry, 11,* 43–53.

Sherwood, P., Given, B., Given, C., Schiffman, R., Murman, D., von Eye, A., Lovely, M., Rogers, L., & Remer, S. (2007). The influence of caregiver mastery on depressive symptoms. *Journal of Nursing Scholarship, 39*(3), 249–255.

Shields, C., & Ownsworth, T. (2013). An integration of third wave cognitive behavioural interventions following stroke: a case study. *Neuro-Disability and Psychotherapy, 1,* 39–69.

Silva, J., Ownsworth, T., Shields, C., & Fleming, J. (2011). Enhanced appreciation of life following acquired brain injury: posttraumatic growth at 6 months post-discharge. *Brain Impairment, 12,* 93–104.

Silverman, M. (2011). The dignity of struggle. *Topics in Stroke Rehabilitation, 18,* 134.

Simmond, M., & Fleming, J. (2003). Occupational therapy assessment of self-awareness following traumatic brain injury: A literature review. *British Journal of Occupational Therapy, 66,* 447–453.

Simmons-Mackie, N., Raymer, A.S., Armstrong, E., Holland, A.L., & Cherney, L.R. (2010). Communication partner training in aphasia: A systematic review. *Archives of Physical Medicine and Rehabilitation, 91,* 1814–1837.

Simpson, G., & Jones, K. (2013). How important is resilience among family members supporting relatives with traumatic brain injury or spinal cord injury? *Clinical Rehabilitation, 27,* 367–377.

Simpson, G., Tate, R., Whiting, D., & Cotter, R. (2011). Suicide prevention after traumatic brain injury: a randomized controlled trial of a program for the psychological treatment of hopelessness. *Journal of Head Trauma Rehabilitation. 26,* 290–300.

Singer, G.H.S., Glang, A., & Nixon, C. (1994). A comparison of two psychosocial interventions for parents of children with acquired brain injury: An exploratory study. *Journal of Head Trauma Rehabilitation, 9,* 38–49.

Snell, D.L., Siegert, R.J., Hay-Smith, E.J.C., & Surgenor, L.J. (2010). An examination of the factor structure of the revised illness perception questionnaire in adults with mild traumatic brain injury. *Brain Injury, 24*, 1595–1605.

Snodgrass, C., & Knott, F. (2006). Theory of mind in children with traumatic brain injury. *Brain Injury, 20*, 825–833.

Sohlberg, M.M., Mateer, C.A., Penkman, L., Glang, A., & Todis, B. (1998). Awareness Intervention: Who needs it? *Journal of Head Trauma Rehabilitation, 13*, 62–78.

Soo C., & Tate R. (2007). (Cochrane review) Psychological treatment for anxiety in people with traumatic brain injury. *Cochrane Database of Systematic Reviews*. Issue 3, DOI: 10.1002/14651858.CD005239.pub2.

Spitz, G., Schönberger, M. & Ponsford, J. (2013). The relationship between cognitive impairment, coping style, and emotional adjustment following traumatic brain injury. *Journal of Head Trauma Rehabilitation, 28*, 116–125.

Stake, J.E., Huff, L., & Zand, D. (1995). Trait self-esteem, positive and negative events, and event-specific shifts in self-evaluation and affect. *Journal of Research in Personality, 29*, 223–241.

Stancin, T., Drotar, D., Taylor, H.G., Yeates, K.O., Wade, S.L., & Minich, N.M. (2002). Health-related quality of life of children and adolescents after traumatic brain injury. *Pediatrics, 109*, e34.

Stanton, A.L., Danoff-Burg, S., Cameron, C.L., & Ellis, A.P. (1994). Coping through emotional approach: Problems of conceptualization and confounding. *Journal of Personality and Social Psychology, 66*, 350–362.

Stefanacci, L., Buffalo, E.A., Schmolck, H., & Squire, L.R. (2000). Profound amnesia after damage to the medial temporal lobe: A neuroanatomical and neuropsychological profile of patient E.P. *Journal of Neuroscience, 20*(18), 7024–7036.

Stergiou-Kita, M., Dawson, D., & Rappolt S. (2012). Inter-professional clinical practice guideline for vocational evaluation following traumatic brain injury: a systematic and evidence-based approach. *Journal of Occupational Rehabilitation, 22*, 166–181.

Stern-Gillet, S. (1995). *Aristotle's philosophy of friendship*. Albany, NY: State University of New York Press.

Stets, J.E., & Burke, P.J. (2000). Identity theory and social identity theory. *Social Psychology Quarterly, 63*, 224–237.

Strang, S., & Strang, P. (2001). Spiritual thoughts, coping and 'sense of coherence' in brain tumour patients and their spouses. *Palliative Medicine, 15*, 127–134.

Strauman, T.J. (1990). Self-guides and emotionally significant childhood memories: a study of retrieval efficiency and negative emotional content. *Journal of Personality and Social Psychology, 59*, 869–880.

Stuss, D.T. (2007). New approaches to prefrontal lobe testing. In B. Miller & J. Cummings (Eds), *The human frontal lobes: Functions and disorders* (2nd edn.). New York: Guilford Press.

Stuss, D.T., Picton, T.W., & Alexander, M.P. (2001). Consciousness, self-awareness and the frontal lobes. In S. Salloway, P. Malloy, & J. Duffy (Eds), *The frontal lobes and neuropsychiatric illness* (pp. 101–109). Washington, DC: American Psychiatric Press.

Stuss, D.T., Alexander, M.P., Floden, D., Binns, M.A., Levine, B., McIntosh, A.R., ... Hevenor, S. (2002). Evidence from focal lesions in humans. *Principles of Frontal Lobe Function* (pp. 392–407). Oxford: Oxford University Press.

Sullivan, H.S. (1953). *The interpersonal theory of psychiatry*. New York: Norton.

Suls, J., Martin, R., & Wheeler, L. (2002). Social comparison: Why, with whom, and with what effect? *Current Directions in Psychological Science, 11*, 159–163.

Svoboda, E., & Richards, B. (2009). Compensating for anterograde amnesia: A new training method that capitalizes on emerging smartphone technologies. *Journal of the International Neuropsychological Society, 15*, 629–638.

Svoboda, E., Richards, B., Leach, L., & Mertens, V. (2012). PDA and smartphone use by individuals with moderate-to-severe memory impairment: Application of a theory-driven training programme. *Neuropsychological Rehabilitation, 22*, 408–427.

Tajfel, H., & Turner, J. (1979). An integrative theory of intergroup conflict. In W.G. Austin & S. Worchel (Eds), *The social psychology of intergroup relations* (pp. 33–48). Monterey, CA: Brooks-Cole.

Tan, L. (2008). Psychotherapy 2.0: MySpace blogging as self-therapy. *American Journal of Psychotherapy, 62*, 143–163.

Tangney, J.P., Niedenthal, P.M., Covert, M.V., & Barlow, D.H. (1998). Are shame and guilt related to distinct self-discrepancies? A test of Higgins's (1987) hypotheses. *Journal of Personality and Social Psychology, 75*, 256–268.

Tate, R.L. (2010). *A Compendium of Test, Scales, and Questionnaires: The Practitioner's Guide to Measuring Outcomes after Acquired Brain Impairment*. New York: Psychology Press.

Tate, R.L. & Broe, G.A. (1999). Psychosocial adjustment after traumatic brain injury: What are the important variables? *Psychological Medicine, 29*, 713–725.

Tate, R.L., Harris, R.D., Cameron, I.D., Myles, B.M., Winstanley, J.B., Hodgkinson, A.E., … Harradine, P.G. (2006). Recovery of impairments after severe traumatic brain injury: Findings from a prospective, multicentre study. *Brain Impairment, 7*, 1–15.

Taylor, H.G., Yeates, K.O., Wade, S.L., Drotar, D., Stancin, T., & Minich, N. (2002). A prospective study of short- and long-term outcomes after traumatic brain injury in children: behavior and achievement. *Neuropsychology, 16*, 15–27.

Taylor, S.E. (1983). Adjusting to threatening events: A theory of cognitive adaptation. *American Psychologist, 38*, 653–662.

Teasdale, J.D., & Barnard, P.J. (1993). *Affect, cognition and change: Remodelling depressive thought*. Hove, UK: Laurence Erlbaum.

Teasdale, T.W., Emslie, H., Quirk, K., Evans, J., Fish, J., & Wilson, B. (2009). Alleviation of carer strain during the use of the Neuropage device by people with acquired brain injury. *Journal of Neurology Neurosurgery and Psychiatry, 80*, 781–783.

Tedeschi, R.G., & Calhoun, R.G. (1996). The Posttraumatic Growth Inventory: Measuring the positive legacy of trauma. *Journal of Traumatic Stress, 9*, 455–471.

Teng, J., Mayo, N.E., Latimer, E., Hanley, J., Wood-Dauphinee, S., Cote, R., & Scott, S. (2003). Costs and caregiver consequences of early supported discharge for stroke patients. *Stroke, 34*, 528–536.

Thickpenny-Davis, K., & Barker-Collo, S. (2007). Does memory performance of adults with brain injury improve following participation in a structured memory rehabilitation group? *Journal of Head Trauma Rehabilitation, 22*, 303–313.

Thomas, S.A., Walker, M.F., Macniven, J.A., Haworth, H., & Lincoln, N.B. (2013). Communication and Low Mood (CALM): A randomised controlled trial of behavioural therapy for stroke patients with aphasia. *Clinical Rehabilitation, 27*, 398–408.

Thompson, H.J., McCormick, W.C., & Kagan, S.H. (2006). Traumatic brain injury in older adults: Epidemiology, outcomes, and future implications. *Journal of the American Geriatrics Society, 54*, 1590–1595.

Thompson, S.C. (1991). The search for meaning following a stroke. *Basic and Applied Social Psychology, 12*, 81–96.

Tiersky, L.A., Anselmi, V., Johnston, M.V., Kurtyka, J., Roosen, E., Schwartz, T., & Deluca, J. (2005). A trial of neuropsychologic rehabilitation in mild spectrum traumatic brain injury. *Archives of Physical Medicine and Rehabilitation, 86*, 1565–1574.

Todis, B., & Glang, A. (2008). Redefining success: results of a qualitative study of postsecondary transition outcomes for youth with traumatic brain injury. *Journal of Head Trauma Rehabilitation, 23*, 252–263.

Todis, B., Sohlberg, M.M., Hood, D. & Fickas, S. (2005). Making electronic email accessible: Perspectives of people with acquired cognitive impairments, caregivers and professionals. *Brain Injury, 19,* 389–401.

Togher, L., McDonald, S., Tate, R., Power, E. & Rietdijk (2013). Training communication partners of people with severe traumatic brain injury improves everyday conversations: A multicenter single blind clinical trial. *Journal of Rehabilitation Medicine, 45,* 637–645.

Toglia, J., & Kirk, U. (2000). Understanding awareness deficits following brain injury. *Neurorehabilitation, 15,* 57–70.

Topolovec-Vranic, J., Cullen, N., Michalak, A., Ouchterlony, D., Bhalerao, S., Masanic, C., & Cusimano, M.D. (2010). Evaluation of an online cognitive behavioural therapy program by patients with traumatic brain injury and depression. *Brain Injury, 24,* 762–772.

Trexler, L.E. (2000). Empirical support for neuropsychological rehabilitation. In A. Christensen & B. Uzzell (Eds), *International Handbook of Neuropsychological Rehabilitation: Critical Issues in Neuropsychology* (pp. 137–150). New York: Kluwer Academic/Plenum.

Trombly, C.A., Radomski, M.V., & Davis, E.A. (1998). Achievement of self-identified goals by adults with traumatic brain injury: Phase I. *American Journal of Occupational Therapy, 52,* 810–818.

Tsaousides, T., Ashman, T.A., & Gordon, W.A. (2013). Diagnosis and treatment of depression following traumatic brain injury. *Brain Impairment, 14,* 63–76.

Tsaousides, T., Ashman, T.A., & Seter, C. (2008). The psychological effects of employment after traumatic brain injury: Objective and subjective indicators. *Rehabilitation Psychology, 53,* 456–463.

Tsaousides, T., Matsuzawa, Y., & Lebowitz, M. (2011). Familiarity and prevalence of Facebook use for social networking among individuals with traumatic brain injury. *Brain Injury, 25,* 1155–1162.

Tulving, E. (1985). How many memory systems are there? *American Psychologist, 40,* 385–398.

Turner, B., Fleming, J., Ownsworth, T., & Cornwell, P. (2011). Perceptions of recovery during the early transition phase from hospital to home following acquired brain injury: a journey of discovery. *Neuropsychological Rehabilitation, 21,* 64–91.

Turner, B., Ownsworth, T., Cornwell, P., & Fleming, J. (2009). Reengagement in meaningful occupations during the transition from hospital to home for people with acquired brain injury and their family caregivers. *American Journal of Occupational Therapy, 63,* 609–620.

Turner-Stokes, L. (2008). Evidence for the effectiveness of multi-disciplinary rehabilitation following acquired brain injury: A synthesis of two systematic approaches. *Journal of Rehabilitation Medicine, 40,* 691–701.

Tyerman, A. (1987). Self-concept and psychological change in the rehabilitation of the severely head injured person. Unpublished Doctoral Thesis. University of London.

Tyerman, A., & Humphrey, M. (1984). Changes in self-concept following severe head injury. *International Journal of Rehabilitation Research, 7,* 11–23.

Tyerman, A.T. & King, N.S. (Eds) (2008). *Psychological approaches to rehabilitation following traumatic brain injury.* Blackwell. Oxford.

Uysal, S., Hibbard, M.R., Robillard, D., Pappadopulos, E., & Jaffe, M. (1998). The effect of parental traumatic brain injury on parenting and child behaviour. *Journal of Head Trauma Rehabilitation, 13,* 57–71.

Vaccaro, M., Hart, T., Whyte, J., Buchhofer, R. (2007). Internet use and interest among individuals with traumatic brain injury: A consumer survey. *Disability & Rehabilitation: Assistive Technology, 2,* 85–95.

Vickery, C.D., Gontkovsky, S.T., & Caroselli, J.S. (2005). Self-concept and quality of life following acquired brain injury: A pilot investigation. *Brain Injury, 19,* 657–665.

Vickery, C.D., Gontkovsky, S.T., Wallace, J.J., & Caroselli, J.S. (2006). Group psychotherapy focusing on self-concept change following acquired brain injury: A pilot investigation. *Rehabilitation Psychology, 51*, 30–35.

Wade, S.L., Carey, J., & Wolfe, C.R. (2006). An online family intervention to reduce parental distress following pediatric brain injury. *Journal of Consulting and Clinical Psychology, 74*, 445–454.

Wade, S.L., Cassedy, A., Walz, N.C., Taylor, H.G., Stancin, T., & Yeates, K.O. (2011). The relationship of parental warm responsiveness and negativity to emerging behavior problems following traumatic brain injury in young children. *Developmental Psychology, 47*, 119–133.

Wade, S.L., Michaud, L., & Brown, T.M. (2006). Putting the pieces together: preliminary efficacy of a family problem-solving intervention for children with traumatic brain injury. *Journal of Head Trauma Rehabilitation, 21*, 57–67.

Wade, S.L., Oberjohn, K., Burkhardt, A., & Greenberg, I. (2009). Feasibility and preliminary efficacy of a web-based parenting skills program for young children with traumatic brain injury. *Journal of Head Trauma Rehabilitation, 24*, 239–247.

Wade, S.L., Walz, N.C., Carey, J.C., & Williams, K.M. (2008). Preliminary efficacy of a Web-based family problem solving treatment program for adolescents with traumatic brain injury. *Journal of Head Trauma Rehabilitation, 23*, 369–377.

Wade, S.L., Walz, N.C., Carey, J., Williams, K.M., Cass, J., Herren, L., Mark, E., & Yeates, K.O. (2010). A randomized trial of teen online problem solving for improving executive function deficits following pediatric traumatic brain injury. *Journal of Head Trauma Rehabilitation, 25*, 409–415.

Wade, S.L., Wolfe, C.R., Brown, T.M., & Pestian, J.P. (2005). Can a Web-based family problem-solving intervention work for children with traumatic brain injury? *Rehabilitation Psychology, 50*, 337–345.

Walker, A.J., Nott, M.T., Doyle, M., Onus, M., McCarthy, K., & Baguley, I.J. (2010). Effectiveness of a group anger management programme after severe traumatic brain injury. *Brain Injury, 24*, 517–524.

Wall, S.E., Williams, W., Morris, R.G., & Bramham, J. (2011). The development of a new measure of social-emotional functioning for young adolescents. *Clinical Child Psychology & Psychiatry, 16*, 301–315.

Walsh, S., Fortune, D.G., Gallagher, S., & Muldoon, O.T. (2012). Acquired brain injury: combining social psychological and neuropsychological perspectives, *Health Psychology Review*, 1–15, first preview.

Ward, J. (2012). *The student's guide to social neuroscience*. Hove, UK: Psychology Press.

Warschausky, S., Cohen, E.H., Parker, J.G., Levendosky, A.A., & Okun, A. (1997). Social problem-solving skills of children with traumatic brain injury. *Developmental Neurorehabilitation, 1*, 77–81.

Watkins, C.L., Auton, M.F., Deans, C.F., Dickinson, H.A., Jack, C., Lightbody, C.E., ... Leathley, M. (2007). Motivational interviewing early after acute stroke. *Stroke, 38*, 1004–1009.

Watkins, C.L., Wathan, J.V., Leathley, M.J., Auton, M.F., Deans, C.F., Dickinson, H., ... Lightbody, C.E. (2011). The 12-month effects of early motivational interviewing after acute stroke. *Stroke, 42*, 1956–1961.

Weinstein, E.A., & Kahn, R.L. (1955). *Denial of illness: Symbolic and physiological aspects*. Springfield, IL: Charles C. Thomas.

Whittaker, R., Kemp, S., & House, A. (2007). Outcome in mild traumatic brain injury: A longitudinal study. *Journal of Neurology Neurosurgery & Psychiatry, 78*, 644–646.

Whyte, J., & Hart, T. (2003). It's more than a black box; it's a Russian doll: Defining rehabilitation treatments. *American Journal Physical Medicine & Rehabilitation, 82*, 639–652.

Wilcock, A.A. (1998). Reflections on doing, being, and becoming. *Canadian Journal of Occupational Therapy, 65*, 248–257.

Willer, B.S., Allen, K., Anthony, J., & Cowlan, G. (1993). *Circles of support for individuals with acquired brain injury: Manual.* State University of New York at Buffalo, Buffalo, NY: Rehabilitation Research and Training Center on Community Integration of Persons with Traumatic Brain Injury.

Williams, W.H., Evans, J.J., & Fleminger, S. (2003). Neurorehabilitation and cognitive-behaviour therapy of anxiety disorders after brain injury: an overview and a case illustration of obsessive-compulsive disorder. *Neuropsychological Rehabilitation, 13*, 133–148.

Wilson, B.A. (2011). Cutting edge developments in neuropsychological rehabilitation and possible future directions. *Brain Impairment, 12*, 33–42.

Wilson, B.A., & Watson, P.C. (1996). A practical framework for understanding compensatory behaviour in people with organic memory impairment, *Memory, 4*, 465–486.

Wilson, B.A., Emslie, H.C., Quirk, K., & Evans, J.J. (2001). Reducing everyday memory and planning problems by means of a paging system: A randomised control crossover study. *Journal of Neurology, Neurosurgery, and Psychiatry, 70*, 477–482.

Wilson, B., Evans, J., Emslie, H., & Malinek, V. (1997). Evaluation of NeuroPage: A new memory aid. *Journal of Neurology, Neurosurgery, and Psychiatry, 63*, 113–115.

Wilson, B., Gracey, F., Evans, J., & Bateman, A. (2009). *Neuropsychological rehabilitation: Theory, models, therapy and outcome.* New York: Cambridge University Press.

Wilson, B.A., Kopelman, M.D., & Kapur, N. (2008). Prominent and persistent loss of past awareness in amnesia: delusion, impaired consciousness or coping strategy? *Neuropsychological Rehabilitation, 18*, 527–540.

Wilson, K.R., Donders, J., & Nguyen, L. (2011). Self and parent ratings of executive functioning after adolescent traumatic brain injury. *Rehabilitation psychology, 56*, 100–106.

Withall, A., Brodaty, H., Altendorf, A., & Sachdev, P.S. (2009). Who does well after a stroke? The Sydney Stroke Study. *Aging & Mental Health, 13*, 693–698.

Wolfe, C.D.A., Crichton, S.L., Heuschmann, P.U., McKevitt, C.J., Toschke, A.M., Grieve, A.P., & Rudd, A.G. (2011). Estimates of outcomes up to ten years after stroke: analysis from the prospective South London Stroke Register. *PLoS Medicine, 8*, e1001033.

Wood, R.L., & Yurdakul, L.K. (1997). Change in relationship status following traumatic brain injury. *Brain Injury, 11*, 491–501.

Woods, D.T., Catroppa, C., Giallo, R., Matthews, J., & Anderson, V.A. (2012). Feasibility and consumer satisfaction ratings following an intervention for families who have a child with acquired brain injury. *NeuroRehabilitation, 30*, 189–198.

World Health Organisation. (2001). *International Classification of Functioning, Disability and Health (ICF).* Geneva: WHO.

Wright, J.C., & Telford, R. (1996). Psychological problems following minor head injury: a prospective study. *British Journal of Clinical Psychology, 35*, 399–412.

Yeates, G.N., Gracey, F., & Collicutt McGrath, J.C. (2008). A biopsychosocial deconstruction of 'personality change' following acquired brain injury. *Neuropsychological Rehabilitation, 18*, 566–589.

Yeates, G., Hamill, M., Sutton, L., Psaila, K., Gracey, F., Mohamed, S., & O'Dell, J. (2008). Dysexecutive problems and interpersonal relating following frontal brain injury: Reformulation and compensation in cognitive analytic therapy (CAT). *Neuropsychoanalysis, 10*, 43–58.

Yeates, K.O., Taylor, H., Walz, N.C., Stancin, T., & Wade, S.L. (2010). The family environment as a moderator of psychosocial outcomes following traumatic brain injury in young children. *Neuropsychology, 24*, 345–356.

Yihong, G., Ying, C., Yuan, Z., & Yan, Z. (2005). Self-identity changes and English learning among Chinese undergraduates. *World Englishes, 24*, 39–51.

Ylvisaker, M., & Feeney, T. (2000). Reconstruction of identity after brain injury. *Brain Impairment, 1*, 12–28.

Ylvisaker, M., & Feeney, T. (2007). Pediatric brain injury: Social, behavioral, and communication disability. *Physical Medicine and Rehabilitation Clinics of North America, 18*, 133–144.

Ylvisaker, M., Feeney, T.J., & Szekeres, S. (1998). Social-environmental approach to communication and behavior. *Traumatic Brain Injury Rehabilitation: Children and Adolescents* (revised edition pp. 271–302). Boston: Butterworth-Heinemann.

Ylvisaker, M., McPherson, K., Kayes, N., & Pellet, E. (2008). Metaphoric identity mapping: Facilitating goal setting and engagement in rehabilitation after traumatic brain injury. *Neuropsychological Rehabilitation, 18*, 713–741.

Ylvisaker, M., Todis, B., Glang, A., Urbanczyk, B., Franklin, C., DePompei, R., ... Tyler, J.S. (2001). Educating students with TBI: Themes and recommendations. *Journal of Head Trauma Rehabilitation, 16*, 76–93.

Ylvisaker, M., Turkstra, L., & Coelho, C. (2005). Behavioral and social interventions for individuals with traumatic brain injury: a summary of the research with clinical implications. *Seminars in Speech & Language. 26*, 256–267.

Yonelinas, A.P., Kroll, N.E., Quamme, J.R., Lazzara, M.M., Sauvé, M.-J., Widaman, K.F., & Knight, R.T. (2002). Effects of extensive temporal lobe damage or mild hypoxia on recollection and familiarity. *Nature Neuroscience, 5*, 1236–1241.

Yoshii, H., & Yoshimatsu, Y. (2003). Self-understanding, understanding of others, and affective understanding in adolescents with autism. *Japanese Journal of Special Education, 41*, 217–226.

Young, Y., Frick, K.D., & Phelan, E.A. (2009). Can successful aging and chronic illness coexist in the same individual? A multidimensional concept of successful aging. *Journal of the American Medical Directors Association, 10*, 87–92.

Zeman, A. (2002). *Consciousness: a user's guide*. New Haven: Yale University Press.

Zhu, Y., Zhang, L., Fan, J., & Han, S. (2007). Neural basis of cultural influence on self-representation. *NeuroImage, 34*, 1310–1316.

Author index

Adams, H.F. 41
Adler, A. 11
Alderman, N. 72
Allport, G.W. 17
Altendorf, A. 41
Anderson, C.S. 124, 126
Anderson, S. 42
Anderson, V. 45, 172
Andrews, T.K. 47
Anson, K. 89–90
Arango-Lasprilla, J.C. 163
Aristotle 7
Asarnow, R. 44
Ashman, T. 126
Ashworth, F. 133
Azulay, J. 123

Babikan, T. 44
Backhaus, S.L. 146
Backhouse, M. 178–9
Bäckman, L. 68
Baltes, P. 67
Bandura, A. 20
Barker, D. 69
Barnard, P.J. 32
Bartha, M. 47
Batson, M. 146
Beardmore, S. 47
Beck, A.T. 21
Bédard, M. 123, 132
Ben-Yishay, Y. 147
Bergenheim, A.T. 58
Berry, E. 135–6
Bigler, E.D. 41
Black, S.E. 69
Blake, H. 146
Blasey, C.M. 41
Bok, H. 6
Bombardier, C. 42, 123, 125
Boschen, K. 167–8

Bouwens, S.F.M. 120
Bowen, C. 169–70
Boyd, R. 177
Braga, L.W. 174
Brandy, C. 167–8
Brinthaupt, T.M. 79–81
Brodaty, H. 41
Brown, F.L. 177
Burkhardt, A. 175
Bye, R.A. 49

Cantor, J.B. 72, 73, 97–9
Capo, M. 134
Cardillo, J.E. 119–20
Caroselli, J.S. 72
Carroll, E. 72, 73, 97, 100, 101
Catroppa, C. 172
Cattelani, R. 148
Choban, G. 67
Cicerone, K.D. 144–5, 148
Clare, L. 37, 112
Clarke, P. 69
Cloute, K. 70
Coetzer, R. 72, 73, 97, 100–1, 149
Cole, W.R. 172–3
Conrad, N. 72
Conway, M.A. 31
Cooley, C.H. 22
Cooper-Evans, S. 72, 73–4
Corrigan, J.D. 38
Cott, C. 69
Couchman, G. 146
Crowe, S. 67
Csikszentmihalyi, M. 18
Culley, C. 135
Curran, C.A. 67
Cusick, A. 49

Dalrymple-Alford, J.C. 45
Damasio, A.R. 26–7, 27, 31

Damasio, H. 42
D'Argembeau, A. 29
Dawson, D. 150
Dawson, D.R. 67
Dewar, B.K. 127
Dirette, D. 60
Dixon, R.A. 68
Doering, B.K. 72, 74
Donnellan, C. 90
Douglas, J. 49, 75, 152
Dyson, M. 152

Egan, J. 158
Ellis-Hill, C. 69, 72, 73, 96
Ergh, T.C. 166
Erikson, E.H. 12–13
Erwin, L.J. 79–81
Evans, J. 120, 127, 135
Exner, C. 72

Feeney, T.J. 45, 133–4, 177, 181
Feinberg, T.E. 26, 27, 27, 30, 60
Fergusson, D.M. 45
Fickas, S. 138
Fleming, J. 114–16
Fleminger, S. 39, 127
Fletcher-Janzen, E. 173
Foreman, P. 152
Foucault, M. 24
Freeman, M. 19
Freud, Sigmund 9–10

Gainotti, G. 32
Gan, C. 167–8
Gargaro, J. 167–8
Gerber, G. 167–8
Gertler, P. *125*
Glang, A. 180
Goffman, E. 22–3
Goldstein, K. 66
Gontkovsky, S.T. *72*
Gracey, F. 74, 76–7, 107–8, 127, 135
Greenberg, I. 175

Hackett, M.L. *124*, 126
Halteh, C. *124*, 126
Hamberg, K. 58
Hanten, G. 47
Harter, S. 15
Haslam, S.A. *72*, 74, 138
Haun, J. 75
Hawley, C.A. 47, 103
Haworth, H. *125*
Henriksson, R. 58

Hillary, F.G. 66
Hodgson, J. *125*
Hoen, B. 141
Hood, D. 138
Hoogduin, C.A.L. 106
Horn, S. *72*, 73, 96
Horney, K. 11–12
Horwood, L.J. 45
House, A. 88, *124*, 126
Howard, K.L. 107
Hsieh, M. *125*
Humphrey, M. 69, 71, *72*, 94–6

Ibarra, S.L. 146

Jacobs, H.E. 153
James, William 8–9
Jetten, J. *72*, 74
Johnson, D.A. 47
Jones, C. 67, 74
Jones, J.M. *72*
Jones, K. 165
Jones, S.J. 60
Judd, D. 108–9
Jumisko, E. 71
Jung, Carl 10–11

Kade, H.D. 173
Keenan, J.P. 27
Keijsers, G.P.J. 106
Kelly, A. 146
Kelly, G.A. 20
Kemp, S. 88
Kendall, E. 62, 89, 90–1
Kennedy, M.R.T. 49
Kesler, S.R. 41
Kilov, A.M. 158, 181
Kiresuk, T.J. 119–20
Klonoff, P.S. 107
Klyce, D. 146
Knight, C. *72*
Kosciulek, J.F. 165
Koski, P.R. 71
Krause, M.O. 49
Krefting, L. 59, 61
Kreutzer, J. 168–9
Kristensen, O.S. 60
Krpan, K. 67

Lamb, S.A. 141
Lannin, N. 114–16
Leavitt, M.B. 141
Lebowitz, M. 158
Levack, W.M.M. 138–9

Levin, H.S. 46, 47
Levine, B. 67
Li, L. 44
Lincoln, N.B. *125*
Liu, J. 44
Llewellyn, G.M. 49
Locke, John 7
Lorenz, L.S. 70

Macniven, J.A. *125*
Malec, J.F. 146
Marcantuono, J.T. 173
Marcia, J.E. 16
Markus, H. 12
Marsh, N.V. 165
Maslow, A.H. 18
Mathews, D.J.H. 6
Matsuzawa, Y. 158
McDonald, S. *125*
McKay, A.J.D. *125*
McKinlay, A. 45
McKinlay, L. 177
McPherson, K.M. 121–2
Mead, G.H. 22
Mealings, M. 49
Medd, J. *125*
Medley, A.R. 67
Mitchell, A. 70
Morris, R. *72*, 74
Moss-Morris, R. 88
Mulla, F. 101

Nalder, E. 39, 40
Neiss, M.B. 28
Nick, T.G. 41
Nochi, M. 65, 70
Northoff, G. 29
Nurius, P. 12

Oberjohn, K. 175
O'Callaghan, C. 60
Oddy, M. *72*
Orlinsky, D.E. 107
Orth, U. 17
Ownsworth, T. 76–7, 112, 114–16, 127, 142, 144
Oyebode, J. 60

Payne, S. 69
Pepping, M. 40
Plaisier, B.R. 60
Pleydell-Pearce, C.W. 31
Ponsford, J. 39, 67, 89–90, *125*, 146
Powell, T. 60, 67, *125*

Prigatano, G.P. 59, 173

Rabins, P.V. 6
Radford, K. 152
Ramanathan, D.M. 66
Rappolt, S. 150
Reid, D. 69
Rief, W. *72*
Riley, G.A. 88
Rittman, M.R. 75
Rochette, A. 62
Rodger, S. 178–9
Rogers, Carl 19, 34
Rose, F.D. 47
Roueche, J.R. 40
Ruddle, J.A. 100, 101

Sachdev, P.S. 41
Salander, P. 58
Sale, P. 150–1
Sambuco, M. 163
Saroyan, S. *72*, 74
Schaap, C.P.D.R. 106
Schmidt, J. 114–16
Schönberger, M. *125*
Secrest, J.R. *72*, 73, 99–100
Sedikides, C. 28
Shadden, B.B. 71
Sharp, N.L. 49
Sherer, M. 41
Sherron, P. 150–1
Sherwood, P. 165
Simpson, G. 165
Slocomb, J.E. 66
Smith, A. 119–20
Sofronoff, K. 177
Sohlberg, M.M. 138
Soo, C. *124*
Stancin, T. 49
Stergiou-Kita, M. 150
Stevenson, J. 28
Stuss, D.T. 33, 67
Sullivan H.S. 11

Taffe, J.R. *125*
Tate, R.L. 39, *124, 125*
Taylor, H.G. 45, 46
Taylor, S.E. 63, 65
Teasdale, J.D. 32
Telford, R. *72*, 73, 96
Terry, D. 62, 89
Thelander, M. 141
Thomas, S.A. *125*, 126
Todis, B. 138, 157

Topolevec-Vranic, J. 123
Tranel, D. 42
Trexler, L.E. 146
Tsaousides, T. 126, 158
Tulving, E. 30–1
Turkstra, L.S. 49
Tyerman, A.T. 69, 71, *72*, 94–6

Vaughan, F.L. 100
Vickery, C.D. *72*, 96, 145
Voss, B.S. 141

Wade, S.L. 45, 175, 176, 179
Walker, M.F. *125*
Ward, C. 69
Wardecker, M.M. 66
Watkins, C.L. 126
Wehman, P. 150–1
Wells, A. 141

West, M. 150–1
Whittingham, K. 177
Williams, W.H. *72*, 74, 127
Wilson, Barbara 2
Wilson, K.R. 49
Wilson, S.L. 108–9
Withall, A. 41
Wolfe, C.D.A. 39
Wong, D.K. *125*
Worsley, J. 141
Worthington, A. 67
Wright, J.C. *72*, 73, 96

Yates, P. 70
Yihong, G. 25
Ylvisaker, M. 45, 120–1, 133–4, 177, 181

Zeller, R. *72*, 73, 99–100

Subject index

Bold page numbers indicate figures, *italic* page numbers indicate tables.

ABC exercise 127–8, **129**
Acceptance and Commitment Therapy (ACT) 131–2
adolescence/adolescents: assessment of self-concept 101–5; brain injury in 48–50; case study of injury 52–4, **54**; developmental psychology of 15–16; interventions for 178–82; social media 181–2; transition to work/higher education from school 180–2
adulthood, developmental psychology in 16–17
affect mirroring 11
age: maturity, developmental psychology in 17; and outcome of injury 40, 43–4; severity of injury 45 *see also* adolescence/adolescents; childhood/children
analytic psychology 10–11
anima archetype 10
anxiety: and coping 67; due to self-appraisal 62; incidence of after injury 57
aphasia: adjustment to 71; communication with people with 169
appearance, changes in 69–70
Appraisal of Threat and Avoidance Questionnaire (ATAQ) *83*, 88–9
appraisals, self-: accurate, benefits of 61; and coping strategies 67; emotional distress due to 61–2; sense-making 62–5, 86–9; threat 62–3
archetypes 10–11
Asian cultures 24
assessment of changes to self: Appraisal of Threat and Avoidance Questionnaire *83*; Awareness Questionnaire *82*, 84; Baycrest Psychosocial Stress Test (BPST) 91; Brain Injury Grief Inventory *93*, 100–1, 190–1; children and adolescents 101–5; Continuity/Discontinuity of Self Scale *93*, 99–100; Coopersmith Self-Esteem Inventory (CSEI) *92*, 94, 103; Coping Scale for Adults (CSA) *83*, 89–90; coping strategies *83*, 89–91; Head Injury Semantic Differential Scale *93*, 94–7, **189**; Illness Perceptions Questionnaire - Revised (IPQ-R) 87–8; measurement of self, issues concerning 79–81; Patient Competency Rating Scale (PCRS) *82*, 84; Perceived Control Scale for Brain Injury (PCS-BI) 87; performance-based measures 90–1; Piers-Harris Children's Self-Concept Scale (CSCS) 102–3; Robson Self-Concept Questionnaire *92*; Rosenberg Self-Esteem Scale (RSES) 91, *92*, 94; self-awareness *82*, 84–6; Self-Awareness of Deficits Interview *82*, 85; self-efficacy 86–7; Self-Efficacy for Symptom Management Scale 86–7; self-report methods 80–1, *82–3*, 84–6; Self-Understanding Interview 104–5; Selves Adjective Checklist 97–9; Selves Interview *93*, 97–9; sense-making appraisals *83*, 86–9; Social-Emotional Questionnaire for Children (SEQ-C) 103–4; Strategies Used by People to Promote Health (SUPPH) 86; Stress Appraisal Measure (SAM) *83*, 87; Tennessee Self-Concept Scale-2 *92*; Ways of Coping Questionnaire (WCQ) *83*, 89, 90
attachment theory 11
autobiographical self 27, *27*, 31
autobiographical system 31
awareness of injury: adolescence 48–9; changes in functioning 57–62; children's 46–7; concealment of problems 59–60; and coping strategies 67; development 60–2; impairment of 58–60 *see also* self-awareness

Subject index

Awareness Questionnaire *82*, 84
Awareness Support Programme (ASP) 142–4, 156

Baycrest Psychosocial Stress Test (BPST) 91
behavioural/emotional self-regulation 33
behavioural outcomes of injury: adolescents 49–50; children 44–5
blind spots 65–6
bodily self 26, *27*
brain injury: in adolescence 48–50; causes of 37–8; in childhood 43–8; and development of the brain 43; factors influencing outcomes 40–3, **41**; outcomes of 38–40
Brain Injury Family Intervention (BIFI) 168–9, 179
Brain Injury Grief Inventory (BIGI) *93*, 100–1, 190–1

Canadian Occupational Performance Measure (COPM) 118–19
caregiver stress 165–6 *see also* family
childhood/children: assessment of self-concept 101–5; brain injury during 43–8; case study of injury 50–2, **53**; Coopersmith Self-Esteem Inventory (CSEI) 103; developmental psychology of 13, *14*, 15; holistic rehabilitation 173–4; interventions 170–8, *176–7*; knowledge of injury 46–7; parents, impact of child's injury on 162; parents as the injured person 164; Piers-Harris Children's Self-Concept Scale (CSCS) 102–3; self-concept 46–8; Self-Understanding Interview 104–5; Social-Emotional Questionnaire for Children (SEQ-C) 103–4; younger children 174–5, *176–7*, 177–8
Circles of Support 152
Classification of Functioning, Disability and Health (ICF framework) 38–9
Clubhouse model 153
cognitive adaptation, theory of 63, **64**
Cognitive Awareness Model (CAM) 33–4
cognitive behavioural therapy (CBT): in brain injury 127–33, **129**, *130–1*; depression 126; internet-delivered 123; stroke victims 126–7; third wave cognitive and behavioural therapies 131–3
cognitive neuroscience 27–8
cognitive theories on self and identity 20–2
Collaborative Model of Psychotherapy after Brain Injury 107
collective self *27*

collective unconscious 10
communication with people with aphasia 169
community participation initiatives 152–6, *154–5*
community rehabilitation: holistic 147–9; main approaches 140
community reintegration 39
comparator mechanisms 33–4
Compassion Focused Therapy (CFT) 132–3
compensation 67–8
concealment of problems 59–60
conceptual self *27*
context-sensitive interventions 134
Continuity/Discontinuity of Self Scale (CDSS) *93*, 99–100
Coopersmith Self-Esteem Inventory (CSEI) *92*, 94, 103
Coping Scale for Adults (CSA) *83*, 89–90
coping strategies 65–8; measurement of *83*, 89–91
core beliefs 21–2
core self 26–7, *27*, 31
cultural/collective self *27*
cultural conceptions of self 24–5

defensive personality style 59, 66–7
depression: cognitive behavioural therapy (CBT) 126; and coping 67; due to self-appraisal 61–2; incidence of after injury 57
Descartes, René 7
development of the brain 43
developmental psychology 12–13, *14*, 15–17

ecological self *27*
education: and outcome of injury 41; re-integration of adolescents 49–50; support at school 179–81; transition to work/higher education 180–2
ego 9–10, 12–13
Ego and the Id, The (Freud) 9–10
emotions: and coping 67; distress due to self-appraisal 61–2; impact on cognitive processing 34; and memories 31–2; regulation of 71
ethnicity and outcome of injury 41
executive control system 33
exercise groups 146
existential perspectives on self-identity 18–20
extended self *27*

Facebook 158

family: adolescents, support for 50; caregiver stress 165–6; development of awareness of injury 60–1; environment and outcomes from injury 44–5; I-InTERACT (Internet-based Interacting Together Everyday: Recovery After Childhood TBI) 175, *176*, 178; identity, impact of injury on 159–65; interventions for members 167–8; involvement in group interventions 146; and outcome of injury 45–6; parents, impact of child's injury on 162; parents as the injured person 164; partner of injured person 162–3; problem-solving 175, *176*; relationships after injury 39–40; resilience of 164–5; sexual relations after injury 163; siblings of injured person, impact of injury 163; system interventions 168–70; therapy involvement of 166–7
fear processing 31–2
feedback 23; development of awareness of injury 60; and psychoeducation 114–16; and self-awareness 113–14
flow 18
freedom *versus* determinism debate 8
functioning, changes in: awareness of 57–62; and coping 67–8
future research 188

gender and outcome of injury 41
Generic Model of Psychotherapy 107
genetics and outcome of injury 40
Goal Attainment Scaling (GAS) 119–20, *121*
goal-directed interventions 112–22, *116*, **118, *121***
group interventions: brain injury support groups 141–2; developing support networks 149–56, *154–5*; exercise groups 146; family involvement 146; holistic rehabilitation 147–9; self-concept 145; self-esteem 145–6; structured 142–6; use of 139
group membership: changes in 74–5; and wellbeing 137–40, **139** *see also* social identity
growth, personal, due to injury 63–5

Head Injury Semantic Differential Scale *93*, 94–7, **189**
heredity 28
hiding of problems 59–60
hierarchy of human needs 18
higher education, transition to from school 180–2

holistic rehabilitation 147–9, 173–4
humanistic perspectives on self-identity 18–20

I-InTERACT (Internet-based Interacting Together Everyday: Recovery After Childhood TBI) 175, *176*, 178
ICF framework 38–9
id 9–10
idealised/real self 11–12
identity: conditions for changes in 22; defined 6; historical perspectives 7–8; statuses during adolescence 16; transition as dynamic and cyclical 57
Identity Oriented Goal Training (IOT) 121–2
Illness Perceptions Questionnaire - Revised (IPQ-R) 87–8
illusions 65–6
implicational meanings 32
independence, return to 39
injury to the brain. *see* brain injury
internet 123, 156–9
interpersonal self 27
IQ and outcome of injury 41

jobs, return to 150–2

knowledge of injury: adolescence 48–9; changes in functioning 57–62; children's 46–7

lifecycle framework 12–13, *14*, 15–16
locus of control 21

Making Sense of Brain Tumour (MSoBT) Project 166–7
maturity, developmental psychology in 17
measurement of self: Appraisal of Threat and Avoidance Questionnaire *83*; Awareness Questionnaire *82*, 84; Baycrest Psychosocial Stress Test (BPST) 91; Brain Injury Grief Inventory *93*, 100–1, 190–1; children and adolescents 101–5; Continuity/Discontinuity of Self Scale *93*, 99–100; Coopersmith Self-Esteem Inventory (CSEI) *92*, 94, 103; Coping Scale for Adults (CSA) *83*, 89–90; coping strategies *83*, 89–91; Head Injury Semantic Differential Scale *93*, 94–7, **189**; Illness Perceptions Questionnaire - Revised (IPQ-R) 87–8; issues concerning 79–81; Patient Competency Rating Scale (PCRS) *82*, 84; Perceived Control Scale

for Brain Injury (PCS-BI) 87; performance-based measures 90–1; Piers-Harris Children's Self-Concept Scale (CSCS) 102–3; Robson Self-Concept Questionnaire 92; Rosenberg Self-Esteem Scale (RSES) 91, 92, 94; self-awareness 84–6; Self-Awareness of Deficits Interview 82, 85; self-efficacy 86–7; Self-Efficacy for Symptom Management Scale 86–7; self-report methods 80–1, 82–3, 84–6; Self-Understanding Interview 104–5; Selves Adjective Checklist 97–9; Selves Interview 93, 97–9; sense-making appraisals 83, 86–9; Social-Emotional Questionnaire for Children (SEQ-C) 103–4; Strategies Used by People to Promote Health (SUPPH) 86; Stress Appraisal Measure (SAM) 83, 87; Tennessee Self-Concept Scale-2 92; Ways of Coping Questionnaire (WCQ) 83, 89, 90
memory systems 30–2; impairment 70; technology-based aids 135–6
mentalisation 11
Metacognitive Awareness System (MAS) 34
metaphoric identity mapping (MIM) 120–2
mindfulness 19
minimal self 27
mirror neuron system 29

narrative, personal 70–1
narrative self 26, 27
nature *versus* nurture debate 8
networks of support 149–56, 154–5
NeuroPage service 135
neuropathologies of the self 30
neuropathology, underlying, and outcomes of injury 42
neuropsychological and social processes, model of 76–7
neurorehabilitation: technology used in 135–6 *see also* psychotherapy
neuroscience: brain damage and the self 30; cognitive 27–8; connectivity supporting self 28–30; neuropathologies of the self 30; neuropsychological processes and changes to self 33–4; neuropsychological processes supporting self 30–3; social 26–8, 27
non-Western conceptions of self 25–6

object relations theory 11
observation 80
occupational therapy 19
occupations, return to 150–2

Subject index 231

ongoing self 27
optimism, dispositional 66
OZC User Group 156

paediatric rehabilitation. *see* childhood/children
parents: active involvement in rehabilitation 174; impact of child's injury on 162; as the injured person 164; styles of and outcomes from injury 44–5, 46
partner of injured person 162–3
Patient Competency Rating Scale (PCRS) 82, 84
peak experience 18
Perceived Control Scale for Brain Injury (PCS-BI) 87
performance-based measures 90–1
person-centre principles 19
persona archetype 10
personal agency 20–1
personal construct theory 20
Personal Data Base (PDB) 33–4
personal narrative 70–1
personality and coping style 66–7
phenomenology 19–20
philosophical assumptions 7–8
physical appearance, changes in 69–70
Piers-Harris Children's Self-Concept Scale (CSCS) 102–3
positive behavioural supports (PBS) 174–5, 177
positive psychology 18
possible selves 12
post-traumatic growth 63–5
premorbid IQ and outcome of injury 41
Principles of Psychology, The (James) 8–9
private self 27
problem-solving, family 175, 176
project-based interventions 133–4, 153–4
propositional meanings 32
proto-self 26, 27
psychoeducation and feedback 114–16
psychological adjustment to injury: awareness of changes in functioning 57–62; coping strategies 65–8; depression 57; neuropsychological and social processes, model of 76–7; overview of process 55–7, **56, 58**; research on changes to self-identity 69–78, 72
psychological perspectives on self-identity: cognitive theories 20–2; cultural conceptions of self 24–5; developmental psychology 14, 15–17; early 8–9; existential 18–20; humanistic 18–20; non-Western

conceptions of self 25–6; psychoanalytic theory 9–12; social psychology 22–4
psychotherapy: Acceptance and Commitment Therapy (ACT) 131–2; agreement to 109–10, *111*; Canadian Occupational Performance Measure (COPM) 118–19; cognitive behavioural therapy (CBT) 123, 127–33, **129,** *130–1*; Collaborative Model of Psychotherapy after Brain Injury 107; Compassion Focused Therapy (CFT) 132–3; context-sensitive interventions 134; engagement in 108–12, *110, 111*; Generic Model of Psychotherapy 107; Goal Attainment Scaling (GAS) 119–20, *121*; goal-directed interventions 112–22; individual 122–34, *124–5,* **129,** *130–1*; metaphoric identity mapping (MIM) 120–2; project-based interventions 133–4; psychoeducation and feedback 114–16; SenseCam 136; SMART goal setting 117–18; for stroke victims 126–7; suitability of 109; therapeutic relationship 106–8; third wave cognitive and behavioural therapies 131–3; values, identifying 116–17, **118**; Y-shaped model 107–8

questionnaire-based measures: coping strategies 89–90; self-awareness *82*, 84–6; sense-making appraisals 86–9; Social-Emotional Questionnaire for Children (SEQ-C) 103–4

real/idealised self 11–12
reconstructed self-narratives 65
Relational Approach to Rehabilitation 169–70
relational self 26, *27*
religion 25–6
remembering-imaging system 3131
Robson Self-Concept Questionnaire *92*
role identity 23
Rosenberg Self-Esteem Scale (RSES) 91, *92*, 94

schemas 21–2
school: re-integration of adolescents 49–50; support at 179–81; transition from to work/higher education 180–2
self: conditions for changes in 22; defined 5; possible 12; real/idealised 11–12*see also* assessment of changes to self
self-appraisals: accurate, benefits of 61; and coping strategies 67; emotional distress due to 61–2; sense-making 62–5

self archtype 10–11
self-awareness: assessment of *82*, 84–6; defined 5; and feedback 113–14; and goal-directed interventions 112–22, *116*, **118,** *121*
Self-Awareness of Deficits Interview *82*, 85
self-body split 69
self-categorisation 23
self-concept 16; adolescents 49–50; after injury 71, *72*, 73–7; after stroke 73; assessment of for children and adolescents 101–5; and children 46–8; defined 5–6; group interventions 145
self-discrepancy theory 24, 73, 77, 97, 108
self-efficacy 21; defined 6; measurement of 86–7
Self-Efficacy for Symptom Management Scale 86–7
self-esteem 17; after injury 73–4; of children, and interventions 171; children's 47; defined 6; group interventions 145–6
self-identity: defined 6; historical perspectives 7–8; research on changes after injury 69–78, *72*; schematic representation 35, **35***see also* psychological perspectives on self-identity
self-limiting belief systems 63
self-memory system 31
self-narratives reconstructed 65
self-report methods: advantages and issues with 80–1; coping strategies 89–90; self-awareness 84–6
self-reported cognitive deficits 74
self-schemas 21–2
Self-Understanding Interview 104–5
Selves Adjective Checklist 97–9
Selves Interview *93*, 97–9
sense-making appraisals 62–5, *83*, 86–9
SenseCam 135–6
sensorimotor self *27*
severity of injury: age 45; life satisfaction 74, 77; and outcome of injury 43
sexuality, changes in 70, 163
shadow archtype 10
short messaging service (SMS) 135
siblings of injured person, impact of injury 163
Signposts for Building Better Behaviour programme *177*
Skills To Enable People and communitieS (STEPS) 153
SMART goal setting 117–18

Subject index   233

SMS texts 135
social biofeedback model 11
social comparison 23
social constructionist theory 24
Social-Emotional Questionnaire for Children (SEQ-C) 103–4
social environment: awareness impairment 58–60; development of awareness of injury 60–2; group membership, changes in 74–5; redefinition of concepts 61
social factors and outcome of injury 45–6
social group membership 39–40
social identity: brain injury support groups 141–2; community participation initiatives 152–6, *154–5*; defined 6; developing support networks 149–56, *154–5*; group interventions 139; holistic rehabilitation 147–9; rehabilitation approaches 139–40; Social Identity Model of Identity Change 139–40; structured group interventions 142–6; and wellbeing 137–40, **139**; work, return to 150–2
social identity theory 23
social media 156–9, 181–2
social neuroscience 26–8, *27*
social psychology 11, 22–4
social skills: changes in 71; children's development 47
socio-cognitive theory of personality 20–1
Specific Activities and Avoidance Questionnaire (SAAQ) 88–9
spirituality 25–6
spouse of injured person 162–3
Stepping Stones *177*, 177–8
Strategies Used by People to Promote Health (SUPPH) 86
Stress Appraisal Measure (SAM) *83*, 87
stroke: cognitive behavioural therapy (CBT) 126–7; incidence of 37–8; outcomes of 39–40; and physical impairment 69–70; psychotherapy for 126–7; self-concept after 73

strong-tie expressive support 75
superego 9–10
support: brain injury support groups 141–2; Circles of Support 152; development of awareness of injury 60–1; development of networks 149–56, *154–5*; at school 179–81; strong-tie expressive 75

technology: internet 123, 156–9; in neurorehabilitation 135–6
Teen Online Problem Solving (TOPS) *176*, 179
Tennessee Self-Concept Scale-2 *92*
texting 135
therapeutic milieu 147
therapeutic relationship 106–8
therapy. *see* psychotherapy
third wave cognitive and behavioural therapies 131–3
threat appraisals 62–3
traumatic brain injury (TBI): incidence of 38; outcomes of 39–40
tumours 42

uniqueness *versus* universality debate 8

values, identifying 116–17, **118**
vocational rehabilitation 150–2

Ways of Coping Questionnaire (WCQ) *83*, 89, 90
Western/non-Western conceptions of self 25–6
Whittaker, R. 88
women and outcome of injury 41
work: return to 150–2; transition to from school 180–2
working self 31

Y-shaped model 107–8

Zen Buddhism 25–6

Printed in Great Britain
by Amazon